Developmental
and
Adapted
Physical Education

H. HARRISON CLARKE, Ed.D.

Research Professor
School of Health, Physical Education, and Recreation
University of Oregon

DAVID H. CLARKE, Ph.D.

Assistant Professor
Department of Physical Education
University of California, Berkeley

1963

Developmental
and
Adapted
Physical Education

PRENTICE-HALL, INC.

Englewood Cliffs, N. J.

Developmental and Adapted Physical Education

Clarke and Clarke

© 1963

PRENTICE-HALL, INC.

Englewood Cliffs, N. J.

LIBRARY OF CONGRESS CATALOGUE CARD NO.: 63-7165
PRINTED IN THE UNITED STATES OF AMERICA 20837-C

PRENTICE-HALL INTERNATIONAL, INC.
London · Tokyo · Sydney · Paris
PRENTICE-HALL OF CANADA, LTD.
PRENTICE-HALL DE MEXICO, S.A.

To

parents and grandparents

ISABEL BUCKLIN and HENRY ELLIOT CLARKE

Preface

Never before in the history of physical education in the United States during peacetime has this field been so positively challenged to improve the physical fitness of all youth. Exercise as a way of life is becoming accepted as a basic need for adults. The necessity for improving fitness through proper physical activity is critical due to the demands of a strong and enduring populace for national survival, to the results of medical research showing the necessity for a physically active life in the reduction of the incidence of degenerative diseases, and to the demonstrated general fitness inferiority of our youth.

President John F. Kennedy wrote in the December 26, 1960, *Sports Illustrated:* "For the physical vigor of our citizens is one of America's most precious resources. If we waste and neglect this resource, if we allow it to dwindle and grow soft, then we will destroy much of our ability to meet the great and vital challenges which confront our people. We will be unable to realize our potential as a nation." Subsequently, The President's Council on Youth Fitness proclaimed the following basic feature of a youth fitness program: "Pupils who have a low level of muscular strength, agility, and flexibility should be identified by a screening test as part of health appraisal. Pupils so identified should be required to participate in a program of developmental exercises and activities designed to raise their physical performance to desirable levels."

As a consequence of these considerations, this comprehensive book on developmental and adapted physical education is most timely. It is intended for physical educators in schools and colleges, although applications to physical reconditioning and corrective therapy in hospitals and rehabilitation centers can readily be made. Both authors have had extensive experience in this field in the armed forces and in schools and colleges. They have consistently advocated, conducted, and promoted such programs throughout their professional careers.

In addition, each has done extensive research related to this field.

In the efforts of physical educators to plan programs that will be completely effective in realizing educational objectives, the necessity for meeting individual needs becomes readily apparent. Thus, developmental and adapted processes were devised—not as a separate entity, but evolving from the over-all purposes and potentialities of this field. The following definition is proposed: "The purpose of developmental and adapted physical education is to meet, through physical education methods and activities, the individual needs of boys who are handicapped in some respect, who have functional defects or deficiencies amenable to improvement through exercise, or who possess other inadequacies which interfere with their successful participation in the diversified and vigorous activities of the general physical education program."

As shown in chapter 1, developmental and adapted physical education in the United States has a rich heritage extending over a century in time. Much of the early leadership was provided by physicians attracted to physical education because of its preventive medicine potentialities. Two world wars saw physical educators recruited for rehabilitation and physical reconditioning to speed the recovery of battle casualties. Chapter 2 is devoted to the place of developmental and adapted physical education in schools and colleges. Consideration is given to the ways in which physical education may best serve individual boys and girls; a broad approach to this problem is taken, involving physical, emotional, and social conditions.

In chapter 3 a number of factors essential to practice of developmental and adapted physical education are discussed. These considerations include the need for a scientific approach to content and method, the desirable characteristics and training of teachers in this field, the utilization of effective motivational techniques, and the adoption of proper organizational and administrative procedures. Chapter 4 is devoted to the presentation of tests and other evaluative measures related to the subject. In chapter 5 the value of exercise and its effects upon the organism are reviewed.

The procedures for meeting the needs of individual boys and girls who are subpar in basic physical fitness components are presented in chapter 6. A basic feature of this process is the identification of the causes of unfitness through a case-study approach; once the cause or causes are identified, appropriate individual follow-up procedures can be effectively applied. Chapter 7 is devoted to exercise for the physically unfit. Eight principles of exercise are presented as guides in devising an activity program for any unfit individual. Specific conditioning exercises, weight training, individual and group contests, and circulatory-respiratory activities are described; in respect to these activities, the principles of exercise tolerance, overload, and progression are systematically applied. In chapter 8, the identification and improvement of posture and foot faults and functional back pain are discussed.

The last four chapters are devoted to the adapted phase of physical education—work with handicapped boys and girls. Chapter 9 deals with orthopedic disabilities, including various joint conditions, congenital deformities, bone and disc disorders, and amputations. Chapter 10 considers neurological disabilities, including paraplegia, cerebral palsy, epilepsy, poliomyelitis, multiple sclerosis, and muscular dystrophy. Chapter 11 is concerned with medical, sensory, and surgical conditions, including heart lesions, diabetes, blindness, deafness, and post-surgery and illness. Chapter 12 deals with psychologic disorders, including temporary personality reactions, psychoneuroses, psychotic disorders, psychopathic personalities, and delinquency. In presenting these handicapping conditions, the pathological involvements and the medical, surgical, or psychiatric treatments usually applied are described. This is done so that the adapted physical educator will have, for his purposes, an adequate understanding and insight into the various disabilities. Thus, he should be better able to execute medical prescriptions of exercise for such students and should be better able to assist effectively with their total problem—adjustment to their disabilities. In all instances, the use of exercises and physical activities in the adapted physical education program is considered.

H. H. C.
D. H. C.

Contents

Developmental
and
Adapted
Physical Education

1

Historical Orientation

F ORMAL EXERCISE FOR THERAPEUTIC AND FITNESS BENE-
fits is part of recorded history extending from the time
of primitive man to the present. The application of exercise to develop
the body and to alleviate and improve or correct certain types of physical defects and neuropsychiatric conditions was apparent long before
physical education *per se* was recognized. A brief review of this history
will serve to orient the physical educator to the purposes and contributions of the developmental and adapted aspects of his field.

PRIMITIVE AND ANCIENT TIMES

The needs of primitive man were basic but not complex. As a consequence, his culture was relatively simple. The ability to hunt, fish, care
for crops, and fight the enemy was essential for his survival. The learning of such skills was part of his education; the development and conditioning of the body through vigorous physical activity were vital for
efficient performance. This need to develop the strength and endurance
of the body has been recognized through the ages as essential for effective living. Thus, this basic function of physical education has its origin
in antiquity.

Corrective physical education also had its beginning during the early
history of mankind. Records and drawings have been found presenting
the use of crude corrective gymnastics by the Chinese about 3000-2600
B.C. There is evidence of the use of exercise, massage, and baths by the
early Egyptians, Hindus, Greeks, and Romans. The importance of exercise

in its effect upon mental condition, which today is considered one of its most desirable results, was recognized during an early period of civilization. Pliny sent this thought through the ages when he wrote, "The mind is stimulated by movements of the body." Later, also, Hippocrates used exercise in the treatment of disease at the sanatorium at Cos; Galen also advocated this practice.[1]

An important milestone in the unfolding concept of physical education is found in Athenian education of the fifth century B.C. Physical activities were avowedly employed to develop a beautiful and harmonious body. Balance in physical education, as contrasted with specialization and Spartan brutality, was considered the logical way to assure health, harmony of form, symmetry of movement of all parts of the body, and the natural development of the whole being. Aristotle contended that such a physical rearing would also make the citizens much more adept and confident in martial life. When the Spartans yielded first place in body culture, they became inferior as warriors.[2] Athenian education "saw physical education rise to a place of honor not since achieved in the schools and colleges of the modern world." [3]

In addition to emphasis on symmetrical body development, Greek education recognized the need for balance between mental, social, and physical training. Modern attempts to establish a similar concept have not yet been generally successful.

EUROPEAN INFLUENCES

Following the decline of Athens, physical education went into an eclipse lasting for many centuries. Limited largely to the training of warriors by the Roman Empire, and subjected to the devastating concept of the honored spirit and denounced body of the Middle Ages, physical education did not again achieve cultural significance until the Reformation of the sixteenth and seventeenth centuries. Certain basic philosophies and practices of great importance to modern physical education originated during this latter period.

EDUCATIONAL PHILOSOPHY

Emerging from a void where the principles of antiquity had been buried in the frustrations of the Middle Ages, the voices of France's Rabelais and Montaigne and the Catholic priest J. Baptiste de la Salle could be faintly heard proposing a limited program of physical educa-

---

[1] E. G. Schroeder, *Handbook of Physical Education* (New York: Doubleday, Doran and Company, 1929), pp. 91-93.

[2] Jean E. Chryssafis, "Aristotle on Physical Education," *Journal of Health and Physical Education*, I, No. 1 (1930), p. 3.

[3] Clifford L. Brownell and Patricia E. Hagman, *Physical Education Foundations and Principles* (New York: McGraw-Hill Book Company, 1951), p. 67.

tion for "the gentlemen." During this period, too, England's John Locke [4] propounded this startling thesis:

> A Sound Mind in a Sound Body, is a short, but full description of a happy state in the World. He that has these two, has little more to wish for; and he that wants either of them, will be little better for anything else. . . . He, whose mind directs not wisely, will never take the right Way; and he whose body is crazy and feeble, will never be able to advance it.

In the second book of his *Emile*, Rousseau specified a program of physical education for Emile to follow not only for the development of the body but also for the mind. Rousseau's belief was that a sane body should be accompanied by a sane mind: *mens sana in corpore sano.* He thought of physical education as having two purposes: wealth of body and wealth of mind. As his reasoning is followed, a third purpose is found—"the strengthening of morality." Rousseau believed, too, that: "Women ought to be healthy but not coarse robustness like men, in order that men who shall be born of them may be healthy and robust also." [5]

From the philosophies of Locke, Rousseau, and others sprang certain fundamental concepts of education basic to present-day physical education. Emerging is the concept of the whole child; he cannot be separated into mental, social, and physical aspects, but is a unity with action and interaction among all parts. He is an entity rather than a trichotomy of forces.

PHYSICAL EDUCATION PRACTICES

During the period of the sixteenth and seventeenth centuries, physical education emerged formally in Europe. Toward the end of this period, definite systems of physical education flourished, largely associated with military preparedness. Two of these systems in particular, the German and Swedish, had profound influences on the early development of this field in America.

In Germany, physical education had been introduced into the curriculum of the schools in order to harden the body and discipline the mind. Eventually, the German interest culminated in the *Turnverein,* under the inspiring leadership of Frederich Jahn (1778-1852). This system of exercise was aimed at developing the body, mind, and character of youth through heavy apparatus gymnastics, mass drills, and games of skill. Jahn strove to unify and prepare Germany for successful resistance against the persistent onslaughts of Napoleon's France.

The Swedish system of physical education, like the German system, rose from an impulse for patriotism. However, in the hands of Per

---

[4] John Locke, *Some Thoughts Concerning Education,* 2nd ed. (Cambridge: University Press, 1898).

[5] B. L. Henin, "Jean Jacques Rousseau on Physical Education and Study of the Child," *Education* (April, 1912).

Henrick Ling, its scholarly founder, it became much more refined as a gymnastic system. Ling's work developed along three distinct lines: educational, military, and medical. Out of the medical aspect came corrective exercises, of special import for this text, which were used to overcome physical weakness and alleviate or correct certain defects in children.

Thus, during the eighteenth and nineteenth centuries in Europe, basic philosophy was expressed and systems of physical education were developed which were to play a vital role in the initiation and evolution of similar programs in that new and unsettled country across the ocean to the west, the United States of America. Locke and Rousseau presented the need for physical training in education; historians and students of ancient art kept alive the knowledge of Greek gymnastics; formal systems of physical education were developed in Germany and Sweden; exercise for corrective purposes became a definite phase of the physical education process; and a number of medical writers directed attention to the importance of bodily exercise in the preservation and restoration of health. The consideration of the child as an entity in education, the utilization of physical education activities to improve mental, social, and physical processes, and the recognition of the therapeutic value of physical activity are of special import in understanding and appreciating the growth of developmental and remedial physical education in this country.

PRIOR TO WORLD WAR I

As has been indicated, the earliest formal physical education in the United States was patterned after European systems. The first two school and college gymnasia, both of them outdoors, were opened in 1825 at the Round Hill School, Northampton, Massachusetts, and in 1826 at Harvard University. They were headed by two well-trained Germans, Charles Beck and Charles Follen. The apparatus, activities, and methods were exact transplants from the Jahn system. During these early days, the German system of gymnastics had the most energetic promotion and greatest acceptance in this country.

While Swedish medical gymnastics were first utilized by physicians in America around 1850, little was known of the aims, content, and method of the Ling system until much later. Not until 1889 were the claims for this system brought forward with sufficient clearness and cogency to attract general attention.[6]

Although remnants of these systems still exist in physical education, neither one of them, nor others introduced from abroad, was generally

---

[6] Fred E. Leonard and George B. Affleck, *A Guide to the History of Physical Education*, 3rd. ed (Philadelphia: Lea and Febiger, 1947), p. 329.

adopted or gained more than a temporary foothold in educational institutions of the United States. A new culture was being formed here in a land of tremendous potential growth; a new country was being explored, settled, and developed; a new and powerful nation was being created. If physical education was to become firmly established, it must eventually reflect and support this unfolding culture. Although certain beginnings can be traced to this earlier period, the emergence of a culturally oriented physical education did not become apparent until after World War I.

European physical education had two major aims: to prepare men for war and to develop the physical organism. In respect to the first of these aims, American culture never has accepted preparation for war as an objective of education, except during short periods of armed conflict. In fact, *until recently,* such preparation has not been a national necessity. The United States has not had powerful enemies on its borders, and it has not engaged in territorial aggrandizement for many decades. Great oceans have been effective barriers to invasion by major powers elsewhere in the world. Thus, a prime purpose for the promotion of physical education in European countries has not been of significance here. As a consequence, the presentation of physical education in educational institutions as preparation for national defense has not been effective and programs designed to achieve this end have not survived.

However, the second European aim, the development of the physical organism, became the basic purpose of physical education in early America and has continued with varying degrees of emphasis to the present day. Between the Civil War and World War I, physical education was primarily engrossed in the development and maintenance of adequate levels of physical fitness for boys and girls, men and women. With few exceptions, the physical education leaders of this era were trained in medicine.[7] Undoubtedly, these men and women were attracted to physical education because of the potential health values of proper physical activity—a form of preventive medicine. As expressed in 1878 by Hitchcock in the Tenth Annual Report of the Massachusetts Board of Health, the sole objective of physical education at Amherst College was to "keep bodily health up to normal standards so that the mind may accomplish the most work, and to preserve the bodily powers in full activity for both the daily duties of college and the promised labor of a long life."

---

[7] To name a few, all with M.D. degrees: Edward Hitchcock, Amherst College; Dio Lewis, Boston; Dudley A. Sargent, Harvard University; W. G. Anderson and Jay W. Seaver, Yale University; Fred E. Leonard and Charles W. Savage, Oberlin College; Luther H. Gulick and James H. McCurdy, Springfield College; R. Tait McKenzie, University of Pennsylvania; Kate C. Hurd, Bryn Mawr College; Alice J. Hall, Goucher; William Skarstrom, Boston Normal School of Gymnastics; Thomas A. Storey and Clark W. Hetherington, Stanford University; Thomas D. Wood, Columbia University.

Logically, formal school corrective physical education programs were inaugurated during this period. Building upon the Swedish exercise system, specialized programs, facilities, and personnel were utilized to correct postural defects, alleviate various organic conditions, and develop weak musculatures. Special courses in "correctives" were included in teacher-training courses of study. Many special devices and testing instruments were invented during this period. In particular, Sargent introduced many items of apparatus and designed activity programs to meet the needs of the individual, after examinations and tests had revealed those needs.

Thus, these physicians gave major direction to physical education for a half century during its formative years. They recognized more clearly than is generally true today, that a primary function of physical education should be the care and development of the body. Furthermore, they felt that such care and development was not only valuable by itself, but contributed dynamically to the individual's mental, emotional, and social effectiveness. In a sense, then, the thinking of Locke, Rousseau, and other European philosophers was gaining expression from an entirely different direction and as a result of an entirely different approach.

Other voices were also being heard on the American scene advocating the values of physical education and suggesting the direction it should take. Around 1850, Horace Mann argued that the care of the physical body should be given consideration in the schools along with academic and intellectual efforts. These thoughts were echoed by such great educators as Henry Bernard and Herbert Spencer. Such insistence, increasing as time went on, coupled with a growing dissatisfaction within the profession over the limited scope of physical education, effectively set the stage for realistic changes following World War I. These changes were accompanied by a reconsideration of the developmental and therapeutic values of physical education, a process still much in evidence at the present time.

BETWEEN WORLD WARS

The tragic lesson of World War I, when many of our youth were found physically unfit to defend the nation against a powerful enemy, resulted in a tremendous expansion of physical education in American schools. Prior to this time, physical education did not appear generally in public school curriculums. Only two states, North Dakota and Idaho, had state laws requiring this subject in their schools. By 1932, however, 36 states, representing 90 per cent of the population, had enacted such laws.[8] In 1948, all but eight states had statutes requiring physical education in their schools.

---

[8] J. F. Rogers, *Statewide Trends in School Hygiene and Physical Education* (Washington: Department of the Interior, Office of Education, 1934).

Such a growth, as would be expected, resulted in many changes affecting American physical education. Only those developments most relevant to the purpose of this text will be discussed here.

First, the influence of medical leadership in physical education waned. With rare exceptions, no longer did physicians enter this field. In more recent years, this leadership has come from men and women holding Doctor of Philosophy or Doctor of Education degrees. The change from leaders trained primarily in medicine to those trained primarily in philosophy, psychology, pedogogy, and, frequently, in the biological sciences resulted in a re-evaluation of objectives and procedures in this field.

Second, emphasis on the individual as an entity was recognized. In 1920, the Society of Directors of Physical Education in Colleges approved the concept that physical education was more than systematic exercise of the neuromuscular system and the development of correct motor habits. Their report stated:

> A usage more in conformity with the present conception of man's nature as a unit is that which sees in measures insuring bodily health and the right kind and amount of motor activity an avenue of approach through which the whole individual may be influenced for good, in mind and character as in body; it employs the word physical to denote the means, and not the end.

Social relations and character values were considered of great importance, and rightfully so, but underlying such aims, the report continues, "must be the purpose to promote the normal growth and organic development of the individual, conserve his health and provide a fair degree of strength and endurance, and to secure an erect and self-respecting carriage of the body and the neuromuscular control required for prompt and accurate response and graceful and effective movements." This is a good statement. Unfortunately, however, for the realization of the full potentialities of physical education, this concept was largely ignored in practice during the next two decades.

Third, a consistent effort was made to align physical education with total school purposes. During this period, American culture was undergoing a terrific upheaval. Many forces were at work: urbanization and industrialization of the country, interdependence of the population, increased communication of many kinds, monotony of labor, socio-economic conflicts, increase in amount of leisure time, support and defense of the democratic way of life, to mention a few. At the close of this period, the United States was to emerge as the most powerful nation on earth with accompanying worldwide responsibilities for leadership. Education was hard pressed to meet this challenge, and physical education leaders of the time struggled constantly to keep pace.

Fourth, although variously stated, physical education recognized three broad objectives: physical fitness, social efficiency, and recreational competency. Methods, materials, and precedures were developed to realize these objectives based upon physiological, psychological, and sociological principles. As a consequence, physical education underwent radical changes. As propounded by David K. Brace [9] in his 1949 address before the American Academy of Physical Education, these changes were described as follows:

> The formal calisthenics and artificial exercises transported from foreign countries have largely disappeared from our school programs. In their place have been substituted the natural activities of play, sports, games, and dance. The massed class instruction under the military type of command of the teacher has been replaced by a class organized into groups with a student leader. There has been a change from prescribed exercises, in the main purposeless to children and youth, to units of instruction comprising pupil activities of value in life and so graded and presented as to call forth physiologically sound effort and social participation.

Fifth, following World War I, college after college throughout the United States inaugurated training programs to meet the increased demands for personnel trained in health, physical education, and recreation work. The following statistics, giving the number of institutions providing such training, indicate the rapidity and extent of this growth: in 1918, 20 institutions; in 1929, 139 institutions; in 1944, 295 institutions; in 1947, 361 institutions; and in 1954, well over 500 institutions. As is well recognized today, the quality of instruction from college to college ranges from very demanding and superior to meager and inadequate. In fact, it may be stated that the type of training a physical educator receives depends largely upon the institution he attends. This situation has affected the courses offered in the training programs, which are of essential value to developmental and adapted physical education. In one questionnaire survey, in which 192 institutions replied, only 53 per cent required a course in corrective physical education; 49 per cent, in tests and measurements; and 34 per cent, in physiology of exercise.[10]

Sixth, while important progress was made during this between-war period, certain inadequacies were apparent, including the following:

1. In general, physical education abandoned its biological heritage. The understandings and tested processes developed over a century were largely rejected in the rush to adopt new ideas and procedures. Much

---

[9] David K. Brace, "The Contribution of Physical Education to Total Education," *Journal of the American Association for Health, Physical Education, and Recreation,* 20, No. 10 (1949), p. 636.

[10] H. Harrison Clarke, "Select Your Physical Educator with Care," *Education,* 68, No. 8 (April, 1948), p. 463.

of the new was vital, and was a great credit to those who sought to improve the services of physical education during this hectic period. However, much of the old was also vital for realization of the full potentialities of this field. A sifting and re-evaluation are essential, in order that activities and processes from all available sources may be selected and utilized in an expanded and effective program;

2. Too frequently, the improvement of physical fitness became a concomitant of an activity program designed to realize other educational objectives. Data are lacking that such an outcome occurs under these conditions. Contrarily, considerable evidence is available to indicate that the activity program designed to meet the physical fitness objective of physical education must be planned as carefully and specifically as any other;

3. Largely, the individual needs of boys and girls were not considered during this period, despite the existence of a dynamic educational philosophy to support and quantities of physiological and psychological evidence to justify the practice. Physical educators quite generally became engrossed in coaching athletic teams, teaching sports activities, and developing leisure skills. Valuable as these activities are, adequate time and effort, unfortunately, were not devoted to the application of appropriate procedures for identifying students with personal needs and for adapting program content and method to meet the needs thus identified.

Seventh, despite extensive criticism of physical education during this period, a number of realistic physical educators maintained an interest in the physical, psychological, emotional, and social needs of individual boys and girls. They conducted professional programs designed to alleviate, improve, and correct such deficiencies as were described. Evidence of this development is as follows:

1. A number of excellent texts on *corrective* physical education appeared during this time and subsequently, written by such physical educators as: George T. Stafford, Josephine L. Rathbone, Ivalclare Sprow Howland, Ellen D. Kelly, Arthur S. Daniels, Eleanor B. Stone, Mabel Lee, and Eleanor Metheny. Books on kinesiology, closely associated with this field, were produced by other physical educators, especially Gladys Scott, Gertrude Hawley, Katherine Wells, and Leon G. Kranz. Texts on physiology of exercise were published by other nonmedical people, Laurence Morehouse and Arthur Steinhaus. Numerous researches have also been completed by competent workers in this field;

2. Beginning in 1928 under the stimulus of Frederick Rand Rogers, then New York state director of physical education, a new type of physical fitness program gradually emerged. This program ideally consisted of the following seven steps, as described by Rogers: "medical, dental, and psychological examinations; followed by PFI tests (gross strength related to norms based on sex, age, and weight); followed by

analysis of results of the above; followed by recommendations of rest, diet, exercise, medical treatment; followed by individual action in accord with such advice; followed by repeated PFI tests (to determine results); followed by appropriate individual re-direction in the light of test results."[11] Perfected by many physical educators through actual use in schools and colleges of New York State, New England, and elsewhere, this type of program proved unusually successful;

3. Consistent recognition of the place of developmental and remedial physical education was evident in the structure of the American Association for Health, Physical Education, and Recreation. The national and several of the district organizations provided Therapeutic Sections. These sections met annually to conduct business and present professional programs.

Eighth, new therapeutic applications of exercise were developed between the wars, not only in physical education, but in medicine. From World War I, two technical specialties in medicine, occupational therapy and physical therapy, emerged. Gradually, too, a new medical specialty evolved, which eventually became recognized as physical medicine. The full recognition of this field came to dramatic fruition in World War II. As will be seen below, the utilization of many physical education activities for therapeutic purposes became a definite part of this development.

Ninth, while not evident in this country until the outbreak of World War II, a number of European countries focused attention on the physical training of youth as an obligation of the state in safeguarding national integrity. In evidence were several movements, particularly: *Hitler Jugend* and the *Kraft durch Freude of the Deutsches Arbeitsfront of Germany;* the Ready for Labor Defense of Russia; the Keep Fit Campaign of England; the *Sokel* and the *Orel* of Czechoslovakia; and the *Balilla* and *Aranguardisti* of Italy. Some of the movements had a strong military stamp; in the main, they combined disciplined physical training of the masses with patriotism; stress was placed forcefully on the inculcation of a desire to be fit.[12] Once mobilization started in the United States, "Fitness for Defense" programs sprang up throughout this country, sponsored by federal, state, community, and military organizations.

DURING AND AFTER WORLD WAR II

With the advent of World War II, great vistas opened for the developmental and remedial applications of physical education. Nearly every activity known to physical education was utilized for some phase of hospital and convalescent care. This understanding and growth, how-

---

[11] Frederick Rand Rogers, *A Basic Program for National Defense,* Bulletin Eleven (Monterey, Calif.: North American Physical Fitness Institute, 1950), p. 7.

[12] F. A. Hellebrandt, "Medical Implications of the British National Fitness Campaign," *War Medicine,* 2, No. 3 (1942), p. 230.

ever, did not take place in the schools and colleges. It began in the medical services of the armed forces during the war and has been carried on since in Veterans Administration hospitals and community rehabilitation centers. Under the direction of physicians, physical activities were applied by personnel trained basically in physical education.

PHYSICAL RECONDITIONING IN THE ARMED FORCES

The first convalescent reconstruction program of the Medical Department of the United States Army was developed during World War I. Based upon prior efforts of the British, medically designed and prescribed exercises were introduced into the hospitals in order to hasten the recovery of convalescent patients. Extensive use was made of physical therapy, occupational therapy, and physical retraining.

Following this war, no sustained effort to continue this form of convalescent service was evidenced by the armed forces. Only a few of the larger Army hospitals provided such services, and these were on a conservative basis with only nominal medical supervision. When World War II broke out, again the prior experience of the British[13] furnished the example for establishing similar programs by the United States which were eventually conducted separately by the Army Air Forces, the Army, and the Navy.

Army Air Forces. The first branch of the armed forces to provide formally for special convalescent services was the Army Air Forces. A Convalescent-Rehabilitation Program was inaugurated in December, 1942, by Dr. Howard A. Rusk at Jefferson Barracks, Missouri. In January, 1943, he was transferred to the Air Surgeon's Office in Washington and was placed in charge of the administration of the program in all AAF hospitals. Initially, convalescent services were made available at station hospitals; later, special convalescent centers were established throughout the United States. The programs in these hospitals were designed to recondition patients and send them back to duty in a shorter time and in better physical condition than had been the case formerly, to improve their morale, and to teach skills that would make them more effective members of the Air Forces. Physical reconditioning was an essential phase of this process, conducted by physical education personnel. Physical activities were utilized as follows: therapeutic exercise and adapted sports, for physical retraining of orthopedic patients; conditioning exercises, for maintenance and improvement of the strength of bed and ambulatory patients during the early reconditioning process; gymnastics and tumbling, for the development of strength and agility during later stages of reconditioning; climbing, running, and activities necessitating

---

[13] Due to the insistence of British labor unions, rehabilitation services for men and women injured in industry were continued in England between the wars.

sustained running, for improvement of circulatory-respiratory endurance, especially as the patient approached return-to-duty status; competitive sports, for advanced reconditioning and for emotional release and diversionary purposes in neuropsychiatric cases; and recreational sports, such as skiing, fishing, riding, boating, golf, and the like, for diversionary and morale values and for the acquisition of desirable leisure skills, especially for those receiving disability discharges.[14]

United States Army. Following the example of the Air Forces, the Army Service Forces established convalescent programs in all but the smallest station hospitals of the military services both overseas and in the Zone of the Interior. A distinctive type of rehabilitation hospital was originated for advanced patients. The emphases in these hospitals were primarily upon the early return to duty of the sick and injured, and, for those with disabling conditions, upon return to effective civilian life.

A vital factor in the establishment of rehabilitation and reconditioning services in the European Theatre of Operations was the significant percentage of military personnel unable to carry on their former duties after discharge from general hospitals because of physical and mental deterioration occurring during hospitalization. The seriousness of this loss of manpower led to the inauguration of convalescent services in this theater. The basis for the procedures involved in this program was planned exercise. The practices were successful beyond expectations, both in the excellence of the physical capacity and mental status of the fighting man returned to his duties and in the economy of medical personnel and facilities required for effective convalescence.[15]

United States Navy. A directive from Vice-Admiral Ross T. McIntire was issued on April 12, 1944, ordering that physical training for patients "be included in the daily routine of the hospital and considered a part of the general treatment plan."[16] The Navy's convalescent program was similar to those in the AAF and the Army in that special emphasis was placed upon expediting recovery and return to duty of as many patients as possible, and to prepare those whose disabilities necessitated their discharge to civilian life for maximum adjustment to their conditions.

Post-War Developments. Since the war, the Army has been the most active of the armed forces in the utilization of convalescent services. A Physical Medicine Consultants Division was organized in the Office of

---

[14] *Physical Reconditioning Manual*, AFPDC Manual 25-26-1 (Louisville, Ky.: Headquarters, AAF Personnel Distribution Command [Prepared by Major Arthur S. Daniels and Major H. Harrison Clarke], 1945).

[15] Captain Frank Rathauser, M.D., "Rehabilitation and Reconditioning in the European Theatre of Operations during World War II," Report, Office of the Surgeon General, Department of the Army.

[16] "Rehabilitation Program of the Medical Department of the United States Navy," Bureau of Medicine and Surgery, Bu Med. J-JS, P-4-4/P 3-2 [081], (Department of the Navy, Washington, D. C., April 12, 1944).

the Surgeon General with three branches: Physical Therapy, Occupational Therapy, and Physical Reconditioning. Thus, physical reconditioning continued as a definite phase of convalescent care. In 1949, the Army announced a new-type Convalescent Center.[17] This installation is designed to provide convalescent care and physical reconditioning for casualties requiring less than three week's treatment for return to duty within the Combat Zone. The whole psychology and activity of the center is geared to conditions favoring the patient's return to combat with his own unit.

VETERANS ADMINISTRATION

The Veterans Administration's hospital program increased tremendously following World War II. By 1951, 150 hospitals of various kinds cared for 123,134 patients; 60 regional offices treated veterans on an out-patient basis; 33 additional hospitals were under construction.[18] As corrective therapy, many of the activities of physical education are utilized extensively and effectively in the treatment of patients. The application of physical and motor activities in therapy reached a new all-time high in the Veterans Administration, especially in the treatment of severely handicapped and chronically ill patients.

In addition, as was true in the armed forces, special services' activities are carried on in Veterans Administration hospitals. This program is separate from the physical medicine rehabilitation services. Recreational elements include: sports and athletics, music, drama, motion pictures, entertainment, radio, hobby and other group activities, social events, tours, outings, and others.[19] The functions of this program are to provide recreation for the patients in the hospital and to contribute to improved morale.[20]

CIVILIAN HOSPITALS AND REHABILITATION CENTERS

While post-war rehabilitation, as so far described, has centered in the dramatic developments of the armed forces and the Veterans Administration, the problem is no less acute in the civilian population. With vivid clarity, Rusk has pointed out that, while disabled veterans are numbered in the thousands, they constitute only a fraction of our handicapped and disabled people. Prior to the onset of World War II, the

---

[17] *Convalescent Center, Army,* TC No. 7 (Department of the Army, Washington, D.C., 26 March 1951).

[18] A. B. C. Knudsen, "Present Needs of the Veterans Administration in Physical Medicine and Rehabilitation," *Archives of Physical Medicine,* XXXII, No. 10 (1951), p. 632.

[19] "Recreation in Veterans Administration Hospitals," *Recreation,* XLV, No. 2 (1951), p. 72.

[20] B. E. Phillips, "The Veterans Administration Athletic Program," *Journal of Health and Physical Education,* 18, No. 6 (1947), p. 368.

U. S. Public Health Service estimated that there were 23 million persons in this country who were handicapped by disease, accidents, maladjustments, or former wars. As expressed by Rusk:

> Between Pearl Harbor and V-J Day, there were approximately 17,000 amputations in the Army, but during this same period there were over 120,000 major amputations from disease and accidents among our civilian population. In the first ten days after D-Day, 11,000 soldiers were wounded on the beaches of Normandy, yet, even with curtailed traffic, automobile accidents alone accounted for more than twice that many civilian casualties in the same ten days. During World War II, 260,000 veterans were permanently disabled as a result of combat wounds, but during the same four years 1,250,000 civilians suffered permanent disabilities from accidents.[21]

The new concept of rehabilitation in medicine, which Dr. Rusk has termed "the third phase of medical care," has become a phase of treatment in some civilian general hospitals. The "first comprehensive, total, medical rehabilitation program" in any community hospital in this country was started in the spring of 1947 at Bellevue Hospital in New York City.[22] By 1949, there were approximately 150 communities in the nation which had expressed interest in establishing similar centers.[23] Most of these are following the recommendations of the Baruch Committee on Physical Medicine that such centers be medically directed and be associated with civilian hospitals and medical schools.[24]

The place of physical education as a technical specialty in medicine is still not clear. However, there is a definite tendency to utilize personnel trained in physical education and recreation in community hospitals and rehabilitation centers. In the functional plan of rehabilitation centers prepared by the Baruch Committee, physical education is included as a therapeutic adjunct; "corrective physical rehabilitation" and "planned recreation" are provided at the Institute of Physical Medicine and Rehabilitation of New York University.

SCHOOLS AND COLLEGES

In general, school and college physical educators were slow to respond to the new developments in convalescent services and rehabilitation affecting their field. A glance at the programs of the various national

---

21 Howard A. Rusk, "Rehabilitation and Early Ambulation," *Modern Medicine* (January 1, 1948).

22 Howard A. Rusk, "Rehabilitation," *Journal of the American Medical Association*, 140 (May 21, 1949), p. 286.

23 *Annual Report of the Baruch Committee on Physical Medicine* (New York: The Baruch Committee on Physical Medicine, 1947), p. 164.

24 *A Community Service and Center* (New York: The Baruch Committee on Physical Medicine, 1946).

and district Therapeutic Section meetings of the American Association for Health, Physical Education, and Recreation will show that these physical education specialists are still primarily concerned with body mechanics and posture and "restricted" activities for the handicapped. Even the title adopted for the sections gives a narrow functional connotation.

From available literature, too, one must conclude that considerable lethargy exists in regard to the potentials of this service, particularly in the public schools. For 25 states studied in a national co-operative survey of health and physical education, Bookwalter[25] reported that only 4 per cent of the high schools included "corrective" work in their physical education programs. Thus, concern for developmental and adapted physical education in the high schools of these states is apparently so slight as to be virtually non-existent.

The prevalence of corrective physical education for boys in the high schools of Pennsylvania, however, is considerably greater than for this incomplete national survey, according to a study by Gross.[26] Of 844 high schools of all sizes in the state, 220, or 26 per cent, maintained a program of this kind. Approximately, 40 per cent of the large and very large schools (enrollments of 500 and above) provided corrective physical education for their atypical students.

The college situation has been quite different, with the prevalence of corrective physical education, being related to the size of the college or university. The larger institutions generally maintained programs of this type, as shown in an early survey: enrollments 5000 and over, 87 per cent; enrollments between 2000 and 5000, 59 per cent; enrollments under 2000, 38 per cent. In general, too, the larger colleges had finer corrective programs, better prepared teaching personnel, and more equipment and facilities for this service.[27].

Physical education needs to take stock of its full developmental and therapeutic potentialities. For the first time in the history of physical education in the United States, primary leadership in this specialty has been lost by the schools and colleges. Personnel, basically trained in physical education but engaged in non-educational institutions such as Veterans Administration and Army hospitals and various rehabilitation centers, are developing this field far beyond the narrow confines of the traditional corrective program. The need for adopting an expanded con-

---

[25] Karl W. Bookwalter, "A National Survey of Health and Physical Education for Boys in High Schools, 1950-1954," *American Academy of Physical Education*, Professional Contributions No. 4, November, 1955, p. 1.

[26] Elmer A. Gross, "A Study of the Present Practices in Corrective Physical Education for Boys in the Public Schools of Pennsylvania" (Doctor's thesis, University of Pittsburgh, 1953).

[27] Port G. Robertson, "A Study of Corrective Physical Education in Sixty-nine Selected Colleges and Universities" (Master's thesis, University of Michigan, 1941).

cept of developmental and adapted physical education in educational institutions is pronounced. The opportunity is present for providing a greater service to boys and girls than ever before, a service which will contribute dynamically to their physical, mental, and social well-being and effectiveness.

In 1955, Kraus and Hirschland[28] published statistics showing that United States children had a great many more failures than did Italian, Switzerland, and Austrian children on the Kraus-Weber Test of Minimum Muscular Fitness. With this disclosure, physical fitness entered the cold war against communism. President Dwight D. Eisenhower turned his attention to this vital problem. He was prompted to do so by his own knowledge, as General of the Armies, of the inadequate fitness of young men reporting for military service; and he treated with respect and concern the Kraus-Hirschland findings. Executive action followed with the establishment of a President's Council on Youth Fitness and a President's Citizens' Advisory Committee.

As a result of President Eisenhower's intervention, a vast public relations program was undertaken to alert America to the dangerously low physical fitness of her youth and to the realization that fitness is essential for national survival. Many leading figures in medicine spoke and wrote on the need for exercise in the maintenance of an organically sound body from birth to old age. The governors of many states called fitness conferences to motivate their people toward strong programs in this area. The physical education profession was mobilized in the interest of a positive emphasis on fitness by the American Association for Health, Physical Education, and Recreation.

In 1961, a new President, John F. Kennedy, immediately took action to deal with the physical fitness of the nation's youth. He appointed Charles B. Wilkinson as his Special Consultant on Youth Fitness. The President's council office, re-formed under Wilkinson, included professional physical education and medical personnel on the staff and/or as consultants. After his election, and before he was inaugurated, President Kennedy wrote forcefully on his views regarding this problem in the pages of *Sports Illustrated:* "For the physical vigor of our citizens is one of America's most precious resources. If we waste and neglect this resource, if we allow it to dwindle and grow soft then we will destroy much of our ability to meet the great and vital challenges which confront our people. We will be unable to realize our full potential as a nation."[29]

The need to improve the physical fitness of those boys and girls who

---

[28] Hans Kraus and Ruth P. Hirschland, "Muscular Fitness and Orthopedic Disability," *New York State Journal of Medicine,* 54 (January 15, 1954), p. 212.
[29] John F. Kennedy, "The Soft American," *Sports Illustrated,* December 26, 1960.

are subpar in basic fitness elements through developmental and adapted physical education is fundamental in this effort. True, vigorous exercise as a way of life is essential for all from birth to old age. However, this does not negate the necessity for identifying and adapting program content and method for those in greatest need; to point the way to a realization of this end is a major function of this book.

SUMMARY

In this chapter, an historical overview of the utilization of physical education methods and materials for developmental and therapeutic purposes has been presented. The strategic landmarks in this process are worthy of review.

1. The use of physical activity to improve and maintain physical fitness dates from antiquity, a practice usually associated with preparing men to fight. Except in time of war, however, this objective has not been effective in the United States.

2. The Greeks believed that physical development was closely associated with mental effectiveness and that physical development was essential for the education of the total individual. Similar relationships were expressed by European philosophers of the sixteenth and seventeenth centuries and were practiced in early formal European physical education systems.

3. Today, educators express this concept in terms of the total individual. Man is not divisible, but is an entity reacting and interacting in many ways. Deficiencies in any of his basic powers will affect performance in the others.

4. The use of exercise as therapy also originated in antiquity. It was practiced by the medical authorities of Greece. It was also advocated by early European physicians.

5. Physical education leadership in the United States between the Civil War and World War I was provided largely by men and women trained in medicine. The physical education of this period was primarily directed toward the development of physical fitness, not only for its own sake but as an essential factor of the well-rounded personality. Therapeutic exercise was widely utilized during this period.

6. After World War I, leadership in physical education became the province of individuals trained in philosophy, psychology, and education. As a result, this field conformed more and more to the broad objectives of education. In general, the physical fitness of boys and girls became somewhat incidental to the program as a whole.

7. In the late 1920's and during the 1930's, physical education programs based upon meeting the individual physical and social needs of boys and girls were inaugurated and developed in a number of schools in New

York State, New England, and elsewhere. In practice, these procedures proved unusually effective.

8. During World War II, the medical departments of the various branches of the armed forces utilized a wide range of physical education activities in the treatment of convalescent patients. The Veterans Administration has carried this practice to a new high point as applied to the acutely disabled.

9. Developmental and adapted physical education in schools and colleges, with certain notable exceptions, has not kept pace with these new understandings and practices. The need for these services in educational institutions, however, is pronounced and constitutes a challenge to physical education.

10. Two presidents of the United States, Dwight D. Eisenhower and John F. Kennedy, have stressed the need to improve the physical fitness of America's youth as essential for national survival. Thus, physical educators have been called to enter the cold war against communism. The basic functions they must perform are to present vigorous exercise as a way of life and to stress the improvement of the physically unfit through developmental and adapted procedures.

SELECTED REFERENCES

Brace, David K., "The Contributions of Physical Education to Total Education," *Journal of the American Association for Health, Physical Education, and Recreation*, 20, No. 10 (1949), 636.

Brownell, Clifford L., and Patricia E. Hagman, *Physical Education: Foundations and Principles*. New York: McGraw-Hill Book Co., Inc., 1951.

Hellebrandt, F. A., "Medical Implications of the British National Fitness Campaign," *War Medicine*, 2, No. 3 (1942), 230.

Kennedy, John F., "The Soft American," *Sports Illustrated*, December 26, 1960.

Knudsen, A. B. C., "Present Needs of the Veterans Administration in Physical Medicine and Rehabilitation," *Archives of Physical Medicine*, XXXII, No. 10 (1951), 632.

Leonard, Fred E., and George B. Affleck, *A Guide to the History of Physical Education*, 3rd ed. Philadelphia: Lea and Febiger, 1947.

Rogers, Frederick Rand, *Tests and Measurement Programs in the Redirection of Physical Education*. New York: Bureau of Publications, Teachers College, Columbia University, 1927.

Rusk, Howard A., "Rehabilitation," *Journal of the American Medical Association*, 140 (May 21, 1948), 286.

Strickland, B. A., and Cecil W. Morgan, "Physical Reconditioning," *Journal of the American Association for Health, Physical Education, and Recreation*, 20, No. 1 (1949), 20.

2

Functions in
Education

THE PRIMARY CONCERN OF THIS BOOK IS THE PROBLEM
of how physical education may best serve individual
boys and girls in schools and colleges. A broad approach to needs is
contemplated, including physical, social, emotional, and psychological
conditions. Many terms have identified this physical education service.
In earlier days, "medical gymnastics" and "corrective physical education"
had common usage. As the field expanded, especially during and after
World War II, other designations were adopted by various organizations,
especially: physical reconditioning, by the Armed Forces; corrective
therapy, by the Veterans Administration; exercise therapy, by the United
States Civil Service Commission.

There is no general agreement on a common name for this field. Dissatisfaction has been widely expressed by school and college physical
educators over the connotations and limitations of the earlier terminology. For example, medical gymnastics implies strict medical supervision of special exercises applied to orthopedic disabilities; corrective
physical education has negative connotations, is too limited in scope, and
does not include the concept of living stressed for the handicapped; the
use of therapy or therapeutic in the name implies definitive care of patients under medical direction.

Actually the service of meeting individual needs through physical
education activities and methods is as broad as the entire basic field,
itself. Theoretically, all pupils may have some needs which may be
helped by physical education. In practice, however, only selected conditions and degrees of involvement are considered, the physical educator

arbitrarily establishing levels to represent minimum standards. Thus, the low physical fitness level may be placed at a Physical Fitness Index of 85 or 90 or 100; the accepted posture level may be at slight, moderate, or marked deviations; the unsatisfactory social adjustment level may include those with disciplinary problems only or may also include those with scores below selected points on a standard test.

Nevertheless, a label to designate this service offers some advantage in identifying it. A single all-inclusive term, satisfactory to all, seems impossible, at least for the moment. So, in this book, *developmental and adapted physical education* has been chosen. Under the aegis of this term are included conditioning activities for low physical fitness, strengthening and stretching exercises for the improvement of posture, adapted skills and the like for the handicapped, and guidance and use of selected activities for social, emotional, and psychological adjustment. A greater delineation of this service follows.

BREADTH OF APPLICATION

In this book, the developmental and adapted physical education service is applied primarily to schools and colleges. However, it will be well at the outset to consider the broad utilization of physical education methods and materials for therapy in many situations. The full scope of this development becomes evident when the variety of institutions including such services is known. Among them are: schools and colleges, neuropsychiatric hospitals, armed forces hospitals and convalescent centers, special schools and classes, public and private hospitals, convalescent homes, camps for crippled children, sheltered workshops, children's hospitals, special organizations, certain social agencies, community rehabilitation centers, and Veterans Administration hospitals.

The therapeutic application of physical education constitutes an essential phase of the newer developments in physical medicine and rehabilitation. A better understanding of this expanding technical specialty will serve to further clarify these relationships. It is within this framework that the fulfillment of developmental and adapted physical education is evident. Krusen[1] has provided the following definitions of physical medicine and rehabilitation.

Physical Medicine: The employment of the physical and other effective diagnostic and therapeutic properties of light, heat, cold, water, electricity, massage, manipulation, exercise, and mechanical devices for diagnosis, for research, and for physical and occupational therapy and physical rehabilitation.

---

[1] Frank H. Krusen, "The Scope and Future of Physical Medicine and Rehabilitation," *Journal of the American Medical Association*, 144, No. 9 (1950), p. 727.

Rehabilitation: The employment of physical medicine technics of psychosocial adjustment and vocational retraining for the purpose of aiding the patient to achieve the maximal function and adjustment and of preparing him physically, mentally, socially, and vocationally for the fullest possible life compatible with his abilities and disabilities.

During the last decade, physicians have broadened their concept of what constitutes complete medical practice. There is a growing realization that the diagnosis of disease and the application of curative measures during the definitive phase of illness are not enough. Rusk[2] states that the practice of rehabilitation "begins with the basic philosophy that the doctor's responsibility does not end when the acute illness is ended or operation completed; it ends only when the patient is retrained to live and work with what is left." This development has resulted in the broadening of the Council on Physical Medicine to the Council on Physical Medicine and Rehabilitation and the creation of the American Board of Physical Medicine and Rehabilitation of the American Medical Association.

The consequences of the development of this "third phase of medicine" have been the recognition of a need for new technical services and the expansion of the older services in physical medicine. Established ways of doing things are being reconsidered; new services and personnel are being evaluated. The activities of physical education are proving vital to this process, especially in the "rehabilitation" phase.

Interestingly, this utilization of physical activities and physical education personnel in medicine is not a radically new practice. After World War I, physical education became the parent body of physical therapy, and still contributes many physical educators for specialized training in this field. In fact, several prominent physicians now working in physical medicine were trained originally in physical education; the same is true for a number of prominent physicians now in psychiatry. Two reasons may be advanced to account for this phenomenon: Medicine has acquired an increased understanding of the values and uses of exercise and physical activities in the treatment and after-care of patients; personnel prepared in physical education have the basic training essential to serve as technicians under medical direction and supervision.[3]

In reviewing statements defining the therapeutic application of physical education, it is found that no, one, accepted definition is available. Each agency or organization has prepared its own—based upon the

---

[2] Howard A. Rusk, "Rehabilitation and General Practice," *Journal of the American Medical Association,* 139, No. 1 (1949), p. 14.

[3] H. Harrison Clarke, "Schools of Physical Education and the Training of Physical Medicine and Rehabilitation Specialists," *Journal of the Association for Physical and Mental Rehabilitation,* 7, No. 2 (1953), p. 44.

specific job to be done. An analysis of these definitions reveals the following characteristics:

First, each definition is written to meet a particular situation, with variations evident in the armed forces, the Veterans Administration, and so forth. This procedure will be necessary until agreement is reached on the specific functions to be performed by this specialty.

Second, there are certain elements common to all the definitions, such as: to maintain and improve physical condition, to allay and prevent deconditioning and physical deterioration, to contribute to psychological readjustment and resocialization, to provide the handicapped with desirable skills within the limits of their disabilities, and to afford opportunities for self-expression and release from physical and emotional stresses.

Third, corrective therapy treatment in Veterans Administration hospitals includes the widest utilization of exercise modalities. Considerable application is made to many patients who are chronically ill with a great variety of medical, orthopedic, neurological, and psychiatric disabilities.

Fourth, in all instances exercise and physical activity applied to patients are medically prescribed. Close medical direction and supervision are standard operating procedures in hospitals and convalescent centers, as well as in other medical establishments.

The situation for developmental and adapted physical education in schools and colleges differs from those in hospitals and convalescent centers. As a consequence, the definition of this field as applied to educational institutions must take these differences into account. In the following section, the potentialities of this physical education service in such institutions will be considered.

BASES FOR DEVELOPMENTAL AND ADAPTED PHYSICAL EDUCATION

In considering the role of developmental and adapted physical education in schools and colleges, the following factors should be taken into account: the essential characteristics of such institutions as contrasted with medical establishments; the objectives of physical education in schools and colleges; the procedures adopted for realizing these objectives. Based on these considerations, the functions of the developmental and remedial service can be formulated.[4]

CONTRAST WITH MEDICAL ESTABLISHMENTS

Developmental and adapted physical education must be structured around certain essential characteristics of educational institutions. Five

---

[4] Reference is not intended here to schools for crippled children or other special schools and classes for children with various types of chronic physical, social, and mental handicaps.

such characteristics may be mentioned specifically.

1. As the school is obviously not a hospital or convalescent center, exercise and physical activity are not needed for bed patients. However, infirmary care in colleges may have significance for developmental and adapted physical education.

2. Furthermore, the care of ambulatory patients is not a problem, as it is in hospitals. However, following illnesses, accidents, and operations, advanced convalescent care is appropriate for students before returning to the vigorous activities of the regular physical education program.

3. Contrasted with the large number of chronic disabilities of all kinds in Veterans Administration hospitals, the number of severely disabled in any one school or college is relatively small. The larger the institution, of course, the greater this number. The need for help, on the part of those disabled who do attend, however, is very great. Developmental and adapted physical education can provide vital services for these individuals.

4. In schools and colleges, physical educators have primary responsibility for developmental and adapted physical education; thus, this program is not under the direction of medical personnel. As practiced in educational institutions, most activities of this service are educational and conditioning in nature and do not require medical supervision. There are times, however, as will be shown later, when consultation with the school and/or family physician may be essential in dealing with individual cases.

5. Traditionally, developmental and adapted physical education has been concerned with the improvement of postural defects and the physical development and conditioning of individual students. While posture correction may be recognized as a proper function of comparable programs in hospitals and convalescent centers, the emphasis is usually not nearly so great. Also, special techniques, procedures, and testing instruments have been devised and are used by physical educators to identify and improve sub-strength and low-fitness individuals. In general, this process is little understood or practiced by corrective therapists in hospitals and convalescent or rehabilitation centers.

PHYSICAL EDUCATION OBJECTIVES [5]

Developmental and adapted physical education should emerge as an essential service of the physical education program as a whole. Justification for this service rests on its contribution to the realization of the basic objectives of this field. Therefore, a logical statement of purposes for the developmental and adapted program must be based upon clearly

---

[5] These objectives are developed from those proposed by H. Harrison Clarke in: *Application of Measurement to Health and Physical Education,* 3rd ed. (Englewood Cliffs, N. J.: Prentice-Hall, Inc., 1959), chap. I.

defined objectives of physical education; and must be a part of the procedures formulated for achieving these objectives.

The danger in presenting objectives of physical education is that the teacher will make the common error in education of separating the individual into parts, each part related to a stated objective. For administrative purposes, however, the determination of objectives is the only convenient way of identifying areas of fundamental importance. Such designations should be considered only as a method of analysis; any tendency to accept them as mutually exclusive categories should be avoided. In operation, the approach to the individual should be in terms of his total being. With these factors in mind, therefore, three physical education objectives are presented.

> *Physical fitness:* The development and maintenance of a strong physique and soundly functioning organs, to the end that the individual realizes his capacity for physical activity, unhampered by physical drains or by a body lacking in strength and vitality.

This definition implies that physical fitness is more than "not being sick" or merely "being well." It is different from resistance to or immunity from disease. It is a positive quality, extending on a scale from death to "abundant life." All living individuals, thus, have some degree of physical fitness which varies considerably in different people and in the same person at different times.

In accordance with this concept, boys and girls who are not sick, who are free from defects and handicaps, and who are adequately nourished, may still exhibit physical deficiencies. For physical education, such deficiencies may be observed in pupils who are muscularly weak for their sex, age, weight, and somatotype, and pupils who are lacking in circulatory-respiratory endurance. In addition, the physical educator is able to correct functional postural defects, increase body flexibility as needed, and improve the general physical condition of those with handicaps.

> *Social efficiency:* The development of desirable standards of behavior and the ability to get along well with others.

The term *social efficiency* indicates those traits usually included in the concepts of character and personality. It has a definite social implication, since in our democratic society the effect of one's actions upon others is of primary concern. An individual's social behavior is dependent upon: (1) individual traits, such as courage, initiative, morality, perseverance, integrity, and self-control; (2) group traits, such as sympathy, courtesy, loyalty, and co-operation; and (3) their interaction for the common good. *A socially efficient individual is one who functions harmoniously within himself, in his relationship with others, and as a member of the society of which he is a part.*

Individuals vary in social characteristics and needs as widely as they do in physical characteristics and needs. Effective physical education procedures in this area should include the identification of boys and girls with personality conflicts, undesirable character traits, or anti-social tendencies. It is important that such an individual be located early—while his condition is in its incipient stages. The possibility of successful treatment through physical education and other processes is, thus, much greater. For handicapped individuals, resocialization and personal psychological adjustment can be greatly enhanced through developmental and adapted physical education.

Culture: The enrichment of human experience through physical activities that lead to better understanding and appreciation of the environment in which boys and girls find themselves, and the development of recreational competency for leisure.

In this interpretation, culture is interpreted broadly as "one's stock of appreciations," including all aspects of living that will improve one's understanding and enjoyment of people and events in his civilization. Examples from physical education are: the grace, rhythm, and creative expression of the dance; a biological and aesthetic understanding and appreciation of the human body; appreciation of skilled performance; the historical background and cultural associations of many physical education activities.

Physical education is one of the many education fields that contributes to the recreational competency of boys and girls. Many sports such as swimming, tennis, golf, and the like, have value as leisure time activities.

The developmental and adapted physical education service has definite potentialities for the development of the cultural appreciations and recreational competency of handicapped children. Their spectator enjoyment of many physical education activities can be greatly enhanced; they can be taught skills and activities in which they may participate within the restrictions imposed by their disabilities.

Emphasis for Girls. In this report, the objectives of physical education are considered to be fundamentally the same for girls as for boys. They differ, however, in emphasis and in essential motivation. Basic strength is essential for each sex to realize its own purposes: for girls, sufficient strength means effortless bodily control reflected in poise, grace, and pleasing posture; for boys, adequate strength permits satisfying participation in sports and athletics; for both, minimum strength levels contribute to the efficient functioning of vital processes.

As Dorothy La Salle has so aptly expressed it: "Women have always needed to be fit for the biological and traditional purposes of our society. Child-bearing and rearing require healthy women."[6] Attention to their physical welfare is necessary and is recognized by women themselves, as shown in the findings of Eleanor Metheny at the University of Southern California.[7] Analyzing the responses of a random sample of 300 college women at that institution, she found that 68.3 per cent of this favored group believed that they did not have sufficient health to profit completely from the opportunities of university life; and approximately half of them stated they were under some medical and professional care. Among the conditions regarded as unfavorable by these young women were: chronic fatigue, faulty body mechanics, frequent colds, overweight, undesirable mental attitudes, and dysmenorrhea.

Girls and women need to participate in activities that will contribute to their personal and social growth and adjustment. Social patterns should be developed which "permit women to like being women in fulfilling the various roles our society calls upon them to play—wife, mother, wage-earner, and home-maker."[8] They need opportunities to make friends, to develop democratic conduct and ideals, and to acquire social skills that will add to their popularity and social adjustment. These factors, and others, should be given basic consideration not only in planning developmental and adapted physical education programs for girls but in providing proper and effective motivation for the participants.

FUNCTIONS OF DEVELOPMENTAL AND ADAPTED PHYSICAL EDUCATION

In the efforts of physical educators to plan programs that will be completely effective in realizing educational objectives, the necessity of meeting individual needs of boys and girls becomes readily apparent. Children differ in innumerable ways. For example: their muscular strength varies from weak and puny to physically powerful; their ability to learn skills ranges from neuromuscularly inept to well-coordinated and highly skilled; their nutritional status ranges widely from undernourished to obese; their somatotypes are of many variations; some individuals have serious handicaps of various kinds while others are free from all defects; the differences in social adjustment and mental health are obvious to any astute observer. Program adaptations for such factors must be provided if physical education is to be fully effective in the lives of all individuals.

As a consequence of these realizations, developmental and adapted

---

[6] Dorothy La Salle, "Fitness Today on the Home Front," *Journal of Health and Physical Education,* 15, No. 10 (1944), p. 535.

[7] Eleanor Metheny, "Some Health Problems of College Women," *Journal of Health and Physical Education,* 17, No. 4 (1946), p. 205.

[8] Hilda Clute Kozman, ed., *Group Process in Physical Education* (New York: Harper & Brothers, 1951), p. 35.

processes were devised—not as a separate entity, but evolving from this complex situation. This program should be a vital phase of the total physical education program. Its justification should be in terms of basic growth and development of the individual. Simply stated, then, *the purpose of developmental and adapted physical education is to meet, through physical education methods and activities, the individual needs of boys and girls who are handicapped in some respect, who have functional defects or deficiencies amenable to improvement through exercise, or who possess other inadequacies which interfere with their successful participation in the diversified and vigorous activities of the general physical education program.*

In presenting specific functions of developmental and adapted physical education, the many related developments affecting physical education from all sources should be brought together and applied. This process should include the early experiences of physical education, the basic concept of the unity of the individual, and the relationship of the physical aspect to that entity, the successful practices of physical education since its inception in the United States, and the broad utilization of physical education as therapy during and following World War II. Specific procedures should be devised and materials selected in accordance with the needs of school and college populations. As will be discussed later, the capabilities of physical education personnel to practice therapy must necessarily constitute a limitation to the program attempted at particular institutions.

Based on these considerations, then, the specific functions of the developmental and adapted program in school and college physical education include the following factors.

1. *General developmental and conditioning activities for individuals free of handicaps but of low physical fitness status.*

Many individuals in any school or college population, who are organically and structurally sound and who are well nourished, are still deficient in basic strength and endurance elements. These individuals should be identified by tests and examinations, studied for causes of their low fitness status, and provided with individual programs to eliminate such causes and improve their general fitness.

Mild, progressing to vigorous exercise regimens should be provided for boys and girls returning to school after devitalizing illnesses and operations before they are permitted to participate in the strenuous activities of the general physical education program. In this way, such students can gradually and systematically return to desirable physical fitness levels without the danger of over-exertion from prematurely vigorous athletic activities. Where feasible, pre-operative general body conditioning would prove beneficial. In some colleges, too, it would be possible to provide bed and ambulatory exercises for convalescent students in health-service infirmaries.

2. *Body mechanics training for individuals with non-pathological conditions.*

Among the demonstrated accomplishments of physical education is the development of correct body mechanics and the prevention and correction of postural and bodily defects. The responsibility for improving postural and weak foot conditions has long been recognized by this field in schools and colleges.

The extent of the need for posture training, proper use of the feet, and body mechanics teaching is widespread. Fundamentally, posture work should be included in childhood education, as it is during these formative years of life that proper attitudes and habits can best be developed. Also, during this period, the detection and correction of slight deviations from normal may be most effective, often resulting in the prevention of structural deformities. General agreement, therefore, places emphasis on this phase of developmental and adapted physical education in the elementary school. However, functional postural defects and weakened foot conditions should be treated at any level where found.

3. *Adaptation of physical education and recreation activities for the handicapped.*

Although physical educators for many years have conducted "restricted" activities for students with all sorts of physical handicaps, the experiences with reconditioning in the hospitals of the armed forces and in corrective therapy in Veterans Administration hospitals have added a new chapter in understanding the potentialities of this phase of the program. Basically, physical education should strive to accomplish the following with handicapped individuals: to develop strength, stamina, and skill within the limits of individual disabilities; to provide and adapt sports and recreational activities for use during leisure time in accordance with individual capabilities; to aid these students in the acceptance of their disabilities and to motivate them to live most effectively with their handicaps.

In this statement, the use of therapeutic exercise is not included, primarily for the following three reasons: First, schools and colleges are not now generally established as medical treatment centers; second, physical therapy training, or its equivalent in foundations and practices of therapeutic exercise, is essential for this function; third, the functions proposed are primarily educational and are within the capabilities of properly trained physical educators. It should not be forgotten that developmental and adapted physical education in schools and colleges is not primarily therapeutic, although there will be therapeutic values realized from the program, but is basically educational in nature.

4. *Psychological and social adjustments of "normal" individuals with atypical tendencies.*

Studies of the childhood backgrounds of psychiatric casualties in World War I emphasize the need for certain personality traits, without which men find it difficult to stand the rigors of war. Emmanuel Miller[9] presented data which show that those who lacked psychological stamina in the first World War were characterized by childhood backgrounds of nervousness, fussiness, over-evaluation of their egos, sensitive dispositions, over-attachment to their mothers, rigid personalities, and marked lack of aggressiveness. Our accelerated mode of living, the emotional pressures of everyday life, and the change from interesting and challenging to monotonous and routine employment which generally involves small-muscle rather than large-muscle activity, necessitates less psychological stamina than was demanded during war.

These same conditions have resulted in placing a premium on social adjustment. Not only must the individual in our civilization be conscious of his obligations to society, but he must be able to work co-operatively and well with others for the common good.

In developmental and adapted physical education it is imperative to consider the psychological and social deviates. The program itself should provide activities in which individuals can participate together and in which they are afforded opportunities for expression, thus helping to diminish physical and emotional tensions. Physical activities should be conducted to improve the psychological and social condition of maladjusted individuals. This program should also develop, create, or re-create a positive mental attitude toward the use of activities as a means for further total growth and development of the individual.

5. *Relaxation activities for individuals suffering from chronic fatigue and neuromuscular hypertension.*

Chronic fatigue and neuromuscular hypertension are closely associated, and are recognizable, as is true fatigue, by a definite increase of tension in the neuromuscular system. This tension is reflected in the tenseness of the skeletal muscles of the individual. Rest and specially devised relaxation activities are needed to counteract and alleviate this condition. Similar programs are needed for post-operative cases, tuberculosis suspects, and undernourished students. Rest and relaxation are also fre-

---

[9] Emmanuel Miller, *The Neuroses of War* (New York: The Macmillan Company, 1943), chap. V.

quently desirable for many low-fitness individuals at the start of, and at different times during their developmental and conditioning process.

6. *Counseling, guidance, and assistance with physical fitness, personal adjustment, and social problems.*

Permeating the developmental and adapted physical education program is the need for counseling, guidance, and assistance for individuals with physical fitness, personal adjustment, and other problems. The handicapped must understand the nature of and be motivated to accept his disability; the socially maladjusted may need guidance toward desirable inter-personal and democratic relationships; the individual with a personality conflict needs considerate help.

In his counseling relationships, the physical educator will frequently need the assistance of other school personnel. For example: the home economics teacher may help if serious dietary problems are encountered; the school doctor is essential if organic drains are present; the school nurse is invaluable when parental co-operation in dealing with health problems is desired; the guidance officer will be needed if personality conflicts need study and counsel. As a consequence, relationships with many other school personnel will be necessary in conducting developmental and adapted physical education. If an all-school guidance program exists, the physical educator may logically become a participant; it may even be feasible to merge his counseling function with this over-all institutional program.

Developmental and adapted physical education, thus, undertakes the difficult task of dealing with the individual and with individual needs far more specifically and intensively than do other phases of physical education. As aptly expressed by Rosalind Cassidy: "Research has shown this to be a necessity if democratic values and the facts of biology are to be respected."[10] Physical educators do not disagree on the principle that individual needs should be met; however, they may not all accept the manner in which this goal is to be accomplished. In this book, details relative to a basic approach to this problem are presented.

PREPARATION OF PERSONNEL.

As intimated before, the amount and nature of developmental and adapted education attempted in any school or college should depend upon the qualifications of the physical educators involved. The basic training of these individuals should be the four-year major in physical education. Inasmuch as undergraduate programs in this field vary

---

[10] Rosalind Cassidy, "New Directions in Physical Education," *Journal of Health and Physical Education,* 11, No. 7 (1940), p. 409.

considerably within the several hundred colleges and universities throughout the country, however, the prospective teacher should select an institution offering a strong sequence of studies for this work. The following training program is proposed from recommendations made by Blesh[11] and may be considered desirable in accordance with present thought and best practice (reference to the usual liberal arts or general education requirements for the bachelor's degree is omitted):

1. Foundation sciences, including biology, human anatomy, kinesiology, human physiology, and physiology of exercise;

2. General psychology;

3. Professional education, including history of education, principles of education, educational psychology, methods of teaching, and student teaching;

4. Technical training, including measurement and evaluation, physical examinations, corrective exercise, normal growth and development, nature and function of play, training and first aid, school programs in physical education, recreation leadership, camping, administration of physical education, and physical skills and coaching techniques.

The well-trained physical educator must have a thorough grounding in foundation sciences, must understand the learning process and the effective application of his activities to the education and development of the individual, must have great versatility in teaching many activities in a physical education program, and must be able to administer, supervise, and evaluate a varied program of physical education and athletics. That it is difficult to achieve the objective of preparing physical educators adequately within the limits of a four-year college program and still provide for the liberal-cultural education of the student is not to be denied. As a consequence, specialization in developmental and adapted physical education is not feasible in the four-year program under these circumstances. To be sure, related courses (basic sciences, correctives, measurement, etc.) are included, to provide the physical educator with an initial acquaintance with this specialty.

Physical educators who wish to become fully qualified to carry on the developmental and remedial functions in hospitals and rehabilitation centers should have postgraduate study at institutions providing specialized programs in this field. The trained physical educator should take more courses in anatomy, kinesiology, physiology, physiology of exercise, and psychology than he had as an undergraduate and must know their relationships to pathological conditions. He needs to understand the pathology of the various disabilities he will encounter and the utilization of physical activity in surgical, orthopedic, neurologic, and psychiatric conditions. He must be thoroughly acquainted with the modalities of

---

[11] T. E. Blesh, "Evaluative Criteria in Physical Education," *Research Quarterly,* 17, No. 2 (1946), p. 114.

exercise, adapted sports, aquatics, and recreational activities and should have extensive supervised clinical and field experience.[12]

Although physical educators in schools and colleges do not work with patients *per se* and although their objectives and program of activities are largely educational in nature, nevertheless, specialized training is advantageous if they are to be completely effective in their efforts to meet the individual needs of boys and girls. However, until the need for such training is generally recognized and provided, physical educators must, necessarily, perform only those functions for which they are specifically qualified. They definitely need to recognize their professional limitations in this respect.

RELATIONSHIPS WITH SCHOOL HEALTH SERVICES

Today, the school physician is becoming a medical educational consultant as related to the presence in children of physical defects, physical and mental retardation, psychological maladjustment, and the like.[13] In carrying out this responsibility, it is logical to expect that he should familiarize himself with the nature and purposes of the physical education program and understand the potentialities of its adaptation to individual needs.[14] In many instances, the physician is an indispensable part of the developmental and adapted physical education effort; he should consistently be considered a medical and health consultant.

In the public schools, too, full-time nurses are frequently found. Their duties may include assisting the school medical supervisor and other school officials in protecting the health of school children; assisting in health appraisals of school children; visiting homes in order to confer with parents regarding the health habits of children, securing the treatment of defects, and investigating the illness absences of children; inspecting the sanitary condition of the school plant; assisting in the maintenance of first-aid service; advising teachers, principals, and the superintendent of schools with regard to all matters affecting the health of school children.

Occasionally, school dental treatment is also provided, as well as the part-time services of personnel trained in the treatment of nervous and mental diseases, visual, hearing, orthopedic, and other conditions which may necessitate service to individual children.

In colleges and universities, the health service practices are usually

---

[12] H. Harrison Clarke and Earl C. Elkins, "Evaluation of Training of Physical Educationists for Reconditioning and Rehabilitation," *Archives of Physical Medicine,* XXIX, No. 2 (1948), p. 99.

[13] C. Morley Sellery, "Role of the School Physician in Today's Schools," *Journal of School Health,* XXII, No. 3 (March, 1952), p. 69.

[14] Delbert Oberteuffer, *School Health Education* (New York: Harper & Brothers, Inc., 1954), p. 409.

much more extensive and complete than those found in the public schools. An important reason for this difference is that much less reliance can be placed on the family and the family physician in colleges, where many students are living away from home. As a consequence, many institutions of higher learning provide complete infirmary services and are ready through their own facilities or those of nearby medical centers to care for many types of health problems affecting their students.

As is readily seen from the foregoing, responsibility for developmental and adapted physical education is not a direct function of the school or college health service. In effect, the relationship of the health service to this program is the same as that of any other educational program in the school: to provide medical and other health consultation and assistance as needed. Generally, the physical educator should seek this assistance by direct approach to the school health personnel.

Although there are many phases of developmental and adapted physical education which can be carried on without the help of health service personnel, nevertheless, their assistance is frequently essential if the complete potentialities of this program are to be realized. Some ways in which the health service is particularly essential are:

1. To discover individuals with serious defects of such a nature that vigorous exercise would be harmful to them;

2. To provide exercise and activity prescriptions for those with physical handicaps of any nature and for those returning to physical education after debilitating illness, surgery, or accidents;

3. To discover physical conditions resulting in physiological disturbances that may be the cause of low physical fitness in those boys and girls so classified by testing techniques employed by the physical educator;

4. To advise individual pupils on health problems beyond the scope of knowledge of the physical educator. These may include serious dietary deficiencies, chronic neuromuscular hypertension, and various types of maladjustments;

5. To visit the homes of public school pupils in the interest of gaining parental co-operation in the correction of physical defects, in the modification of health habits, and in other ways.

The entire school health service may logically participate in phases of developmental and adapted physical education. The school physician is especially vital in this respect. He should serve as adviser to the physical educator, and should be called on for help and guidance in conducting this program.

In making co-operative arrangements with the health services, the physical educator should take the initiative. The school health personnel should be thoroughly briefed on the purposes, functions, and activities of the developmental and adapted program; their importance to this program should be made clear; their guidance and assistance should be sought as essential to its success. Such a partnership can only result in improved health and physical education services to boys and girls in the schools and to men and women in the colleges.

SUMMARY

In this chapter, the potentialities of developmental and adapted physical education in schools and colleges were discussed. A transition was effected from the broader and more strictly therapeutic applications of this therapy in hospitals and rehabilitation centers to educational institutions. Fundamentally, in this latter situation, the role of physical education is largely educational and developmental.

The need for the developmental and adapted services stems directly from the objectives of physical education. Simply stated, the purpose was designated as meeting, through physical education methods and activities, the individual needs of boys and girls who are handicapped in some respect, who have functional defects or deficiencies amenable to improvement through exercise, or who possess other inadequacies which interfere with their successful participation in the diversified and vigorous activities of the general physical education program.

In considering the specific role of developmental and adapted physical education in schools and colleges, the following functions were presented: (1) General developmental and conditioning activities for individuals free of handicaps but of low physical fitness status; (2) Body mechanics and posture training for individuals with non-pathological conditions; (3) Adaptation of physical and recreation activities for the handicapped; (4) Psychological and social adjustment of "normal" individuals with atypical tendencies; (5) Relaxation activities for individuals suffering from chronic fatigue and neuromuscular hypertension; (6) Advice on and assistance with physical fitness, personal adjustment, and social problems of pupils.

The limitations of physical educators in conducting developmental and adapted programs were indicated based on the typical preparation provided in colleges and universities. Specialized training for such personnel was proposed.

Desirable relationships between physical education and the school health service were considered. The advantages to the physical well-being of boys and girls from such a relationship were presented.

SELECTED REFERENCES

Cassidy, Rosalind, "New Directions in Physical Education," *Journal of Health and Physical Education*, 11, No. 7 (1940), 409.

Clarke, H. Harrison, "Schools of Physical Education and the Training of

Physical Medicine and Rehabilitation Specialists," *Journal of the Association for Physical and Mental Rehabilitation*, 7, No. 2 (1953), 44.

—— and Earl C. Elkins, "Evaluation of Training of Physical Educationists for Reconditioning and Rehabilitation," *Archives of Physical Medicine*, XXIX, No. 2 (1948), 99.

Krusen, Frank H, "The Scope and Future of Physical Medicine and Rehabilitation," *Journal of the American Medical Association*, 144, No. 9 (1950), 727.

LaSalle, Dorothy, "Fitness Today on the Home Front," *Journal of Health and Physical Education*, 15, No. 10 (1944), 535.

Metheny, Eleanor, "Some Health Problems of College Women," *Journal of Health and Physical Education*, 17, No. 4 (1946), 205.

Oberteuffer, Delbert, *School Health Education*. New York: Harper & Brothers, 1954.

3

Considerations in
Conducting Programs

D EVELOPMENTAL AND ADAPTED PHYSICAL EDUCATION WAS
defined in Chapter 2 as a service meeting the individual needs of boys and girls who are handicapped in some respect,
who have functional defects and deficiencies amenable to improvement
through exercise, or who possess other inadequacies which interfere with
their successful participation in the diversified and vigorous activities of
the general physical education program. If such individual needs are to
be met by physical education, various considerations are essential for
successful programs, including: a scientific approach to content and
method; the use of adequate measurement and evaluation processes;
employment of teachers with special qualifications and abilities; utilization of effective motivational techniques; adoption of proper organizational and administrative procedures, and the like. The purpose of this
chapter is to deal with such considerations.

THE SCIENTIFIC APPROACH

Physical education has long employed the knowledge developed by
various basic sciences to an understanding of large-muscle activities and
to the application of these activities in the service of the individual.
Particularly important are the sciences of biology, physiology, physiology
of exercise, anatomy, kinesiology, sociology, and psychology. Furthermore, chemistry and physics have contributed helpful facts to this under-

standing. All of these subjects have provided a basic core of scientific knowledge related to body movement in its many physical educative phases.

A thorough understanding of these undergirding sciences is especially important for the teacher engaged in conducting developmental and adapted physical education; he must constantly apply his knowledge and technical skill to individual student problems rather than through a general or group process to the problems of many students as a unit. To qualify as a specialist in this area, he should seek advanced study of these sciences in their relation to pathological conditions.[1] Subsequently, he needs to keep up with advancing knowledge in these fields and to re-evaluate constantly their application to his work.

Much other scientific knowledge of value to developmental and adapted physical education is being developed today through many other sources. Included among these are the fields of physical medicine and rehabilitation, nutrition, health education, child growth and development, educational psychology, mental hygiene, psychiatry, neurology, and the like. In addition, and not to be overlooked, the field of physical education itself is producing a considerable amount of important research, which has definite value for the developmental and adapted program. To master this knowledge and to apply it is a tremendous but challenging task; maximum effectiveness depends upon it.

All areas of human endeavor which have reached a mature perspective and have achieved universal prestige have done so through logical thought processes. Such recognition should be an ultimate goal of physical education. When a fair share of professional activity is based upon known facts or upon well-conceived hypotheses in the absence of sufficient evidence, developmental and adapted physical education will become worthy of ultimate recognition in education and in society. Sensitivity to current research provides a guide to practices for many professions, such as medicine, physiology, psychology, sociology, and economics. A similar sensitivity should serve the physical educator engaged in this specialty.

The words of Dana Atchley, while applied to medicine, are appropriate here: "The art of healing is as old as recorded history; the science of healing is relatively young and only lately stands on its own feet. Medicine as a whole came of age when the stature of the science grew large enough for it to combine with the art in mutual understanding and respect."[2]

---

[1] H. Harrison Clarke, "Schools of Physical Education and the Training of Physical Medicine and Rehabilitation Specialists," *Journal of the Association for Physical and Mental Rehabilitaton*, 7, No. 2 (1953), p. 44.

[2] Dana W. Atchley, "The Healer and the Scentist," *Saturday Review*, XXXVI, No. 2 (January 9, 1954).

MEASUREMENT AND EVALUATION

Rather consistently in developmental and adapted physical education, objective tests have been considered too time-consuming in their application to be worthy of use. Teachers in this area have too frequently relied upon subjective appraisals and hastily conceived testing devices in their measurement efforts. The hypothesis advanced here is that the evaluative process is a vital function in developmental and adapted physical education—upon it depends the selection of students needing such programs, the progress of these students during the period they attend these classes, and their ultimate disposition from time to time. It is inconceivable that such decisions should be carelessly made on the basis of crude and inadequate testing procedures. Instead, these decisions should reflect the science of this field insofar as such science has developed.

As is true in medicine, where a great variety of specific tests are in constant use, physical education needs to draw on its full resources in the evaluation of individual boys and girls in the schools. Certain of these tests and examinations should be given by physicians, psychologists, and guidance personnel where their special qualifications are needed. However, regardless of who gives the tests or interprets the test results, the following six purposes for measurement are of primary importance in developmental and adapted physical education.

1. *To identify individuals with needs which may be improved through physical education.* By medical examinations, individuals with structural handicaps and organic defects are identified; by strength and endurance tests, individuals with low physical fitness may be found; by posture tests, individuals with faulty body mechanics are discovered; and, in other ways, the physical, social, and emotional status of individuals may be determined. Examinations, objective tests, or subjective appraisals may be used in these processes. The more valid and precise the testing instruments, however, the more reliance can be placed upon the results obtained.

2. *To determine the results of developmental and adapted physical education.* Once individuals with needs are identified through tests and other evaluative procedures, periodic re-tests are essential to determine the results of treatment prescriptions. This process is particularly vital where the individual's condition is subject to improvement through physical education activities and methods. In general, if progress is steady, the prescribed treatment can usually be considered satisfactory and should be continued; where progress is not found, steps can be taken promptly to re-study the case and to consider appropriate changes in individual program content.

3. *To provide assistance in the determination of the cause or causes*

of various atypical or sub-par conditions. In dealing with unsatisfactory physical, social, or emotional states, effective treatment depends upon locating causative conditions so that proper steps may be taken for their elimination or alleviation. Thus, for example, such factors as lack of strength and stamina, general debilitation, or faulty posture habits may be basic causes of poor body mechanics. Various examinations and tests may prove useful in ascertaining the presence and extent of involvement of these and other such conditions.

4. *To orient convincingly individuals assigned to developmental and adapted physical education.* In initiating each individual's program, complete orientation to his or her condition and to the procedures to be followed in accomplishing improvement is vital. In no small way, the effectiveness of such programs is dependent upon each individual's acceptance of and wholehearted participation in the activities prescribed. Objective evidence, based on the results of valid examinations and tests, serves as convincing proof of individual status and need.

5. *To motivate individual students.* In the method of developmental and adapted physical education, the individual must be motivated to co-operate fully in the exercise and other prescriptions made out for him. Successful orientation, as mentioned above, is an essential factor in this process. However, once the program is under way, motivation can well be judged in terms of the individual's progress. The determination of such progress is most realistic to the subject when based upon periodic re-examinations and re-tests of the basic conditions involved.

6. *To determine the final disposition of the individual.* The final disposition of each boy or girl assigned to developmental and adapted physical education can be determined through terminal examinations and tests. Thus, the decision can be properly made as to when the individual should be transferred to other physical education activities. Also, the strengths and weaknesses in physical activities of the permanently disabled can be judged and the individual acquainted with his capabilities and limitations for future activity.

THE EFFECTIVE TEACHER

The effectiveness of the teacher engaged in developmental and adapted physical education should be appraised in terms of his contributions to the physical, social, and emotional welfare of the boys and girls in his care. The rendering of such services to individuals who are handicapped or who are sub-par in some respect is especially difficult because of the nature of these atypical conditions and their effect upon the total personality. As a consequence, the effective teacher must be superior in all the many characteristics required in successful teaching. Some of these characteristics may be listed as follows.

1. *Have a thorough understanding of developmental and adapted physical education.* The teacher should be well prepared in physical education and should have special training in his technical specialty and the physiological, psychological, and social sciences that undergird this field. Furthermore, he should keep up-to-date on the latest thinking, best practices, and current research through formal courses, professional reading, and attendance at conferences.

2. *Be imbued with a desire to serve others.* Developmental and adapted physical education offers a rich reward in personal satisfaction for those physical educators who wish to devote their lives to the service of boys and girls, because those children who most need their help are in this program.

3. *Consider the whole individual not just the specific involvement under treatment.* With the handicapped particularly, the social and emotional concomitants of a disability may be far-reaching in their implications. In lesser degree, this is also true of many other deficiencies. As a consequence, the physical educator must work with the individual as a totality rather than concentrate his technical ability only on a specific condition.

4. *Obtain personal rapport with each individual assigned to developmental and adapted physical education.* Such rapport is based upon an understanding of the person and his problems. It is obtained by taking a personal interest in him, by knowing something of his family background and current interests, and by maintaining an agreeable and approachable attitude both inside and outside the special exercise room.

5. *Understand each individual's capabilities and provide activities which are within his limitations.* An essential rule in working with sub-par or atypical cases is that individual assignments should be achievable. Consistent successes in assigned tasks build confidence and gradually prepare the individual for more difficult activities. Success experiences may also encourage these persons to tackle many of life's problems, helping to depress inferiority complexes that are frequently manifested by these individuals.

6. *Be patient in dealing with atypical students.* Without doubt, a vital characteristic of the physical educator in this specialty is possession of an abundance of patience. Individuals in his classes usually show a low level of skill. If definitely handicapped in some respect, they may also be sensitive and resentful. By combining understanding and forbearance with good rapport and reasonable activity prescriptions, definite progress in meeting the student's personal problems may be achieved.

7. *Be optimistic and encouraging in the approach to students.* Physical educators should not make the mistake of leading handicapped students to believe that they may ultimately achieve goals beyond the limitations of individual handicaps. However, they should present an optimistic

and forceful attitude toward such individuals, encouraging the
accept their disabilities and to live satisfying and productive lives wit.
their capabilities. For those individuals without chronic conditions, encouragement in some instances may extend to reasonably high levels of
achievement.

8. *Be enthusiastic in presenting the activities of the developmental
and adapted physical education program.* No amount of technical knowledge and finesse can compensate for a dead-pan, uninteresting presentation of activities. Exercises of the most formal type can be made
appealing and challenging when led by a dynamic teacher. Voice,
expression, and attitude should radiate enthusiasm.

9. *Be an example at all times.* The physical educator should personify
good health, proper posture, an energetic being. Personal example should
also include a pleasing appearance, neatness and cleanliness of body and
dress, and an engaging and friendly presence.

10. *Motivate each student toward ever increasing ability to perform
physical activities.* Motivation is possible in many ways and will be considered more completely later in this chapter. Basically, however, students
in developmental and adapted classes should be pressed constantly
toward physiological tolerance limits by progressive exercise prescriptions, challenging encouragement, and a gradually formed concept of
their own powers and capabilities.

11. *Be fully prepared for each class period.* Proper preparation involves definite over-all program planning, adequate lesson plans, individual exercise routines, necessary equipment, and planned administrative
set-up for each period. Ineptitude in this respect results in loss of
class time, ineffective instruction, lack of class interest, and reduced
pupil activity.

12. *Strive constantly to realize social and spiritual goals in life.* The
physical educator should not be content merely to achieve technical
treatment goals and to realize individual adjustments to handicaps. The
ultimate aim should be to lead boys and girls toward living spiritual
lives for the benefit of mankind.

"Stimulate the laggard, encourage the timid, admonish the lazy and
hold back the pupil who wants to work wonders overnight and as a
result works too hard."[3]

APPLICATION TO AGE-GROUP CHARACTERISTICS

The general approach in presenting developmental and adapted
physical education is to relate activities and methods to the basic
characteristics and interests of the age and sex of the individuals in-

---

[3] Mabel Lee and Miriam W. Wagner, *Fundamentals of Body Mechanics and
Conditioning* (Philadelphia: W. B. Saunders Company, 1949), p. 253.

volved. A brief summarization and application of these factors are given below.[4]

MIDDLE CHILDHOOD

Physically, the normal child from six to nine years old has progressed materially, but continues to grow quite rapidly; average annual growth during this period is 5½ pounds in weight and 2 inches in height. However, body growth is not uniform; the chest grows faster than the abdomen and the legs grow faster than the trunk. The resting heart and breathing rates decline, moving toward adult levels; by age nine years, the rate per minute is rarely above 90 for normal pulse and 20 for normal respiration. Smoothness, skill, and sureness of body movement have progressed over early childhood; strength and co-ordination of the various muscle groups are gradually needed for the development of more complex and specialized skills. Children of this age thrive on physical activity; they are on the go constantly. Therefore, physical education, if interesting, is avidly accepted. The emphasis, however, should be upon general body movement with more complex skills being introduced only gradually, but with greater emphasis toward the end of this period.

The child of this age is a hero-worshiper and imitator. Hence, the glamor of being like the "high school quarterback" or the "champion girl swimmer" is an effective motivator. This child is a show-off and likes to be the center of attention. Therefore, activities designed to permit some prominence for each individual are useful. Boys particularly become interested in stunts and self-testing of their physical abilities. Interest in competition develops. Girls have similar, but less marked, interests in such physical activities.

LATE CHILDHOOD

The rate of growth in height and weight gradually falls off; the minimum rate prior to adolescence is reached between 9 and 10 years for the average girl and 11 and 12 for the average boy. Physically, these children are consolidating and rounding off their earlier basic skills and are ready to progress into more complex movements. Development of strength is essential both from the standpoint of interest and the standpoint of improved performances in activities requiring balance, agility, power, and endurance. This child is competitive. Early in the period, competition is self-testing and involves attempts at superiority

---

[4] For a concise chart of these characteristics, consult: Howard V. Meredith, Jennelle V. Moorhead, and Ralph W. Leighton, *Activity, Health, and Personality Development* (Eugene, Oregon: School of Health and Physical Education, University of Oregon, 1951).

over others of his age in individual events; later in the period, it begins to take the form of organized team games.

Pre-adolescent boys and girls are likely to form strong attachments to persons of the same sex, either older or of the same age. Understanding these attachments and directing them toward wholesome personalities provides an effective motivational base. The personal examples of physical educators are particularly vital, although always important, during this formative period, in order that the appeal will be toward fine physical development, good living habits, and a dynamic spiritual outlook on life. Boys and girls who become leaders in school activities also have a special responsibility due to this emulation and should be brought to a realization of its importance in the lives of both those who are younger than they and those who are their peers.

ADOLESCENCE

During the adolescent years, both boys and girls gradually shift attachments from those of the same sex to those of the opposite sex. From 12 to 15 years of age, and frequently beyond, boys especially continue their drive for acceptance and superiority within their sex group, as evidenced by their strong desire for athletic prominence. Several studies have shown that competitive athletic skills are among the chief sources of social esteem for boys in this period preceding maturity. Jones,[5] in the Berkeley Growth Studies attributes this phenomenon not merely "to the high premium which adolescents place upon athletic efficiency, but also to the fact that strength and other aspects of physical ability are closely joined to such favorable traits as activity, aggressiveness, and leadership." The need to belong to a group is vital for this age group, also, as shown by Goodwin Watson.[6] Therefore, the physical educator may logically motivate boys toward a fine physique through their desire to be physically strong and skilled. And, developmental and adapted activities can frequently be conducted on a group basis, basing performance on inter-group contests.

At this age, girls are more prone to continue progressively with interests which make them increasingly attractive to the opposite sex. This drive is manifested in their desire to avoid excess weight, to achieve pleasing posture and appearance, to be graceful and physically well poised, and to acquire skills in sports which may be played with boys. Studies have revealed that physical skills have some importance to girls, but not nearly to the same extent as for boys.[7] Thus, the prime

[5] Harold E. Jones, "Physical Ability as a Factor in Social Adjustment in Adolescence," *Journal of Educational Psychology*, 40 (December, 1946), p. 287.

[6] Goodwin Watson, "Personality and Growth through Athletics," *Journal of Health and Physical Education*, IX, No. 7 (1938), p. 408.

[7] Caroline C. Tryon, *Evaluations of Adolescent Personality by Adolescents*, Society for Research in Child Development, IV, No. 4 (1939).

motivators for girls at this age must point toward the proper realization of these basic feminine interests.

MOTIVATION

An essential phase of developmental and adapted physical education involves the proper and effective motivation of boys and girls in the program. The full voluntary participation of these individuals is vital for efficient results. Their co-operation is needed in carrying out their exercise routines correctly and vigorously, in responding to advice on personal living habits, and in the correction of such remediable defects as they may possess. Consequently, every effort should be made by the physical educator to secure an enthusiastic response to the developmental activities and adapted procedures assigned.

True manly and womanly development should be the basis for the teacher's thought and action in utilizing motivational procedures. Childhood and adolescent interests and desires can, just as easily perhaps, be directed toward antisocial and predatory actions. In fact, the pupil in the developmental and adapted program may more readily turn in this direction as compensation for any obvious deficiencies he may have. As a consequence, methods and motivational procedures should be directed toward the realization of goals which benefit society through the personal development of the individual.

ORIENTATION AND UNDERSTANDING

An essential step in motivating the pupil assigned to developmental and adapted physical education is to give him a thorough understanding of his status and the procedures to be followed in the improvement of his condition. If tests and examinations have been administered, individual results should be presented and interpreted; if the evaluative process is new to the student, the measuring devices should be demonstrated, the values of the tests explained, and an understanding of personal scores provided. A private conference with each pupil should be held for this purpose and to outline the developmental or adapted procedures to be followed. Cogent reasons should be presented for all actions taken and contemplated. The purpose of exercise should be explained to the student; not just a few generalities, but the specific functions of each exercise or physical activity prescribed, the correct way of performing it, and the probable end results. The physical educator must train himself to think logically, prepare lucid explanations of his procedures, and transmit these effectively to his students.

In this program, the teacher must establish rapport with the student before embarking upon explanations of his or her needs and limitations. In many public schools, rapport is easily achieved, especially if the physical educator is well known, liked, and respected by the student body. In large schools and in most colleges and universities, however, this personal conference may be the first face-to-face contact with the student. In this situation, some time should be spent in becoming acquainted before getting down to the business of the conference. An excellent way to do this is to get the student to talk about his interests, hobbies, home town, and the like. If common interests can be found and discussed with some enthusiasm, the student is usually ready to discuss freely his problems and is receptive to suggestions for improving himself. In this process, too, the student should be encouraged to express his views on his particular situation and share in the decisions made. Invariably, a good start in the conduct of individual programs is assured through these procedures.

An effective way to enhance the student's understanding of his condition is to encourage him to do some homework on it. This homework may consist of reading books, articles, or pamphlets. For example, overweight students might read a chapter in a nutrition book dealing with obesity; those with postural defects might well read an article on this subject presented in non-technical language. Homework could also include the preparation of a written paper on the factors involved in each student's condition. Younger children may prepare posters or cutouts or make a collection of clippings dealing with desirable health habits. Co-ordination with other school departments in certain of these efforts may be desirable, such as English, Art, Home Economics, and others. These studies can be combined with group discussions, especially when several students have similar situations.

As a phase of the homework, too, each student could prepare a brief autobiography. These reports, in addition to historical material, should include accounts of current interests and activities and reasons for these interests. Low-fitness individuals especially should be led to speculate on the cause or causes of their conditions. Autobiographies, if well done, will provide the teacher with a better understanding and appreciation of each student's problems; also, the student will better understand himself.

An understanding of various conditions can also be enhanced through motion pictures. Many excellent films on a great variety of subjects are available. Brief descriptions and evaluations of motion pictures which interest the medical profession have been prepared by the Bureau of Exhibits, Committee on Medical Motion Pictures, American Medical Association, 535 North Dearborn Street, Chicago, Illinois. A compilation of these is contained in Reviews of Medical Motion Pictures, published in 1949 with annual supplements since that date. Topics included which are useful for developmental and adapted physical education are anatomy, physiology, and embryology; cardiovascular system; immunology and public health; laity; neurology, psychiatry, and psychology; nutrition; ophthalmology; orthopedics; otorhinolaryngology; and physical medicine and rehabilitation.

Quantities of free and inexpensive publications on subjects pertaining to developmental and adapted physical education are available. A list of such materials has been compiled by the Advisory Council of the Joint Staff Committee of the Oregon State Board of Health, State Board of Education, and State System of Higher Education. The areas included in this listing are structure and function of the human body, personal hygiene, physiology of exercise, nutrition, first aid and safety materials, choice and use of health services and products, communicable and non-communicable diseases, community health and sanitation, and mental health. The establishment of a reading table in the physical education area with a selection of these pamphlets, as well as other material, could be a source of pertinent information related to the conditions encountered in the program. In some instances, too, certain of these items may be distributed to individual students.

At this point, a word of caution should be added. When the individual has a pathological condition, partial knowledge concerning its nature may have negative results, leading him on one hand to a false sense of security or on the other hand instilling fears that disturb him emotionally and deter him from active participation in the developmental and adapted program. In these cases, the physician or other appropriate specialist should supply this information.

Still another feature, which will enhance student understanding and appreciation of personal deficiencies, is to permit them to share in planning the content and method of the program to be followed. Such participation may be achieved by discussions with all involved students or through an elected council or board of representative students. In either instance, considerable care should be exercised in the operation of this procedure, as these students are not competent to make professional decisions. They may, however, give advice and suggest changes, propose activities to make the program more interesting, carry out many organizational and class details, conduct special contests, and be responsible for certain of the motivational processes presented below.

In dealing with students in the formulation of policies for the developmental and adapted program, the physical education teacher should clearly be considered the expert and his decisions must necessarily be final. However, students can participate in the process with benefit to both parties; the teacher may obtain valuable suggestions which will improve the quality of developmental and adapted physical education, and the students may receive a deeper insight into prescribed procedures and realize the inspiration from being part of a program designed for their benefit. In this situation, the teacher should: (1) guide students toward a desire to reach decisions which are right and best for the group, rather than just personally advantageous; (2) provide the students with valid professional information upon which solutions for problems under consideration may be based; (3) see to it that they understand the full implications of any decision they make. Once these criteria are fulfilled, student decisions will invariably reflect a sincere and responsive attitude; the need for the teacher's "veto" will occur infrequently.

MOTIVATIONAL PRACTICES AND DEVICES

Proper motivation for full and enthusiastic participation in developmental and adapted physical education should be based upon the fundamental interests and drives of the different age groups and sexes, proper orientation to and understanding of each student's condition, and student participation in planning the content, method, and organization of the program, as presented above. In addition, however, there are many motivational practices and devices which can be used effectively. Several of the more important of these are presented below.

1. The exercise area should be immaculately clean, well lighted, attractively decorated, and properly ventilated; the equipment should be in order and efficiently arranged for each class period; the teacher should be neatly dressed and should maintain a professional bearing at all times. The whole atmosphere of this area should reflect the highest standards attainable.

2. Insofar as possible, students with like conditions should be grouped together. Not only does this arrangement result in a more effective teaching situation, as the teacher can concentrate attention on one or, at most, a relatively few conditions at a time, but it permits pupils with like deficiencies to exercise together. An *esprit de corps* can frequently be built up in this way, which could seldom be duplicated by heterogeneous grouping. One of the authors well remembers such a group of obese boys, who had a fine time together and carried their interest to the cafeteria line as a "fat-carbohydrates anonymous" club.

3. Relatively frequent (e.g., each five to six weeks) repetition of the tests used in selecting for developmental and adapted physical education is especially important in the motivational process. Between these testing periods, self-testing procedures can be employed as rough checks. Through this process, students are able to gauge their progress from time to time. A powerful motivator is the student's realization of progress made toward desired goals.

4. The effective utilization of a bulletin board can be an important adjunct for the exercise room. This board may be used for the following purposes: (a) essential notices pertaining to schedules, student

assignments, and special events; (b) instructional information, such as exercise descriptions and routines, diet suggestions, and test instructions; and (c) motivational materials, including posters, clippings, slogans, and the like.

5. Competition has great motivational value, but should be used cautiously with these students because of the tendency to over-exert. The safest competition is the self-testing type, where the effort is made to improve personal performance within restrictions that can be regulated by the teacher. For the low-fitness student, who is well along in his development, however, participation in such games as basketball and soccer is not only enjoyable but has definite conditioning value.

6. Exercising to music or singing while performing prescribed drills adds to the enjoyment of developmental and adapted activities. Contests to compose original songs, poems, dramatizations, and so forth, may add to group interest.

7. Assembly programs and demonstrations before local parent-teachers associations and other civic groups may be held. At bazaars and similar events, certain tests can be used, such as grip strength, footprint angles, lung capacity, and posture silhouettes. These activities, when accompanied with appropriate explanations, have considerable public relations value, but also motivate students—especially if they are the participants in the events.

THE TEACHING OF DEVELOPMENTAL AND ADAPTED ACTIVITIES

An essential phase in the preparation of physical education teachers is the required pursuit of methods courses and the experience of practice teaching. Developmental and adapted programs utilize the activities and methods of physical education, applying them in specific ways to meet the individual needs of boys and girls. For the purposes of this book, therefore, this knowledge is assumed. In applying this knowledge to the unique purpose of developmental and adapted physical education, several factors should be kept in mind, as discussed below.

Each teacher should determine his own most effective method of presenting activities. Some teachers achieve best results through a formal approach, while others are more successful when informal. There is no virtue in either method for its own sake. This issue should be resolved by each teacher in terms of the progress of pupils toward their individual goals in developmental and adapted physical education.

Both the formal and informal methods of teaching physical activities have shortcomings which must be guarded against. The formal method frequently results in a command-response situation, which precludes close rapport between teacher and pupils. This method, also, requires the teacher to "lead" the class constantly, thereby, not permitting adequate opportunity for him to work with individual pupils. The informal method may degenerate into slovenly teaching and a disregard of the values and outcomes intended for the exercises and activities conducted. The tendency, today, is toward informality and the elimination of formal terminology. Constant insistence on the proper execution of prescribed classwork, strenuous enough to produce desired results, however, is vital.

Regardless of the basic method used, the physical educator must maintain complete control of his class. This does not mean that discipline must be stern, strict, or severe. Usually, discipline can be friendly and informal, if proper rapport exists between teacher and pupils. Severity to an individual or a group may be essential in emergency situations, but should not be the usual approach of the teacher to disciplinary problems.

The teacher should be able to obtain the strict attention of his entire class at a moment's notice. This is especially important to save time when announcements, instructions, or explanations must be given to the whole class. Some specific signal, such as blowing a whistle or uttering a given command, may be employed for this purpose.

The class period should be so organized as to permit the teacher to move freely about the exercise room in order to work with individual students. To do this, each pupil should be taught the specific exercises prescribed for him, and be allowed to execute them on his own. The teacher may then devote this time to correcting performances, teaching new exercises, changing exercise routines, and counseling, as deemed necessary.

Student leadership provides individual and group responsibilities; moreover, it is a valuable aid to the teacher. For example, students may aid in class organization and in the care of equipment, may serve on committees, and may help to determine and carry out class projects. Students who already know specific exercises thoroughly may teach them to others. The alert teacher will find many other opportunities for student leadership experiences.

ORGANIZATION OF THE PROGRAM

FUNCTIONAL GROUPINGS

If the full potentialities of developmental and adapted physical education are realized, many defects, deficiencies, and sub-par conditions will be encountered. These will vary from time to time and from school to school. In some schools, especially in the smaller ones, few if any students may have serious orthopedic disabilities or organic conditions; while in the large schools and universities, a number of such individuals are always enrolled. Pupils with other deficiencies are always present, including those with low physical fitness, nutritional disturbances, and pronounced postural deviations.

To organize an effective developmental and adapted physical education program, functional grouping of students is desirable. Such groupings should be based upon the types of exercise required and the amount of protective care necessary in individual cases. In some instances, the exercise program will best be conducted entirely in special classes; in other situations, part of the activities should be in special classes and part in regular physical education. In other instances, vigorous exercise may be applied, while in others the dosage must be carefully regulated; some exercise routines may be related to specific conditions, while others are suitable for general body building and conditioning. The groupings to be adopted in a given school situation will depend, of course, upon the types of cases included in the program.

For ease of presentation, the groupings proposed below are arranged as "units." Each unit presented is closely identified with the function it should perform in developmental and adapted physical education. In some instances, the unit has responsibilities in several areas of the program; in others, it is limited to a specific type of condition with a limited application of activities. Furthermore, in scheduling, it is advisable, when possible, to place all students assigned to certain units in the same class or classes; however, the activities of some units are needed in nearly every class. In the presentation below, these relationships are indicated and the applications pointed out.

1. *Measurement and Evaluation Unit.* Some form of measurement and evaluation is constantly needed in developmental and adapted physical education. This unit should be responsible for the administration of all tests, for co-ordination with other personnel and agencies in securing specialized examinations in individual cases (e.g., medical examinations, psychological tests, etc.), and for recording the results of tests and preparing reports. This process is needed in relation to all such physical education classes; the tests, of course, vary for the different conditions.

2. *Counseling Unit.* Counseling is a vital function in developmental and adapted physical education, involving the orientation of students to the program, the exploraton of the causes of various conditions, and the advisement of students relative to desirable activities and practices. For example, the cause or causes of low physical fitness must be determined through case studies, surveys of living habits, and personal conferences; the student with a permanent disability needs to understand his limitations and to accept his handicap with courage and cheerfulness; those who are socially maladjusted must be brought to a realization of their status and must accept guidance designed to aid them; the obese child should be taught desirable dietary practices and

should develop a desire to follow them. All of these situations, and there are many others, involve some form of counseling; thus, counseling has wide implications and is needed throughout the program.

3. *Developmental and Conditioning Unit.* In this unit, two groups of students are included: (a) the usually large number with low physical fitness, who need general strengthening and conditioning activities; and (b) those convalescing from illness, surgery, or injury, who need physical reconditioning before again participating in vigorous activities. Group exercise is possible and usually desirable, especially when exercise routines are comparable; thus students may frequently obtain special strengthening exercises in special classes and endurance activities in regular physical education. Other groups may also benefit from the developmental and conditioning activities of this unit, including the malnourished, the emotionally disturbed, and those with faulty posture.

4. *Special Exercise Unit.* This unit is designed especially for students with functional postural and foot conditions, who would benefit from specific remedial exercises. Also included in this unit are those recovering from injuries or operations, where exercises individually prescribed for alleviating and improving the specific condition are beneficial. In some instances, too, such exercises are needed for students who have orthopedic handicaps, or various organic conditions where exercise must be carefully regulated. This unit is highly specialized in nature; therefore, the time these classes are scheduled should be such as to permit attendance of the largest number of students needing some form of special exercise.

5. *Relaxation Unit.* A unit for the chronically fatigued and hypertensed is needed. Activities designed to relax the neuromuscular system should be provided. As in the foregoing, the functions of this unit should be distributed among the classes in accordance with need and efficient utilization of personnel and facilities.

6. *Adapted Activities Unit.* Many physical education activities can be enjoyed by the orthopedically handicapped and the organically defective if properly selected or adapted for individual use. The adapted activities unit should fulfill this function. As a specialized unit, activities should be scheduled as needed; for some cases, the activities of the regular physical education classes may be utilized.

CONDUCT OF CLASSES

The manner in which developmental and adapted physical education will be conducted depends in large part upon the schedule of classes set up for a given school situation. If it is possible to arrange the classes as desired, the problem is simplified; if all types of cases are in all classes, the job is much more difficult and calls for ingenuity in the organization of the class period. A blueprint of this class organization cannot be drawn to meet all situations. However, the following suggestions are made to help the teacher work out a plan for his local situation.

1. These classes should be kept small when exercise routines must be carefully worked out and controlled for each individual. Thus, classes made up of students requiring special exercises and relaxation and certain of those needing adapted activities should have enrollments limited to approximately fifteen.

2. For other classes, especially those involving developmental and conditioning activities, the classes may be somewhat larger (about twenty-five students), as group activities may be employed effectively. Individual variations in type and intensity of exercise are usually necessary, but may be achieved by sub-groupings within the class.

3. All exercise and other prescriptions should be based upon scores made on the basic tests administered, the recommendation of physicians or other specialists if applicable, the causes of the various conditions as determined through counseling, and exercise-tolerance evaluations conducted from time to time. A file card for each student, containing diagnosis, exercise routine, and any other pertinent data, should be available in the exercise room and accessible to both the instructor and the student.

4. Lesson plans should be worked out in detail before each class for efficient and effective work, although the teacher may find it necessary to depart from these occasionally when the class, or individuals in it, are not ready to progress as rapidly as anticipated. A constant adjustment in lesson plans is usually necessary as the class work develops. This fact, however, does not excuse the teacher from making plans.

5. List equipment and facilities which will be needed for the successful presentation and conduct of each class. These items should be ready for immediate use without loss of class time. Students may be assigned duties to arrange and put away the special apparatus needed.

6. As early in the program as possible, students should be taught their personal exercises and activities, so that they may proceed without command and instruction from the teacher. Thus, the teacher is freed to work with individuals, to conduct case studies, to change individual exercise routines as needed, and to give general supervision to the class. An efficient teacher is one who can conduct classes in which all students carry out proper exercise prescriptions efficiently without constant direction.

7. The physical educator should keep a file of all exercises and activities found effective for various phases of the program. Each of these may be given descriptive names, as an exercise with a name is remembered more easily than an exercise with a number. With smaller children

of elementary school age, attractive names also serve as motivators. A contest might be held to suggest and select appropriate names for these activities. Older students, after they have an understanding of the factors involved, could vie with each other in devising new exercises, stunts, or games to be used for the various conditions encountered.

8. The developmental and adapted program, as will be shown throughout this book, should not be limited to calisthenic-type exercises, although such exercises do have definite value in certain situations. Other activities, including stunts, contests, games, and sports, should be included whenever advisable.

PROGRAM EMPHASES AT DIFFERENT SCHOOL LEVELS

The program emphasis in developmental and adapted physical education coincides with the objectives, procedures, and content normally found at each grade level. The activities of the program are selected from those which are most appropriate for the different age groups. The great difference from physical education in general lies in the application of these activities to meet the physical, social, emotional, and psychological needs of each boy and girl. Each pupil is studied through tests, examinations, and other evaluative procedures; personal conferences are held to determine the cause or causes of sub-par or atypical conditions; definite activities are then chosen to best serve each individual. Thus, these physical education programs are personalized and are directed toward the improvement of specific conditions.

Developmental and adapted physical education is necessary at all grade levels where individual needs exist which may be improved through physical activity. However, it is generally conceded that "a stitch in time saves nine," so that, if more serious later trouble is to be avoided, physical deviates should be identified and treated at the earliest possible age. Thus, the elementary school is the most crucial, although usually the most neglected level for these programs. An early start in the establishment of good growth patterns, strong and enduring physiques, bodies free from organic and structural defects, and a socially and psychologically well-adjusted individual, is vital to the future well-being of the individual. However, despite high-sounding phrases urging the solution of the developmental and adapted physical education problem in the elementary school, those close to this field recognize that this millennium will not occur for many years. So, the need for such programs in educational institutions will continue unabated from the kindergarten through college.

No attempt is made here to present a unique differentiation of developmental and adapted programs for different school levels. For the purposes to be achieved are the same for the elementary school and the college. As presented in Chapter 2, these are general development and conditioning activities for low fitness individuals, body mechanics training, adapted sports for the handicapped, psychological and social adjustment for those with atypical tendencies, relaxation for the hypertensed, and counseling and guidance for pupils with physical fitness and adjustment problems. The testing techniques, the methods, and the program content will obviously be adapted to the age and sex of the individual. Some differences in the percentage of pupils with different conditions will be found, such as the larger number of handicapped in the colleges. These differences, however, will be in degree. In the chapters which follow, the necessary adjustments to school levels will be presented in relation to the content of developmental and adapted physical education.

SUMMARY

Various considerations related to developmental and adapted physical education in educational institutions were presented in this chapter. The need for a scientific approach to the field and the use of objective tests and other evaluative procedures were emphasized. The essential characteristics of the specialized teacher were given. The application to age-group characteristics was considered. Motivational practices were discussed in some detail. Other factors included were the methodology, the organization, and the program emphases at different school levels for the developmental and adapted physical education program.

SELECTED REFERENCES

Atchley, Dana W., "The Healer and the Scientist," *Saturday Review,* XXXVI, No. 2 (January 9, 1954).

Daniels, Arthur S., *Adapted Physical Education,* Chapters 4 and 5. New York: Harper & Brothers, 1954.

Jones, Harold E., "Physical Ability as a Factor in Social Adjustment in Adolescence," *Journal of Educational Psychology,* 40 (December, 1946), 287.

Lee, Mabel, and Miriam M. Wagner, *Fundamentals of Body Mechanics and Conditioning,* Chapters IX and XI. Philadelphia: W. B. Saunders Company, 1949.

Stafford, George T., *Preventive and Corrective Physical Education,* rev. ed., Chapter III. New York: A. S. Barnes and Company, Inc., 1950.

4

Measurement and
Evaluation

ONSIDERABLE CARE SHOULD BE EXERCISED IN THE SELEC-
tion of measurement and other evaluative procedures
for developmental and adapted physical education. This program will
be judged in no small part by the quality of these procedures. One might
venture to state that the use of valid and precise measuring instruments
is an absolute requisite for gaining proper recognition and respect, while
inaccurate and haphazard testing spells mediocrity, ineffectuality, and
worse.

Very frequently in physical education, tests with superior scientific
worth and with a background of practical application in schools have
been bypassed for those below acceptable standards because they require special apparatus, trained technicians, and qualified professional
people to interpret the results and apply them effectively to physical
education programs. From the standpoint of the maturity and stature
of the profession, such action is most unfortunate. Recognizing that
practical limitations frequently must be placed on testing in schools and
colleges, perhaps the dilemma may be resolved by advocating two or
more levels of testing—from minimal to ideal measurement practices. In
this way, at least, the ultimate in physical education measurement is
recognized and held as a desirable goal.[1]

---

[1] H. Harrison Clarke, "Physical Fitness Testing for Professional Physical Educators," *The Physical Educator*, 12, No. 1 (March, 1955), p. 23.

The tests presented in this chapter are drawn from appropriate sources in physical education, medicine, psychology, and other fields. In order not to devote a disproportionate amount of space to the description of tests, however, references to standard physical education measurement books will be made for test techniques. Greater coverage will be given here when essential tests are not available in these sources.

The selected tests are those considered appropriate for developmental and adapted physical education in public schools and colleges, rather than in hospitals and rehabilitation centers. With few exceptions, therefore, these tests are utilized in physical education as a whole. Such tests, however, are largely limited to basic physical, social, and psychological traits. In certain areas, available tests are well developed and may be utilized with considerable confidence; in other areas, they are meager and still rather crude evaluative instruments. These factors will be considered in the presentation which follows.

SELECTION OF EVALUATIVE MEASURES

The value of a test or examination is first judged in relation to the fundamental importance of the factor which it measures; then, appraisal of its scientific worth should be made. Other things being equal, that test is superior which best meets proper test-construction criteria. All things considered, the following factors should be kept in mind when actually selecting evaluative measures to be used in local developmental and adapted programs.

1. *The examinations and tests should be related to the function of developmental and adapted physical education.* The functions of this program were presented in Chapter 2. Treatment of students with the following conditions was proposed: low physical fitness, poor body mechanics, organic conditions and orthopedic handicaps, psychological and social maladjustment, malnutrition, and chronic fatigue and neuromuscular hypertension. The first consideration in selecting tests, therefore, is to select those which will reveal individuals with these deficiencies.

2. *The evaluative process should reflect the particular emphasis of local developmental and adapted physical education programs.* As presently practiced in the schools and colleges of America, the nature of these programs varies with local institutions. Certain programs emphasize faulty body mechanics; some, the physically handicapped; others, the low fitness group. Seldom is balance achieved among all possible functions. Among the reasons for these variations are the influence of tradition, the qualifications of professional personnel, the particular interests and convictions of individual physical educators, and the practical limitations imposed by insufficient local facilities and specially qualified

teachers. Thus, the physical educator may be forced to exercise his prerogative of placing emphasis where he feels it will do the most good. The evaluative techniques selected, therefore, should be based upon such recognized and acknowledged emphases.

3. *Where local programs must be limited in scope, the selection of examinations and tests may be based upon primary and supplementary functions.* Usually, practical exigencies limit developmental and adapted physical education services in local institutions. As a consequence, the number of evaluative techniques applied to all students must be curtailed. Their selection should be in terms of the basic functions to be achieved; these are considered primary measurements. Other tests, known as supplementary measurements, may be used to detect causitive and associative factors among those with deficiencies selected through primary measurements. For example, a strength test may be used to detect those deficient in this basic physical fitness element, nutrition tests and social adjustment inventories may then be applied to the sub-strength groups to determine if deficiencies in these conditions are also present.

4. *Once the type of test needed is determined, the tests with the best scientific bases should be chosen.* The main scientific elements to be considered are validity, accuracy, and norms; the economy of tests must also frequently be reviewed. Greater detail on the criteria for the selection of tests will be found in physical education measurement textbooks; only a brief description of each will be given here.

Validity. A valid test is one that measures what it purports to measure. Validity is determined by relating the tests to a criterion of the element being measured. If the two have a high relationship, the test measures the same quality as does the criterion. In deciding on the validity of tests, therefore, two elements should be evaluated: (a) the degree to which the criterion represents the quality being measured, and (b) the amount of relationship shown between the test and the criterion.

Accuracy. The accuracy of tests refers to their repeatability; the consistency with which the same results are obtained each time a student is tested. In physical education, objectivity coefficients of tests are usually obtained by different testers giving the same test to the same subjects and computing the coefficient of correlation between the results of the repeated tests. Objectivity coefficients of .90 are considered satisfactory, although coefficients as low as .80 may be used if more consistent tests do not exist.

Norms. Norms are points of reference to indicate levels of performance as compared with like groups. They are necessary in order to interpret test scores, to identify those who have deficiencies. In physical education, norms may be based upon various combinations of sex, age, height, and weight. Scales using some form of the standard-score technique (T-scale, Hull-scale, six-sigma scale) are also in common use.

Norm charts must be evaluated to determine their propriety.

Economy. In considering the economy of tests, two factors are involved: (a) money cost, and (b) time required of testers and subjects. In some instances, the cost of apparatus may be prohibitive; in other instances, an exhorbitant amount of time may be required to administer the tests. Ways should be found to surmount these difficulties, if such tests are of *fundamental* importance in conducting an effective developmental and adapted physical education program.

Satisfactory tests may not always be available for desired purposes. And, in some situations, the physical educator may be interested only in extreme cases, where only a rough screening device is needed. In these instances, a crude measuring instrument may suffice or recourse may be had to subjective appraisals. In considering tests of value to developmental and adapted physical education, therefore, evaluative procedures may range from the best scientific instruments known to this field to those techniques which will only identify pronounced atypical cases.

MEDICAL APPRAISALS

The medical examination must necessarily be the starting point for any evaluative process related to developmental and adapted physical education. The primary service realized from this examination is the detection of boys and girls with defects of such a nature that vigorous exercise would be harmful to them. Such defects include organic heart lesions, respiratory involvements, hernia, kidney ailments, malnutrition, orthopedic handicaps, nervous conditions, digestive disturbances, general debility, vision and hearing losses, and the like. Individuals with such defects have frequently been excused from physical education. With an adequate developmental and adapted program, this should rarely if ever be necessary. But, rather, these individuals may be protected from too vigorous physical activity and can be provided with exercise or rest prescriptions adapted to their conditions.

The medical examination, of course, should only be conducted by a physician. Every effort should be made to secure as complete an appraisal as possible; school authorities should recognize this need and be willing to provide for it. Permitted sufficient time, physicians will be able to conduct proper examinations. If the health status of the pupil is to be understood fully, this examination should include medical history; nutritional status; condition of skin, eyes, ears, nose, throat, lungs, heart, abdomen, and blood pressure; orthopedic conditions; laboratory tests of urine and blood (when indicated); tuberculin test and chest X-ray.[2] Referral for more searching appraisal and diagnosis should be

---

[2] Frank S. Stafford and H. F. Kilander, *Teacher Education for the Improvement of School Health Programs,* Federal Security Agency Bulletin No. 16 (Washington: Government Printing Office, 1948), p. 14.

made when deemed desirable in individual cases.

The physical educator should see to it that the school or college physician understands the purpose, nature, and procedures of developmental and adapted physical education. Informed physicians, who understand modern concepts of physical education, believe in its significance for growing children and youth and give enthusiastic support to programs that are well conceived and conducted.[3]

NUTRITION TESTS

GENERAL TESTS

The use of tests to measure the nutritional status of children in schools has been a common practice. The purpose of this measurement is to discover those boys and girls who are undernourished and those who are obese, in order that appropriate adapted procedures may be applied. Such evaluation may be utilized for all school children as a primary measurement or as a supplementary measure to determine causative or associative factors in those boys and girls selected for developmental and adapted physical education for other reasons, such as low physical fitness, organic conditions, faulty posture, and the like.

The physical educator has several objective tests from which to choose in evaluating the nutritional status of his students. For years, age-height-weight tables have been used in the schools as indices of nutritional status, while monthly weighing of children and plotting of their weight curves have been common practices. Recent researches, however, have cast considerable doubt on the reliance that can be placed on this form of nutritional measurement, largely because body build and the proportions of bone, muscle, and fat are not considered in determining these projected weight indices. A number of other nutritional measures are available for use in physical education, and some of these should be briefly described.

Wetzel Grid.[4] The Wetzel Grid is devised as a direct reading control chart on the quality of growth and development of individual boys and girls. Based on age, height, and weight, the individual is plotted in one of nine channels, indicating quality of physique and degree of undesirable weight deviation. Each child's developmental level and his age schedule of development are also obtained from this plotting; repeated plottings from time to time indicate growth and development direction.

---

[3] Dean F. Smiley and Fred V. Hein, eds., *Physicians and Schools* (Chicago: American Medical Association, 1947), p. 16.

[4] Norman C. Wetzel, *The Treatment of Growth Failure in Children* (Cleveland: NEA Service, Inc., 1948). Wetzel Grids and other information pertaining to them may be secured from the NEA Service, Inc., 1200 West Third Street, Cleveland 13, Ohio.

The main weakness of the grid technique is lack of assurance that an age-height-weight combination is an adequate index of physique when initially placing the child in his channel; thus, consequently, the teacher may strive to perpetuate an improper growth pattern.

Meredith Chart.[5] Meredith prepared channels for elementary school boys and girls similar to the Wetzel Grid, but omitting the developmental levels. Five channels are provided for height, short to tall; and five, for weight, light to heavy. When a boy's or girl's height and weight points do not lie in corresponding zones, the discrepancy should be studied to determine if it is due to a normal slenderness or stockiness of build or reflects an undesirable state of health.

Pryor's Width-Weight Tables.[6] Pryor bases weight tables upon the following three anthropometric measures indicating body build: standing height, bi-iliac diameter, and chest breadth. Width-Weight Tables are available for each age and sex from 1 to 24 years.

Sheldon's Age-Height-Weight Tables: In the next section, Sheldon's somatotype concept will be considered. His *Atlas of Men* contains age-height-weight tables for each of 88 somatotypes; ages are from 18 to 63 years. When somatotyping is done, these tables may be used as the norms for proper weight.

Signs of malnutrition are, of course, produced upon the body in various degrees depending upon the extent of the nutritional disturbance. In addition to objective nutrition tests, signs of malnutrition should be observed. These characteristics are undersized and poorly developed body; small and flabby muscles; loose, pale, waxy, or sallow skin; lack of subcutaneous fat; pale mucous membrane of eyelids and mouth; rough and lackluster hair; dark hollows or blue circles under eyes; fatigue posture; nervous indigestion and constipation tendencies; deficient endurance and vigor.[7]

ADIPOSE TISSUE

In 1955, the Committee on Nutritional Anthropometry of the Food and Nutrition Board of the National Research Council met at Harvard University to prepare recommendations concerning body measurements for the characterization of nutritional status.[8] The creation of this com-

---

[5] Howard V. Meredith, *Height-Weight Interpretation Chart for Elementary School Boys* (American Medical Association, 535 North Dearborn Street, Chicago, Illinois).
[6] Pryor's tables, including manual, may be secured from the Stanford University Press, Stanford University, Stanford, California.
[7] L. Jean Bogert, *Nutrition and Physical Fitness*, 5th ed. (Philadelphia: W. B. Saunders Company, 1949), p. 535.
[8] Josef Brozek, ed., *Body Measurements and Human Nutrition* (Detroit: Wayne University Press, 1956).

mittee was prompted by the belief that the evaluation of nutritional status was a major neglected area of human nutrition.

In a report at this meeting, Brozek[9] maintained that the ratio of height and weight may serve as a first but "very rough" estimate of the amount of soft tissue in relation to the size of the skeleton. However, he pointed out that this and other weight-height indices suffer from the basic limitations of all procedures which consider only height as the reference point, thus neglecting the vertical proportions of the body, the lateral dimensions, and the size of the skeletal musculature.

Brozek[10] proposed that the individual's relative leanness-fatness may be obtained directly from adipose tissue measurements, inasmuch as a large proportion of the total amount of adipose tissue is contained in the subcutaneous fat deposits. Such evaluations can be made quantitatively by measuring either the thickness of skinfolds externally with calipers or the actual fat layer internally from X-rays. Though there is some subjectivity in making pinch-caliper measurements, Garn and Gorman[11] obtained a correlation of .88 between this test and fat-shadow measurements from X-rays made at the same sites. Quite obviously, for general use in schools and colleges, there will be only one method available—the use of calipers—for measuring the amount of adipose tissue.

The minimum sites for taking skinfold measures proposed by Brozek[12] are back of the upper arm over the triceps and subscapular position on the back. In addition, he suggests a third site, on the mid-axillary line at the level of the umbilicus. Garn[13] states that the easiest skinfolds to obtain are those just below the scapula, just below the breasts, and along the mid-axillary line at the level of the lowest large rib. Further, he intimates that the fat sites having the greatest degree of communality and the highest correlation with weight are over the iliac crest (for adult females) and over the trochanter.

A number of fatfold calipers are available commercially, although the better ones are quite expensive. The recommended amount of pressure to be applied to the skinfold is 10 grams per square millimeter; the size of the contact surface of the caliper may vary from 20 to 40 square millimeters, depending in part on the shape of the contact surface.[14]

Directions for testing skinfolds are as follows. Grasp the skinfold between the thumb and index finger; the span of the grasp is dependent

[9] Ibid., p. 15.

[10] Ibid., p. 21.

[11] Stanley M. Garn and E. L. Gorman, "Comparison of Pinch-Caliper and Teleoroentgenogrammetric Measurements of Subcutaneous Fat," Human Biology, 28, No. 4 (December, 1956), p. 407.

[12] Brozek, op. cit., p. 22.

[13] Stanley M. Garn and Zvi Shamir, Methods for Research in Human Growth (Springfield, Ill.: Charles C. Thomas, 1958), p. 68.

[14] Brozek, op. cit., p. 10.

on the thickness of the skinfold. The amount of skinfold held should be great enough to include two thicknesses of skin with intervening fat, but not to include muscle or fascia. To insure against including these latter structures in the skinfold when the tester is in doubt, he should instruct the subject to tense the underlying muscles. The caliper is applied above the fingers holding the skinfold; all measurements are made to the nearest millimeter.

Directions for giving three skinfold tests follow; illustrations of these techniques appear in Figure 1.

Back of upper arm. The skinfold is taken at the back of the upper arm, mid-posterior and over the triceps muscle, at a point halfway between the tip of the shoulder (acromial process) and the tip of the elbow (olecranon process). The point is located with forearm flexed to 90 degrees; in making the skinfold measurement, however, the arm should hang free. The fold is lifted parallel to the long axis of the arm.

Subscapular. The skinfold is taken at the inferior angle of the scapula (tip of scapula) with the subject in a relaxed standing position. The fold is lifted in the diagonal plane at about 45 degrees from the vertical and horizontal planes medially upward and laterally downward.

Lateral abdomen. The skinfold is taken on the side of the abdomen at the mid-axillary line at the level of the umbilicus. The fold is lifted parallel to the long axis of the body.

SOMATOTYPE

After extensive research, Sheldon[15,16] described the following three primary components of body build: (1) *endomorphy,* a predominance of soft roundedness throughout the various regions of the body, with mass concentration in the viscera; (2) *mesomorphy,* a heavy, hard, rectangular physique, with rugged, massive muscles and large prominent bones; and (3) *ectomorphy,* a frail, delicate body structure, with thin segments antero-posteriorly, the skeleton is long for the length and breadth of the chest.

Sheldon recognized that all individuals have varying degrees of each component. They were, therefore, designated on a 7-point scale for each component (although subsequently half-point variations permitted a 13-point scale). The first unit in the sequence refers to endomorphy; the second, to mesomorphy; the third, to ectomorphy. Thus, a 4-4-4 describes the constitutional type of an individual with an equal and moderate amount of all three components. Eighty-eight adult male somatotypes have been identified using the 7-point scale; when half-

[15] W. H. Sheldon, S. S. Stevens, and W. B. Tucker, *Varieties of Human Physique* (New York: Harper & Brothers, 1940).

[16] William H. Sheldon, *Atlas of Men* (New York: Harper & Brothers, 1954).

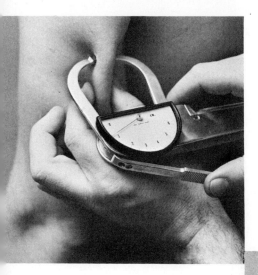

Back of upper arm.

Subscapular.

Lateral abdomen.

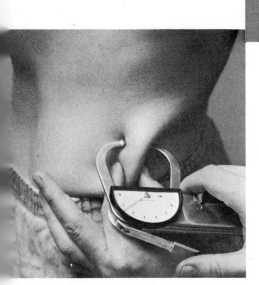

Fig. 1. Skinfold Tests.

points are scored, the number is 505. In *Atlas of Men,* the 505 13-point scale somatotypes are presented, with different examples within the overall frame of the 88 7-point scale.

Somatotyping is *not* basically a test of body status directly related to an atypical condition which can be remedied or alleviated through physical education. Instead, it is a basic frame of reference for the proper understanding and interpretation of the results of other tests. For example, in utilizing the Physical Fitness Index, the average for the dominant endomorph is approximately 85; for the dominant mesomorph, about 110; for the dominant ectomorph, near 100.[17] Likewise, tests of posture, flexibility, endurance, or circulatory-respiratory functions may be understood more clearly against the general background of such a body-build indicator. Furthermore, the individual's reaction to exercise is reflected in part by his somatotype; the extreme mesomorph enjoys strenuous exercise and usually excels in athletics, the extreme ectomorph is prone to fatigue easily, and the extreme endomorph is inclined to avoid physical exertion.

The somatotyping process is complicated and requires specially developed skill to accomplish accurately. By use of the *Atlas,* rough approximations are possible through inspection by experienced observers. Such results, however, indicate dominance and major combinations of components only, rather than a precise description of a somatotype configuration.

LOW PHYSICAL FITNESS DETERMINATION

In Chapter 2, the development of the physical fitness of school children is proposed as a fundamental objective of physical education. In the realization of this objective, standard operating procedure should be the identification of those individuals who are deficient in this basic quality, so that appropriate steps may be taken to improve their condition. The process of insuring for each student a body that has adequate physical strength and is capable of prolonged effort, without efficiency-destroying fatigue, therefore, should constitute a primary responsibility of the physical educator.

Assuming a body free from organic drains and handicapping defects, physical education is concerned with three basic physical fitness components—muscular strength, muscular endurance, and circulatory-respiratory endurance. The construction of tests to measure these components, and others related to physical fitness, has occupied the efforts of researchers in physical education for a century. During World War II, motor fitness tests, so-called, were developed and used by physical educators in evaluating the fitness status of military personnel.

---

[17] Carl E. Willgoose and Millard L. Rogers, "Relationship of Somatotype to Physical Fitness," *Journal of Educational Research,* XLIII, No. 9 (1949), p. 704.

STRENGTH TESTS

Strength tests, although they do not measure all aspects of fitness as the physical educator views the problem, do evaluate basic elements of the individual's general physical status. They have been used successfully in practical school and college situations as a means of selecting students for developmental physical education. A great deal of research has been done in this area, dating from 1880.

The strength test most widely used in physical education to select boys and girls who are sub-par in this quality is the Rogers Physical Fitness Index (PFI).[18] The PFI battery consists of four muscular strength tests (right and left grips, back and leg lifts), two muscular endurance tests (pull-ups, push-ups), and lung capacity. The Strength Index is the gross score from these tests. The PFI is derived from dividing the achieved Strength Index by the normal Strength Index and multiplying by 100; norms are based upon sex, age, and weight. A score of 100 is average; scores of 85 and 115 indicate the first and third quartiles respectively. A number of modifications of this test battery have been posed. The Oregon simplification[19] predicts the Strength Index for boys from a reduced number of test items. Kennedy[20] has successfully proposed substitution of the tensiometer for the dynamometer in back and leg testing.

The selection of individuals with unsatisfactory PFI's for developmental physical education includes at least three groups.

1. *Low scores.* Definitely weak individuals obviously need attention. Many choose 85 as the point below which pupils should be selected; others prefer the national average for the test; still others are governed by practical limitations of time and personnel for follow-up work and include as many of the low PFI's as the local situation permits.

2. *Declining scores.* With the exception of individuals with very high scores, drops in PFI (approximately 10 points or more), regardless of their level, may be a definite danger sign. They usually indicate undesirable changes in physical condition which need to be investigated.

3. *Extremely high scores.* Boys and girls may develop unusual musculatures through extended training in various types of strength-building activities, and, consequently, possess very high PFI scores, which would be a satisfactory status for them. However, in others, an extremely high

---

[18] Present testing techniques and norms appear in H. Harrison Clarke, *Application of Measurement to Health and Physical Education,* 3rd ed. (Englewood Cliffs, N. J.: Prentice-Hall, Inc., 1959), chap. 8.

[19] H. Harrison Clarke and Gavin H. Carter, "Oregon Simplification of the Strength and Physical Fitness Indices," *Research Quarterly,* 30, No. 1 (March, 1959), p. 3.

[20] Frank T. Kennedy, "Substitution of the Tensiometer for the Dynamometer in Back and Leg Lifts for College Men," *Research Quarterly,* 30, No. 2 (May, 1959), p. 179.

PFI (150 and above) may indicate that they are high-strung, over-stimulated, and highly nervous. As a high degree of strength *may* thus be a symptom of such conditions, a PFI reduction becomes an indicator of the success of programs designed to achieve the relaxation of individuals so afflicted.

CIRCULATORY-RESPIRATORY ENDURANCE

Physical education has long been concerned with exercise for the development of circulatory-respiratory endurance. Such exercise requires moderate contraction of large-muscle groups for relatively long periods of time, involving major adjustments of the circulatory and respiratory systems to the activity, as in distance running and swimming. Efforts to measure this component of physical fitness have taken two directions: (1) tests of circulatory-respiratory functions based on the premise that the endurance of the body is dependent upon the efficiency of these systems, hence, a measure of one is a measure of the other; (2) tests of running endurance.

Extensive research has been conducted on the Harvard Step Test, which measures the pulse recovery following stepping up and down on a bench 20 inches high for five minutes at a rate of 30 steps per minute. Adaptations of this test have been made for secondary school boys and for college women and high school girls. Techniques for administering and scoring these tests have also been described by Clarke.[21] The research evidence shows that trained athletes obtain better scores on this test than do untrained athletes and non-athletes.

The best correlations between a step test and motor-fitness criteria were achieved by Russell[22] with college men as subjects. He utilized a 17-inch high bench for stepping and a cadence of 40 steps per minute. Stepping was continued until the subject was no longer able to maintain the cadence due to fatigue. His correlations were .70 with the University of Illinois Motor Fitness Test, .64 with the Air Force's Physical Fitness Test and with the Navy Standard Physical Fitness Test, and .61 with the Indiana Motor Fitness Test. He also obtained the high correlation of .85 between the length of time the step test was continued and the gross oxygen intake on a treadmill run to exhaustion.

A modified form of the step test was found satisfactory by Karpovich, Starr, and Weiss[23] in evaluating the readiness of patients in Army hospi-

---

[21] H. Harrison Clarke, *Application of Measurement to Health and Physical Education*, 3rd ed., pp. 105-110.

[22] Walter L. Russell, "A Study of the Relationship of Performance to Certain Generally Accepted Tests of Physical Fitness and Circulatory-Respiratory Capacity of Normal College Men," (Microcarded Doctoral Dissertation, Louisiana State University, 1948).

[23] Peter V. Karpovich, Merritt P. Starr, and Raymond A. Weiss, "Physical Fitness Tests for Convalescents," *Journal of the American Medical Association*, 126, No. 14 (December 2, 1944), p. 873.

tals recovering from severe respiratory illnesses for participation in physical activity. The regulation 20-inch high bench was used; the cadence was 24 steps per minute. Patients who could perform the test for 30 seconds and had pulse rates less than 100 per minute (double the sitting pulse taken for 30 seconds, beginning one minute after exercise) were considered ready for light calisthenics. For progression in physical activity, both the length of time the patient could continue stepping and his pulse rate after exercise were considered, as shown in Table I. There are three physical training classifications.

Red   mild calisthenics
Blue   calisthenics, games, moderate running, combatives, and "guerilla exercises"
Green   same as blue, with addition of wind sprints and cross-country running

The discharge test, indicating adequate physical stamina for full military duty, required completion of the full Harvard Step Test with a score of 75.

TABLE I

*Scoring Table for Progressive Exercise Based on Modified Harvard Test**

Duration of Exercise	Pulse Rate One Min. after Exercise	Physical Training Classification
Below 2 min.	Regardless of Pulse Rate	Red
2 min. to 2 min. 29 sec.	Below 100	Blue
	Above 100	Red
2 min. 30 sec. to 2 min. 59 sec.	Below 130	Blue
	Above 130	Red
3 min. to 3 min. 29 sec.	Below 100	Green
	100 to 140	Blue
	Above 140	Red
3 min. 30 sec. to 3 min. 59 sec.	Below 110	Green
	110 to 170	Blue
	Above 170	Red
4 min. to 4 min. 29 sec.	Below 130	Green
	Above 130	Blue
4 min. 30 sec. to 4 min. 59 sec.	Below 140	Green
	Above 140	Blue
5 min.	Below 150	Green
	Above 150	Blue

* Reproduced with permission from: Peter V. Karpovich, Merritt P. Starr, and Raymond A. Weiss, "Physical Fitness Tests for Convalescents," *Journal of the American Medical Association*, 126, No. 2 (December 2, 1944) 873.

Circulatory tests. The classical circulatory tests by Schneider, McCurdy and Larson, McCloy, and Tuttle are based on circulatory-respiratory determinations made at rest and after light work loads of short duration. Astrand[24] has contended that it is theoretically incorrect to evaluate the efficiency of the circulatory system by the net pulse, i.e., the pulse rate during work minus the pulse rate at rest. To support this contention, he pointed out that 10 pulse beats at rest with a stroke volume of 60 milliliters are not equivalent to 10 pulse beats at work with a stroke volume of 150 milliliters. For similar reasons, the recovery pulse rate should not be "mixed up" with the work pulse rate. Also, Astrand maintains that, when testing circulatory-respiratory fitness, a type of work must be chosen which engages large groups of muscles and the work levels must be relatively high; the duration of the work must be long enough to permit the adjustment of circulation and ventilation to the level of exercise.

Astrand has proposed further that the individual's capacity for heavy prolonged muscular work will first of all be dependent on the supply of oxygen supplied the working muscle. In types of work which engage large groups of muscles, the limiting factor for the maximum oxygen intake (aerobic capacity) is probably the capacity and regulation of the oxygen transporting system. Direct measurement of aerobic capacity is intricate and requires complex laboratory equipment. Furthermore, maximal tests may frequently be undesirable for untrained subjects, older people, and individuals with certain types of organic conditions.

As a consequence of these considerations, Astrand and his associates[25] studied the possibilities of utilizing submaximal efforts in the measurement of aerobic capacity. From these studies, he reported that the heart rate after about six minutes of work for a group of healthy male subjects averaged 128, when undertaking muscular activity of such severity that the oxygen demand was 50 per cent of maximum intake. The corresponding heart rate for female subjects was 138. When the subjects worked with a load demanding an oxygen intake of 70 per cent aerobic capacity, the average heart beat was 154 for males and 164 for females.

Astrand and Ryhming[26] found that the considerations above could be realized from a single work test with the subject stepping up and down on a bench, cycling on a bicycle ergometer, or running on a treadmill. The best results were obtained when the test work resulted in a steady-state heart rate level between 125 and 170. Within these limits, there was a nearly linear increase in metabolism with heart rate.

---

[24] P. O. Astrand, "Human Fitness with Special Reference to Sex and Age," *Physiological Reviews*, 36, No. 3 (July, 1956), p. 325.

[25] *Ibid.*, p. 326.

[26] P. O. Astrand and Irma Ryhming, "A Nomogram for Calculation of Aerobic Capacity (Physical Fitness) from Pulse Rate during Submaximal Work," *Journal of Applied Physiology*, 7, No. 2 (September, 1954), pp. 218-221.

Comparable results were obtained with the three types of circulatory exercise, stepping, cycling, and running.

The step test utilized in these studies has been described by Ryhming.[27] From the following step-test situation, an oxygen demand of approximately 50 per cent of aerobic capacity was obtained.

1. The height of the bench was 40 cm. (15.75 in.) for young males, 27 cm. (10.6 in.) for males 40 to 70 years of age, and 33 cm. (13 in.) for young females.

2. The cadence was 22.5 complete steps up and down (four count step) on the bench per minute.

3. Stepping continued for five minutes.

4. The pulse rate (radial artery) during work was counted for 15 seconds each minute. In most cases, the pulse rate attained a steady value after the second minute; the steady-value rate for one minute was used in the scoring. If no steady value was found in an individual case, the last value was used.

For scoring this test for physical fitness, Astrand and Ryhming[28] prepared a nomogram, which was subsequently adjusted by Astrand[29] for lower loads. A correction factor for both females and males in older ages was introduced, as shown in Figure 2. The nomogram reveals that the maximum oxygen intake for a male with a weight of 62.0 kg. and a heart rate from the test of 138 is 3.3 1/min., as read from the diagonal line. The same aerobic capacity for a female would be obtained from a body weight of 76.0 kg. and a pulse rate of 138. The oxygen intake can also be estimated from the nomogram, but is not needed for the test. (The "work level" column is used when cycling or running rather than stepping is the exercise medium.) The higher the aerobic capacity on this test the more physically fit is the individual.

Compared with the actual measurement of maximal oxygen intake, the investigators found approximately 6 per cent of error for two-thirds of the subjects. This is a fairly large error when extended over the full range of scores. However, this test may reasonably be used as a gross test of circulatory endurance, especially to identify those who are subpar in this basic physical fitness element and to follow their improvement as a result of conditioning activity. At the opposite extreme, Astrand and Ryhming[30] state that athletes noted for their good results in events calling for endurance, e.g., running and skiing, are characterized by a very high figure for maximum oxygen intake.

Endurance running. So far, the various running indices, such as the

---

[27] Irma Ryhming, "A Modified Harvard Step Test for the Evaluating of Physical Fitness," *Arbeitsphysiologie*, 15 (1954), p. 225.

[28] Astrand and Ryhming, *loc. cit.*

[29] Irma Astrand, "Aerobic Work Capacity in Men and Women with Special Reference to Age," *Acta Physiologica Scandinavica*, 49, Supplement 169, 1960, p. 51.

[30] *Ibid.*, p. 221.

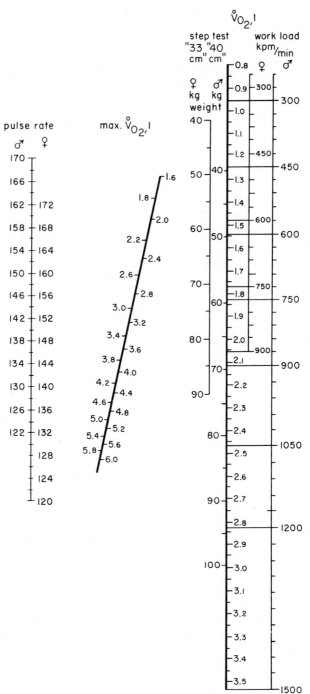

Fig. 2. Nomograph for Scoring Ryhming Step Test.

endurance ratio (proportion between times on short and long runs) and drop-off index (slowing up in seconds for various parts of a long run), have not proven satisfactory as measures of circulatory-respiratory endurance. Potentially, however, they appear to have great possibilities for this purpose in physical education. There are several problems encountered in establishing these measures, such as knowledge of pace, influence of native speed, psychological limitations of the subject to endure fatigue, and inability to establish adequate criteria for the validation of such tests.

KRAUS-WEBER TESTS

The Kraus-Weber Tests of Minimum Muscular Fitness[31] compose a battery of five simple muscular tests and a hip-trunk flexibility test. Kraus and Hirschland have reported a study of 4,000 patients in low back pain clinics at Columbia Presbyterian Medical Center, the Institute of Physical Medicine and Rehabilitation of the New York University-Bellevue Medical Center, and Kraus' private practice. In nearly all cases, the patients were evaluated by a team consisting of an orthopedic surgeon, a neurosurgeon, a radiologist, and a specialist in physical medicine.

The majority of these patients showed a combination of muscle deficiencies and nervous tension. While their complaints were definitely "backache," they were not healthy people suffering from a local difficulty, nor were they simply neurotics somatizing their emotional complaints. They offered a combination of both physical and emotional difficulties. In these people, a minor back strain, either acute or chronic, designated the presence of a much deeper and more complex disease.[32] Of the 4,000 patients, 80 per cent, free from organic disease, were unable to pass one or more of the Kraus-Weber test items.

Descriptions of the six Kraus-Weber tests are briefly presented below.

1. *Strength of abdominal and psoas muscles.* Subject lying supine, hands behind neck, tester holding feet; roll to a sitting position. Scoring: 0 to 10, depending on distance moved unaided in sitting up.

2. *Strength of abdominal muscles without psoas.* Same as Test 1, except the sit-up execution is performed with knees bent.

3. *Strength of psoas and lower abdominal muscles.* Subject lying supine, hands behind neck, legs extended; raise legs off floor ten inches with knees straight, hold for ten seconds. Scoring: 0 to 10, one point for each second feet are held up.

4. *Strength of upper back muscles.* Subject lying prone, pillow under

[31] Hans Kraus and Wilhelm Raab, *Hypokinetic Disease* (Springfield, Ill.: Charles C. Thomas, 1961), p. 12.

[32] Hans Kraus, *et al.*, "Muscular Fitness and Orthopedic Disability," *New York State Medical Journal*, 43, No. 2 (January 15, 1954).

abdomen far enough down to give body the feeling of being a seesaw, hands behind neck; tester holds feet; subject raises chest, head, and shoulders and holds them up for ten seconds. Scoring: 0 to 10, one point for each second upper body is held up.

5. *Strength of lower back muscles.* Same as Test 4, except the tester holds chest down and subject raises legs with knees straight.

6. *Length of back and hamstring muscles.* Subject standing erect in stocking or bare feet, hands at sides, feet together; with knees straight, lean down slowly until fingers touch floor, maintain this position for three counts (seconds). Marking: 10 points when floor touch is held for three counts; deduct one point for each inch away from floor at which position is held for three counts.

MOTOR FITNESS TESTS

Henry[33,34] has discussed problems pertaining to large-muscle learning and performance abilities. In so doing, he challenged the common assumption that gross motor abilities are general or made up of group factors such as strength, speed, and coordination, in disregard of all the other factors available. Henry's belief was formed from studies in his laboratory and elsewhere. In general, these studies resulted in low or insignificant correlations between reaction time and speed of movement, lack of correlation between learning two novel motor tasks initially unpracticed, little if any correlation between speed of arm and leg movements and reaction time involved in a modified baseball throw and football kick, and low correlations in neuromuscular ability for movements and tasks of considerable similarity.

However, tests have been developed which comprise several of the components of motor fitness; certain of these may be of use to the developmental and adapted physical educator. The components frequently included in tests of this sort are muscular endurance, circulatory-respiratory endurance, speed, agility, and power. These tests are designed to secure ease of administration; little training is required to master the testing techniques. With good organization, a large number of individuals can be tested in a short time, and in some instances, self-scoring is encouraged. Much remains to be studied in relation to the effectiveness of motor fitness tests as appraisal instruments. Furthermore, certain of these tests contain extremely exhausting items, which should not be given to unconditioned individuals or to those at the lower fitness levels.

While reports on the use of motor fitness tests in developmental and adapted physical education have not appeared in the literature, investi-

---

[33] Franklin M. Henry, "Motor Learning and Coordination," *Proceedings of College Physical Education Association*, 59 (1956), pp. 68-75.

[34] Franklin M. Henry, "Specificity Vs. Generality in Learning Motor Skills," *Proceedings of College Physical Education Association*, 61 (1958), pp. 126-128.

gations of their use for this purpose might well prove fruitful. Some suggested tests of this type are the Oregon, Indiana, New York, and California motor fitness tests, the AAHPER Youth Fitness Test, and Elder's test for junior high school boys. In most instances, these tests may be applied to both boys and girls at all school levels.[35]

CABLE-TENSION STRENGTH TESTS

In dealing with some postural and orthopedic defects, developmental and adapted physical educators may wish to improve the strength of involved muscle groups. The use of tests to assess the status of weakened muscles at the initiation of exercise and to follow their progress throughout the treatment period is necessary for best results.

Originating during World War II in the AAF convalescent hospital physical reconditioning service, cable-tension tests for measuring the strength of individual muscles groups were proposed and subsequently were perfected by Clarke.[36,37,38,39] Thirty-eight such strength tests were constructed involving movements of the finger, thumb, wrist, elbow, shoulder, neck, trunk, hip, knee, and foot joints. In determining the proper position for the various movements, consultation was held repeatedly with physiatrists at the Mayo Clinic. Objectivity coefficients of .90 and above were obtained when the tests were administered by experienced testers.

TESTING EQUIPMENT

Tensiometer. The aircraft tensiometer,[40] illustrated in Figure 3, is the instrument used in recording muscle strength for the cable-tension tests. This instrument was originally designed to measure the tension of aircraft control cable. Cable tension is determined by measuring the force applied to a riser causing an offset in a cable stretched taut between two sectors. This tension is then converted directly into pounds on a calibration chart supplied with the instrument.

---

[35] Directions and scoring tables for some of these tests and sources for the others appear in Clarke, *Application of Measurement to Health and Physical Education*, 3rd ed., chap. 9.

[36] H. Harrison Clarke, "Objective Strength Tests of Affected Muscle Groups Involved in Orthopedic Disabilities," *Research Quarterly*, 19, No. 2 (May, 1948), pp. 118-147.

[37] H. Harrison Clarke, "Improvement of Objective Strength Tests of Muscle Groups by Cable-Tension Methods," *Research Quarterly*, 21, No. 4 (December, 1950), pp. 399-419.

[38] H. Harrison Clarke, Theodore L. Bailey, and Clayton T. Shay, "New Objective Strength Tests by Cable-Tension Methods," *Research Quarterly*, 23, No. 2 (May, 1952), pp. 136-148.

[39] H. Harrison Clarke, *Manual: Cable-Tension Strength Tests* (West Springfield, N. H.: Stuart Murphy, Publisher, 1953).

[40] Manufactured by Pacific Scientific Company, Bell Gardens, California.

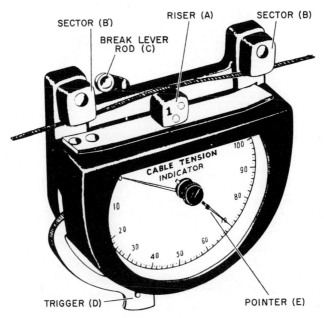

Fig. 3. Tensiometer.

The tensiometer used in strength testing has been adapted by the manufacturers for this purpose by (a) special calibration for an "up-pull" on a cable, rather than placement on a taut cable, (b) addition of a maximum pointer to facilitate reading the subject's score, and (c) deletion of the brake lever rod, as this is needed only to fix the pointer after applying the tensiometer to a taut cable. In the event a brake lever rod is on the instrument, it should not be used in strength testing, as it retards the movement of the pointer, thus recording an inaccurate score. The No. 1 riser shown in the illustration is used with cable sizes of ¹⁄₁₆, ³⁄₃₂, and ⅛ inches, which are adequate for testing the individual muscle groups described here.

When purchasing a tensiometer, it will be necessary to indicate the maximum capacity desired. Instruments with the following capacities are available: 0-200 pounds, 100-400 pounds, and 100-800 pounds. The first two of these are calibrated for use with ¹⁄₁₆″ cable; the third one, for ³⁄₃₂″ cable.

As an aid in deciding upon the tensiometer to obtain, Table II is presented. The low, mean, and high scores obtained by boys seven and 15 years of age on ten of the tests are given. College men will score higher on these tests, as would be expected; the scores for girls will be generally lower. For smaller muscle groups, such as those activating the fingers or thumb, and for testing subjects with severe handicaps, the lowest-capacity instrument will be needed.

TABLE II

Low, Mean, and High Scores on Cable-Tension Strength Tests
for Boys Seven and Fifteen Years of Age°
(Given in Pounds)

Muscle Groups Tested	7 Years			15 Years		
	Low	Mean	High	Low	Mean	High
Elbow Flexors	20	31	47	47	101	150
Shoulder Flexors	18	39	73	61	117	190
Shoulder Inward Rotators	10	23	40	31	58	98
Trunk Flexors	15	33	48	36	105	202
Hip Flexors	14	35	63	50	105	160
Hip Extensors	15	29	55	52	119	197
Knee Flexors	18	34	57	53	101	194
Knee Extensors	25	48	83	62	176	293
Ankle Dorsal Flexors	8	23	35	27	63	106
Ankle Plantar Flexors	25	47	82	72	166	264

° James C. E. Harrison, "The Construction of Cable-Tension Strength Test Norms for Boys Seven, Nine, Twelve, and Fifteen Years of Age," Master's Thesis, University of Oregon, 1958.

Pulling Assemblies. For the cable-tension strength tests presented in this section, the following pulling assembly units are needed (Figure 4).

1. *Cable and chain.* Secure a 12-14″ length of ¹⁄₁₆″ extra-flexible cable. Construct a 1″ loop at each end by turning the cable back on itself and securing with a small clamp of a size to fit the cable; these loops may be reinforced with small thimbles. By use of a 1½″ or 2″ clevis, the cable is attached to a light welded link chain (1″ links). Different lengths of chain are desirable; lengths of 12, 24, and 60 inches are recommended. A second clevis is needed for attachment of the cable to the D-ring of the strap.

2. *Regulation strap.* Construct this strap from 2″ 3-ply belting or nylon safety belt material. Two straps should be made; one to have a loop 9″ long, and the other to have a loop 12″ long. Stitch firmly or rivet around a D-ring. Make a keeper from the same material, folded twice around for stiffness. Form a stirrup in one strap for ankle plantar flexion testing.

3. *Finger strap.* Make this strap from 1″ 3-ply belting 20″ long, forming a 6″ loop. Fold back on itself; stitch firmly or rivet at free end to hold a 1″ D-ring. Construct a keeper.

4. *Trunk strap.* Use two pieces of belting, 4″ x 30″ and 2″ x 30″.

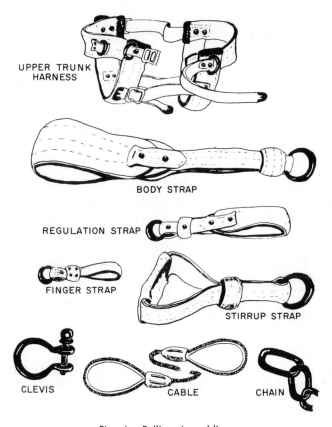

UPPER TRUNK HARNESS

BODY STRAP

REGULATION STRAP

FINGER STRAP

STIRRUP STRAP

CLEVIS   CABLE   CHAIN

Fig. 4.   Pulling Assemblies.

Turn the four corners of the larger piece to fit size of the smaller, which should be drawn through a 2″ D-ring. Rivet to join the two pieces and to secure D-ring; stitching to secure rivets also helps. Construct a keeper for the smaller strap. The loop on this strap will be about 18 inches long; for especially large individuals, a second trunk strap, with loop 24 inches long, will be needed.

5. *Trunk harness.* Obtain the following pieces of webbing: two shoulder straps, each 3″ x 24″; two underarm straps, each 3″ x 12″; and four adjustable straps, each 16″ long, either of 1¼″ cotton webbing or 1½″ luggage belting. Securely sew each shoulder strap at slightly acute angles to each end of underarm strap; bind rough corners with leather to prevent fraying. Attach four adjustable, serrated, lip-type buckles to right shoulder strap as follows: two upper buckles, 5 inches from mid-point of strap, one for chest and one for back; two lower buckles, over junction of shoulder and upper-arm straps. Fasten adjustable straps

to left shoulder piece, directly opposite buckles. At mid-point of each upper-arm strap, attach a 1″ D-ring.

From the appropriate strap and cable-chain, the pulling assembly for any given cable-tension test can be arranged.

Testing Table. As illustrated in Figure 5, a padded table, approximately 78″ long, 24″ wide, and 30″ high, is needed for placing the subject in correct position for most of the cable-tension strength tests. A training-room rubbing table is satisfactory for this purpose. A number of changes in this table must be made.

1. In order to permit attachment of the pulling assembly directly below the subject in trunk and hip strength tests, a slit 7″ x 20″ should be cut lengthwise in the testing table, beginning 10 inches from one end. The edges of this slit should be bound with cover material from the part removed (fold this back when cutting the slit in order to facilitate this process).

2. Stringers, 2″ x 4″, should be attached along each side of the table at floor level. Place sturdy hooks in the upper edges of these stringers as needed for certain of the elbow, shoulder, and trunk tests.

3. A third 2″ x 4″ stringer is needed at floor level; attach horizontally down center of the table. This stringer should have hooks below the

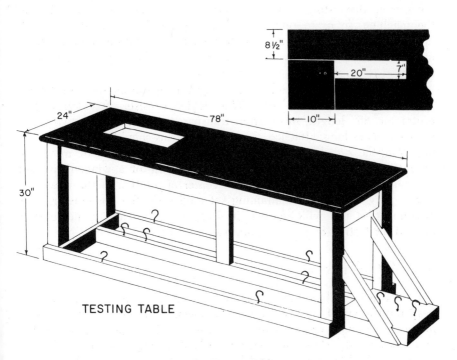

TESTING TABLE

Fig. 5. Testing Table.

table slit for trunk and hip tests, and at the opposite end for knee extension test.

4. At floor level, provide a 20-inch extension of the table at the end opposite the slit; this needs to be very sturdily braced. Place hooks in this extension for neck tests and for knee flexion test.

Wall Hooks. Four-inch, open wall hooks, which will withstand pulls up to 600 pounds, should be screwed into the wall or a firm upright. Usually, it is advisable to attach a 2″ x 4″ joist securely to the wall for these hooks. The lowest hook should be one inch from the floor; others should be placed six inches apart to a height of 43 inches. (A hook at a height of 72 inches is needed if the thumb adduction strength test is to be used.)

Arm-Rest Chair. A school-type chair with a short writing board is needed for strength tests of the fingers and thumb. A ⅜″ hook should be placed low on the leg of the chair below the writing board, and slanted in line with the pull. The back legs of the chair should be built up to level the writing board. A similar arrangement is necessary on the left side if muscles on that side are to be tested.

Supinator-Pronator Machine. A supinator-pronator machine is required for testing supination and pronation of the forearm. Mount 2 feet 9 inches from the floor (measured to center of axle) if the test is to be taken from the testing table. All friction parts should be removed from the machine, so as to permit free movement of the handle. A small hook should be placed at each end of the handle of the supinator-pronator machine. The pulling assembly runs from this hook to another hook placed at the right or left of the machine.

Goniometer. A goniometer is necessary for measuring the joint angles specified for the various tests. This device consists of a 180 degree protractor, 8½″ length, made from transparent material with two arms, each 15 inches long, attached. One of these arms should be fixed extending along the zero line of the protractor; the other should be moveable permitting rotation to the proper angle. The use of a winged nut and bolt placed through an eyelet at the center of rotation of the moveable arm is very helpful in maintaining set angles for the goniometer. This instrument in use will be seen in Figure 10. A small goniometer is needed for testing finger and thumb movements.

General Testing Instructions

1. For each cable-tension test, the position of the subject for the best application of muscle strength is specified. Every effort has been made to eliminate compensatory action of muscles not involved in the joint movement. Thus, the positions of other parts of the body are given and the blocking supplied by the tester is prescribed. Precautions

to be observed in administering the various tests also appear in connection with the test descriptions.

2. The goniometer should be used for measuring the joint angle(s) specified in connection with each test. This process is described later in this chapter.

3. In the test positions described, the pulling assembly is always arranged at right angles to the body part acting as the pulling lever. Zero degrees is a position away from the median line of the body; 180 degrees parallels and is toward the median line.

4. In certain of the tests, the weight of parts of the body is lifted in performing the movement. To record roughly the actual weight lifted by the muscles in these tests, the gravity factor may be added to the test score. To determine the amount of the gravity factor, place the body and its parts in the prescribed position for the test; suspend the part being lifted in the pulling assembly with the strap at the pulling point, at right angles to the part, and determine the amount of tension applied to the cable with the tensiometer when the part being weighed is relaxed.

5. For each test, the tester should adjust the joint being tested in such a way that the angle is approximately correct at the height of the pull.

6. The cable, itself, should be taut at the start of each pull.

DESCRIPTIONS OF CABLE-TENSION STRENGTH TESTS

1. FINGER FLEXION (Fig. 6)

Starting Position. (a) Subject sitting in arm-rest chair; free arm resting on thigh. (b) Forearm and hand on side tested supinated and resting on writing board; towel placed under arm and hand for comfort. (c) Line of metacarpal-phalangeal joints at edge of writing board; finger or fingers being tested fully extended.

Attachments. (a) Finger strap around first phalanx of finger or fingers. (b) Pulling assembly attached to hook on front leg of chair.

Precautions. Prevent palmar flexion and elbow flexion by bracing.

2. FINGER EXTENSION (Fig. 6)

Starting Position. (a) Subject sitting in straight chair; free arm resting on thigh. (b) Upper arm on side tested close to side; forearm and hand pronated and lying flat on arm rest of another chair; finger or fingers just off edge of arm rest, flexed to 80 degrees.

Attachments. (a) Finger strap around first phalanx of finger or fingers. (b) Pulling assembly attached to wall at rear of subject.

Precautions. (a) Prevent wrist dorsal flexion and elbow flexion by bracing. (b) Prevent thumb from interference by extending it.

3. THUMB ADDUCTION (Fig. 6)

Starting Position. (a) Subject sitting in arm-rest chair; free arm resting on thigh. (b) Forearm on side tested in mid-prone-supine position; thumb abducted to maximum; fingers extended.
Attachments. (a) Finger strap around interphalangeal joint of thumb. (b) Pulling assembly attached to wall overhead and at rear of subject.
Precautions. (a) Prevent abduction and elevation of shoulder. (b) Keep wrist and fingers fully extended by bracing.

4. THUMB ABDUCTION

This test is similar to Thumb Adduction with the following exceptions. (a) Thumb on side tested extended in line with extended forefinger at height of pull (place pad under wrist for comfort). (b) Finger strap around phalanx of thumb. (c) Pulling assembly attached to chair-leg hook.

5. WRIST DORSAL FLEXION (Fig. 6)

Starting Position. (a) Subject sitting in chair; free arm resting on testing table. (b) Upper arm on side tested close to side; elbow in 90 degree flexion; forearm in mid-prone-supine position; wrist in mid-position of range of motion; forearm resting on table; free hand bracing wrist being tested.
Attachments. (a) Regulation strap around dorsum of hand above metacarpal-phalangeal joint. (b) Cable attached to wall facing wrist being tested.
Precautions. (a) Prevent shoulder abduction by bracing elbow close to side. (b) Prevent shoulder elevation by bracing.

6. WRIST PALMAR FLEXION

The position for this test is the same as for Wrist Dorsal Flexion. The pulling assembly, however, is attached to opposite side.

7. WRIST ABDUCTION

This test is similar to Wrist Dorsal Flexion with the following exceptions. (a) Hand being tested flat, palm downward, on testing table. (b) Pulling assembly attached to wall next to side being tested. (c) Stabilize arm and elbow and prevent movement of forearm.

8. WRIST ADDUCTION

The position for this test is same as for Wrist Abduction. The pulling assembly, however, is attached to opposite side.

9. FOREARM PRONATION (Fig. 6)

Starting Position. (a) Subject sitting in chair; free arm resting on thigh. (b) Upper arm on side tested close to side; elbow in 90 degrees flexion; forearm resting on testing table at right angle with wall; forearm in 110 degrees supination; hand grasping handle of pronator-supinator machine.

Attachments. (a) Chain attached to wall at right of supinator-pronator machine. (b) Cable hooked to supinator-pronator at upper part of handle for right hand and lower part of handle for left hand. (Reverse these if pulling assembly is attached to left side.)

Precautions. (a) Prevent palmar flexion of wrist. (b) Prevent shoulder abduction by bracing subject's elbow against his side. (c) Prevent lateral flexion of spine by bracing against top of shoulder on side being tested.

10. FOREARM SUPINATION

The position for this test is same as for Forearm Pronation with the following exceptions. (a) Forearm being tested in 80 degrees supination. (b) Pulling assembly is attached in opposite directions to permit supination tests. (c) Prevent dorsal flexion of wrist.

11. ELBOW FLEXION (Fig. 6)

Starting Position. (a) Subject in supine lying position, hips and knees flexed comfortably; free hand resting on chest. (b) Upper arm on side tested close to side; elbow in 115 degrees flexion; forearm in mid-prone-supine position.

Attachments. (a) Regulation strap placed around forearm midway between wrist and elbow joints. (b) Pulling assembly hooked toward subject's feet; hook on table runner.

Precautions. (a) Prevent raising elbow and abducting shoulder by bracing at elbow. (b) Stabilize subject on table by bracing legs.

12. ELBOW EXTENSION (Fig. 7)

The position for this test is same as for Elbow Flexion with the following exceptions. (a) Elbow in 40 degrees flexion. (b) Pulling assembly hooked to wall below subject's head. (c) Prevent shoulder elevation by

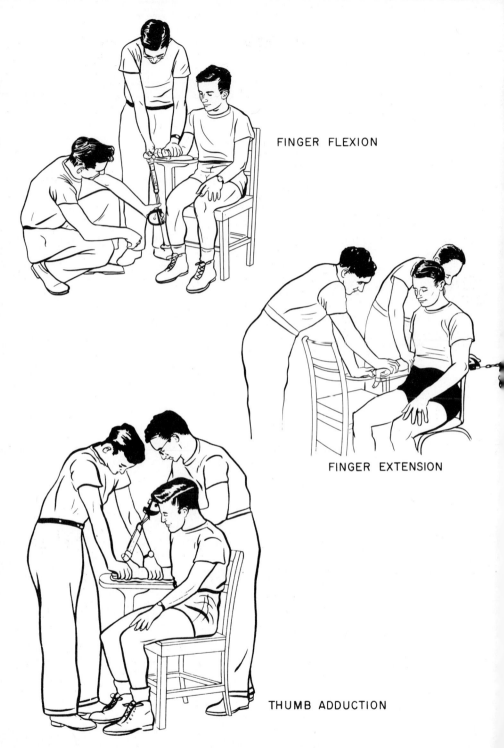

FINGER FLEXION

FINGER EXTENSION

THUMB ADDUCTION

Fig. 6. Cable-Tension Strength Tests.

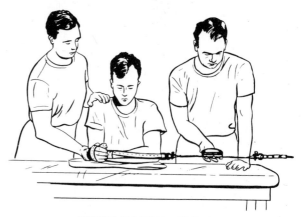

WRIST DORSAL FLEXION

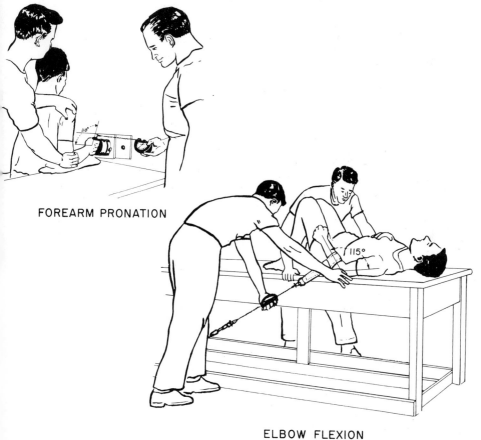

FOREARM PRONATION

ELBOW FLEXION

Fig. 6 (cont.)

83

bracing; require subject to keep his head straight so as to reduce tendency to flex spine laterally.

13. SHOULDER FLEXION (Fig. 7)

Starting Position. (a) Subject in supine lying position, hips and knees flexed comfortably; free hand resting on chest. (b) Upper arm on side tested close to side; shoulder flexed to 90 degrees; elbow in 90 degrees flexion.

Attachments. (a) Regulation strap around upper arm midway between elbow and shoulder joints. (b) Pulling assembly hooked to table runner below subject's arm.

Precautions. Prevent shoulder and hip elevation by bracing.

14. SHOULDER EXTENSION (Fig. 7)

The position for this test is the same as for Shoulder Flexion with the following exceptions. (a) Shoulder on side being tested flexed to 90 degrees; elbow flexed; forearm directly across body. (b) Pulling assembly attached to wall at subject's head. (c) Prevent shoulder elevation by bracing and prevent shoulder adduction by guiding elbow.

15. SHOULDER HORIZONTAL FLEXION (Fig. 7)

The position for this test is the same as for Shoulder Extension with the following exceptions. (a) Knees fully extended instead of bent. (b) Pulling assembly attached to wall away from body. (c) Prevent trunk from lateral flexion and shoulders from lifting by bracing at shoulder and hip; require subject to keep head straight; steady subject's arm in testing position by holding wrist.

16. SHOULDER ABDUCTION (Fig. 7)

Starting Position. (a) Subject in supine lying position, hips and knees flexed comfortably; free hand on chest. (b) Upper arm on side tested close to side; elbow at 90 degrees flexion; forearm in mid-prone-supine position. (c) Pad, or folded towel, under buttocks and another across scapula raising body to permit passage of pulling assembly.

Attachments. (a) Regulation strap around distal end of upper arm, just above olecranon process of elbow. (b) Pulling assembly under subject's back and attached to wall opposite side of limb being tested.

Precautions. (a) Prevent shoulder elevation, raising of elbow, and lateral trunk flexion by bracing. (b) Require subject to keep head straight, so as to reduce tendency to flex spine.

17. Shoulder Adduction (Fig. 7)

Starting Position. (a) Subject in supine lying position, hips and knees flexed comfortably; free hand on chest. (b) Upper arm on side tested adducted to 110 degrees; turn forearm across chest, hand held low, to eliminate effect of biceps muscle.

Attachments. (a) Regulation strap around upper arm midway between shoulder and elbow joints. (b) Pulling assembly attached to wall beyond subject's head.

Precautions. (a) Prevent elevation of shoulder. (b) Brace both shoulders with hands to hold subject in place when pulling.

18. Shoulder Inward Rotation (Fig. 8)

Starting Position. (a) Subject in supine lying position, hips and knees flexed comfortably; free hand on chest. (b) Upper arm on side tested close to side; elbow in 90 degrees flexion, and supported by pad to bring upper arm into position parallel with table; forearm in mid-prone-supine position.

Attachments. (a) Regulation strap around forearm midway between elbow and wrist joints. (b) Pulling assembly attached to wall next to side being tested.

Precautions. (a) Adjust forearm so that it is vertical at height of pull. (b) Prevent "cupping" shoulder by bracing with hand. (c) Prevent raising elbow and abducting upper arm by bracing elbow. (d) Stabilize trunk by bracing hips.

19. Shoulder Outward Rotation

The position of the subject for this test is the same as for Shoulder Inward Rotation. The pulling assembly, however, is attached to wall opposite side being tested.

20. Neck Flexion (Fig. 8)

Starting Position. (a) Subject in supine lying position, hips and knees flexed comfortably, feet and elbows resting on table; hands folded on chest. (b) Occipital lobe of head resting on edge of table.

Attachments. (a) Regulation strap over supra-orbital ridge and forehead (use pad over forehead and bridge of nose for comfort). (b) Pulling assembly attached below head.

Precautions. (a) Require subject to tuck in chin when pulling. (b) Prevent hunching of shoulders.

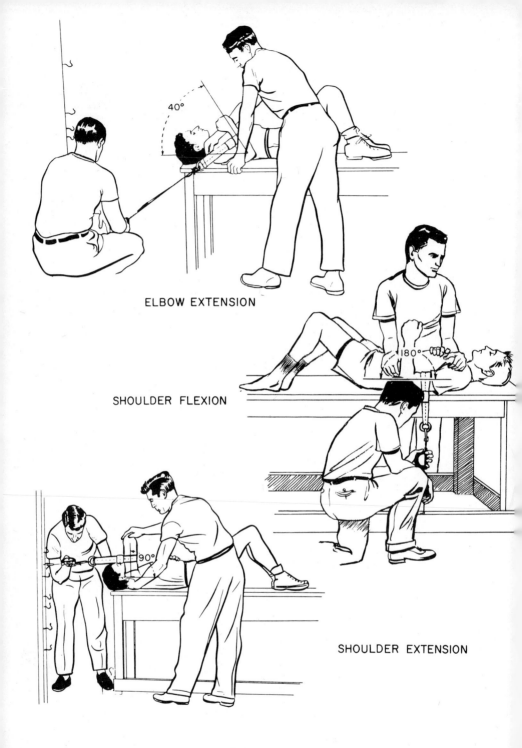

ELBOW EXTENSION

SHOULDER FLEXION

SHOULDER EXTENSION

Fig. 7. Cable-Tension Strength Tests.

86

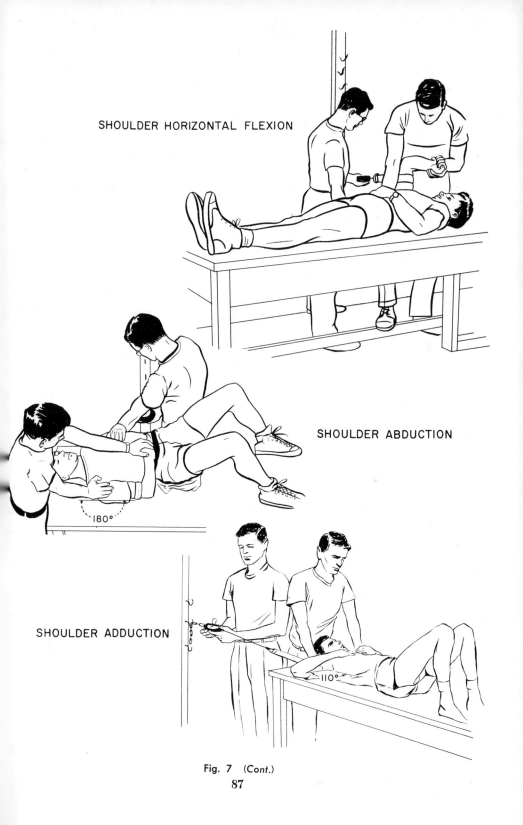

SHOULDER HORIZONTAL FLEXION

SHOULDER ABDUCTION

180°

SHOULDER ADDUCTION

110°

Fig. 7 (Cont.)

87

21. NECK EXTENSION

This test differs from Neck Flexion in the following ways. (a) Subject
in prone lying position, legs extended, and forearms dangling over edge
of table (use pad under clavicle and manubrium areas of chest and
shoulders for comfort. (b) Rest chin on edge of table. (c) Regulation
strap over occipital lobe of head. (d) Insure straight position of head
when pulling; prevent lifting of chest by bracing.

22. NECK LATERAL FLEXION

This test differs from Neck Flexion in the following ways. (a) Subject
in side-lying position; under arm extended to help support head; under
leg flexed at hip and knees to help hold body position; upper leg
extended. (b) Regulation strap over head diagonally from forehead
to occipital lobe. (c) Stabilize trunk and shoulders so that shoulders
are in line with body.

23. TRUNK FLEXION (Fig. 8)

Starting Position. Subject in supine lying position with upper back
over slit in table; legs straight and together; arms folded on chest.
Attachments. (a) Trunk strap around chest, close under armpits. (b)
Pulling assembly attached beneath subject.
Precautions. Prevent raising legs by bracing.

24. TRUNK EXTENSION

This test is performed in same manner as Trunk Flexion except subject
is in prone lying position with hands clasped behind back.

25. TRUNK LATERAL FLEXION

This test differs from Trunk Flexion in the following ways. (a) Subject in side-lying position; lower arm placed through slit in table and
other arm resting at side; head placed on small pad for comfort. (b)
Prevent lifting hips by bracing; maintain lateral plane of body perpendicular to table; be sure hand through slit remains free.

26. TRUNK ROTATION (Fig. 8)

Starting Position. Subject in supine lying position close to edge of
table; legs straight and together; arms folded on chest.
Attachments. (a) Trunk harness strapped firmly to subject. (b) Pulling assembly snapped to D-ring on side of harness and attached below
subject at side of table.

Precautions. (a) Prevent lifting hips by bracing. (b) Do not permit trunk lateral flexion.

27. Hip Flexion (Fig. 8)

Starting Position. (a) Subject in supine lying position; hip and knee of free leg flexed comfortably with foot resting flat on table; arms folded on chest. (b) Hip and knee of leg being tested fully extended over table slit.

Attachments. (a) Regulation strap around thigh, lower third between hip and knee joints. (b) Pulling assembly attached below leg.

Precautions. (a) Prevent lifting shoulders by bracing. (b) Be sure leg below strap is free of table when lifting.

28. Hip Extension

This test is performed in the same manner as Hip Flexion, except subject is in prone lying position with arms along sides. Prevent lifting of hips by bracing. Be sure leg below strap does not touch table.

29. Hip Abduction (Fig. 8)

Starting Position. (a) Subject in side-lying position; lower knee flexed to permit passage of strap; lower arm extended for head-rest; upper arm resting on side with elbow flexed comfortably. (b) Hip of upper leg on side tested fully extended over table slit.

Attachments. (a) Regulation strap around thigh, lower third between hip and knee joints. (b) Pulling assembly attached beneath subject.

Precautions. (a) Prevent lifting of shoulders and hips by bracing. (b) Maintain lateral plane of body perpendicular to table. (c) Prevent free leg from interfering with strap and movement.

30. Hip Adduction

The position of this test is the same as for Hip Abduction with the following exceptions. (a) Subject in side-lying position with both legs fully extended. (b) Upper leg held in slight abduction by tester to avoid interference with movement and to eliminate necessity for lifting in taking test.

31. Hip Inward Rotation (Fig. 9)

Starting Position. Subject in sitting position at end of table; legs hanging free; padded support under knees; arms folded on chest.

Attachments. (a) Regulation strap around leg just above ankle joint. (b) Pulling assembly attached to wall on side away from limb being tested.

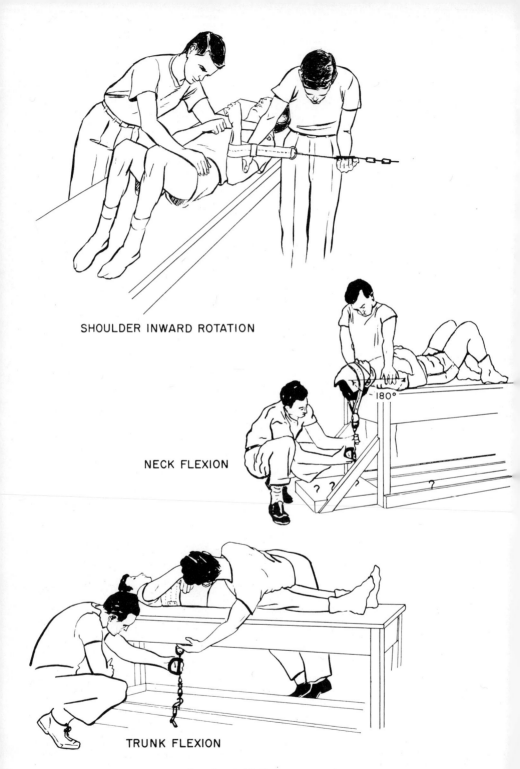

SHOULDER INWARD ROTATION

NECK FLEXION

180°

TRUNK FLEXION

Fig. 8. Cable-Tension Strength Tests.

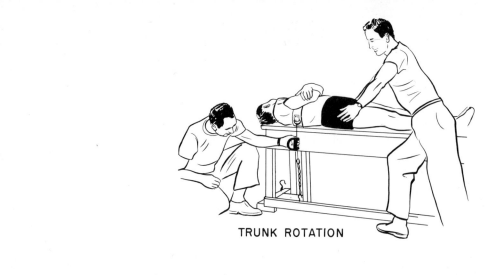

TRUNK ROTATION

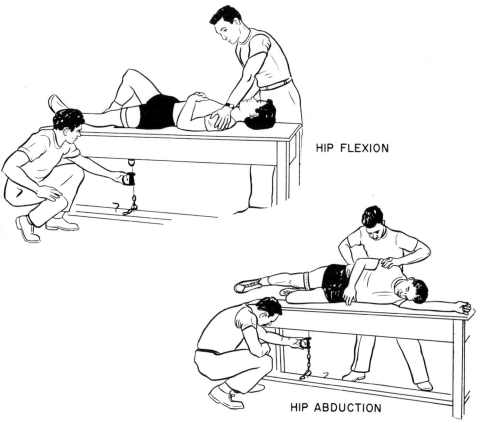

HIP FLEXION

HIP ABDUCTION

Fig. 8 (cont.)

Precautions. (a) Prevent hip adduction and flexion by bracing. (b) Prevent eversion at foot.

32. Hip Outward Rotation

The position of the subject for this test is the same as for Hip Inward Rotation. The pulling assembly, however, is attached to wall next to side being tested.

33. Knee Flexion (Fig. 9)

Starting Position. (a) Subject in prone lying position; patella just at edge of table; head resting on folded arms. (b) Knee on side tested flexed at 165 degrees.

Attachments. (a) Regulation strap around leg midway between knee and ankle joints. (b) Pulling assembly attached to hook below and at lower end of table.

Precautions. Prevent extension of spine by holding chest on table (flexing of hips permissible).

34. Knee Extension (Fig. 9)

Starting Position. (a) Subject in sitting, backward-leaning position; arms extended to rear, hands grasping sides of table. (b) Knee on side tested in 115 degrees extension.

Attachments. (a) Regulation strap around leg midway between knee and ankle joints. (b) Pulling assembly attached to hook at lower end of table.

Precautions. (a) Prevent lifting buttocks. (b) Prevent flexing arms.

35. Ankle Dorsi Flexion (Fig. 9)

Starting Position. (a) Subject in supine lying position with legs fully extended; arms folded on chest. (b) Ankle on side tested in 125 degrees dorsal flexion.

Attachments. (a) Regulation strap around foot above metatarsal-phalangeal joint. (b) Pulling assembly attached to wall at subject's feet.

Precautions. (a) Prevent inversion or eversion of foot. (b) Prevent flexion at metatarsal-phalangeal joint. (c) Prevent flexion at knee by holding leg against table.

36. Ankle Plantar Flexion (Fig. 9)

The position of subject for this test is the same as for Ankle Dorsi Flexion, with the following exceptions. (a) Use stirrup strap for this test. (b) Ankle on side tested is in 90 degrees flexion. (c) The pulling assembly is attached to wall at subject's head. (d) Brace behind shoulders to hold subject in place when pulling. (The results from this test will be improved by constructing shoulder braces to hold subject firmly in position.)

37. FOOT INVERSION (Fig. 9)

Starting Position. (a) Subject in supine lying position; hip and knee of free leg flexed comfortably; arms folded across chest. (b) Leg on side tested fully extended; ankle at 90 degrees dorsi flexion and midposition of inversion and eversion.

Attachments. (a) Regulation strap around ball of foot. (b) Pulling assembly attached to wall at side of limb tested.

Precautions. (a) Prevent movement of knee and hip by bracing. (b) Prevent hip rotation with fist at ankle.

38. FOOT EVERSION

The position for this test is the same as for Foot Inversion. The pulling assembly, however, is attached to wall away from side being tested.

APPLICATIONS

During the formal construction of the cable-tension strength tests, trials of the tests were made by patients with orthopedic disabilities in three hospital situations: U.S. Naval Hospital, Chelsea, Mass.; Veterans Administration Regional Office, New York City; and Bronx Veterans Administration Hospital, New York City.[41] According to medical opinion at these hospitals, the results of these trials corresponded well with opinion of patient status. No complications or sequelae occurred attributable to the testing. The physicians believed that, if such had been the case, it would not mean that the tests were unsuitable but rather that the patients were not ready for heavy exertions.

A number of suggestions were made by the orthopedists for applying these tests to patients, including the following. Where tenderness in the joint area is present, the patient should be instructed not to pull beyond the force he can apply comfortably. If the range of motion in the patient's limb is limited, thus preventing assumption of prescribed joint angles, the tester should make necessary allowances until it improves sufficiently to permit proper positions to be taken; direct comparisons of strength test scores, however, are proper only when like positions are used. Adjustments in position of the pulling strap would also be necessary if the prescribed position is uncomfortable in indi-

---

[41] H. Harrison Clarke, *Manual: Cable-Tension Strength Tests,* pp. 8-10.

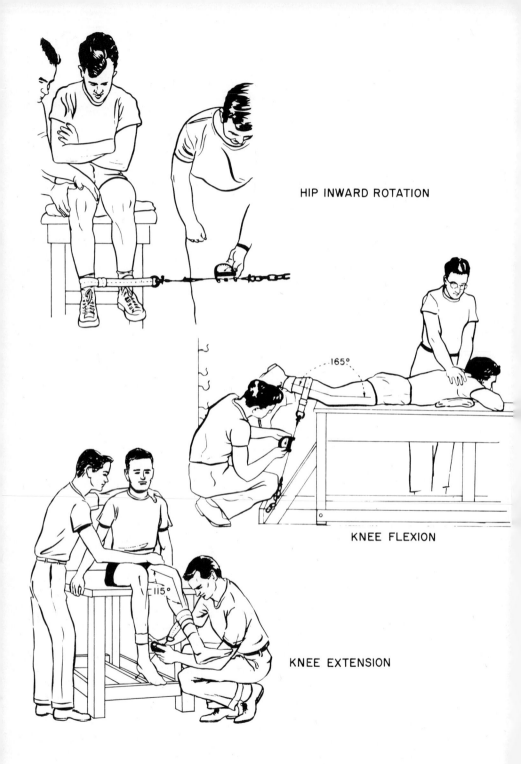

HIP INWARD ROTATION

KNEE FLEXION

165°

KNEE EXTENSION

115°

Fig. 9.   Cable-Tension Strength Tests.

94

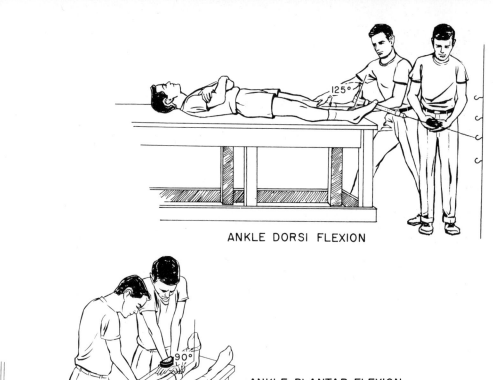

ANKLE DORSI FLEXION

ANKLE PLANTAR FLEXION

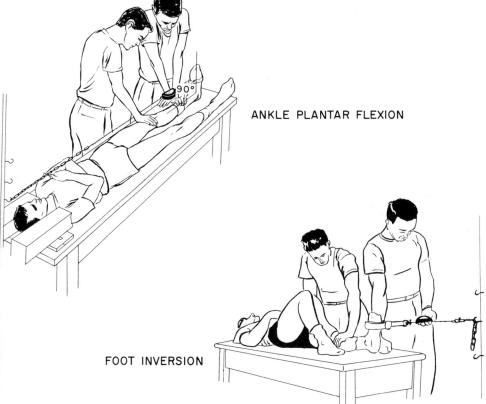

FOOT INVERSION

Fig. 9 (cont.)

vidual cases. And, with patients, of course, strength testing should be done under medical supervision.

For non-pathological conditions, such as faulty posture and body mechanics, the physical educator may apply these tests on his own cognizance.

STRENGTH DECREMENT INDEX

The Strength Decrement Index (SDI)[42] designates the proportionate strength loss of individual muscle groups after exercise. Cable-tension strength tests are given to a particular group of muscles before and immediately after exercise, and the following formula applied:

$$\text{SDI} = \frac{S_b - S_a}{S_b} \times 100$$

in which S_b = Before exercise strength
             S_a = After exercise strength

Studies utilizing the Kelso-Hellebrandt ergograph to fatigue the elbow-flexor muscles revealed a pronounced drop in strength 30 seconds after exhaustive exercise, an initial sharp rise in strength during the next two minutes, and a leveling off with a very gradual rise continuing for some time. The SDI technique has also been used successfully to evaluate the fatigue of muscles involved in carrying packs and in all-out swimming.

The SDI can be used in developmental and adapted physical education to measure the amount of fatigue in exercised muscles. This procedure may be desirable in determining exercise routines for individuals in a convalescent state, upon returning to classes after illnesses, accidents, or operations, and for those with weakened musculatures resulting from various diseases and orthopedic conditions.

FLEXIBILITY AND RANGE OF
JOINT MOVEMENT

Developmental and adapted physical education is concerned with tests of "flexibility" from two points of view—the range of motion in various joints of the body, particularly when related to orthopedic disabilities, and general body flexibility, especially the large central mass of the body involving the trunk and hips. Exercises to increase flexibility in joint movements are indicated when such range of motion is restricted for whatever reason (unless pathologically contraindicated).

---

[42] H. Harrison Clarke, Clayton T. Shay, and Donald K. Mathews, "Strength Decrement Index: A New Test of Muscular Fatigue," *Archives of Physical Medicine and Rehabilitation*, 36, No. 6 (June, 1955), p. 376.

Thus, an instrument to determine the degree of joint movement is needed in the physical educator's kit of measuring devices.

Goniometry, or the use of instruments for measuring the range of motion in joints of the body, has been presented in medical and allied literature since the turn of the century. Moore[43] has published a comprehensive review of this subject. The number of devices proposed have been many; some are quite complicated and impractical while others are simple and easy to apply.

A simple form of the goniometer constructed from a protractor with attached extended arms was previously described. The application of goniometry is simple, as illustrated in Figure 10, in which the range of motion of the knee joint is being tested. The arms of the goniometer are placed parallel to the leg and thigh, with the center of motion at the knee joint. Readings in degrees of a circle are taken with the knee flexed as fully as possible, as in the illustration, and again with full extension; the difference between the two readings represents the range of motion.

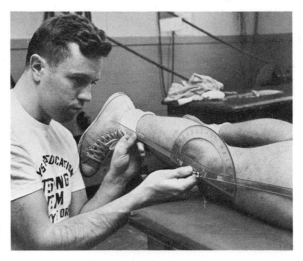

Fig. 10. Use of Goniometer for Testing Range of Motion of Knee Joint.

The Leighton flexometer,[44] illustrated in Figure 11, has also been designed to measure range of joint motion. This instrument is equipped with a rotating flat circular dial, marked off in degrees of a circle, and a moveable pointer; both the dial and the pointer are balanced to always point upward. The flexometer is strapped on the moving part

[43] Margaret L. Moore, "The Measurement of Joint Motion, Part I, Introductory Review of the Literature," *Physical Therapy Review*, 29, No. 5 (1949), p. 1.

[44] Jack R. Leighton, "An Instrument and Technic for the Measurement of Range of Joint Motion," *Archives of Physical Medicine and Rehabilitation*, 36, No. 9 (September, 1955), p. 571.

being tested. The dial is locked in position at one extreme position of the range of motion and the pointer at the other; a direct reading of the pointer on the dial gives the range of motion. Twenty-one range of motion tests have been devised, involving movements of both trunk and extremities. Reliability coefficients for the various tests range from .89 to .997.

Leighton has computed the average range of motion for his tests with the flexometer. These are presented in Table III.

TABLE III
*Leighton's Range of Joint Motion**
(Listed in Degrees)

Location	Joint Movement	Mean Ranges of Joint Motion
Wrist	Flexion-Extension	160-165
Elbow	Flexion-Extension	148-150
Shoulder	Flexion-Extension	243-248
Head	Flexion-Extension	140-141
	Rotation	175-176
Trunk and Hip	Flexion-Extension	172-173
	Sideward Flexion-Extension	103-104
Hip	Flexion-Extension	109-110
Knee	Flexion-Extension	123-124
Ankle	Flexion-Extension	62-63

* Jack R. Leighton, "A Simple Objective and Reliable Measure of Flexibility," *Research Quarterly,* 13, No. 2 (May, 1942), 205.

POSTURE AND BODY MECHANICS

Inasmuch as one of the authors has devoted a chapter in another book primarily to posture measurement, this material will not be duplicated here. The reference is Chapter 8, "Measurement in Remedial Work," *Application of Measurement to Health and Physical Education,* published by Prentice-Hall, Inc. Both subjective posture appraisals and objective posture tests are presented.

SOCIAL, EMOTIONAL, AND PSYCHOLOGICAL ADJUSTMENT

An objective commonly designated in physical education is social efficiency, the development of desirable standards of conduct, and the ability to get along with others. Physical education has typically dealt with social, emotional, and psychological behavior patterns related to sportsmanship, co-operation, leadership, courage, initiative, persever-

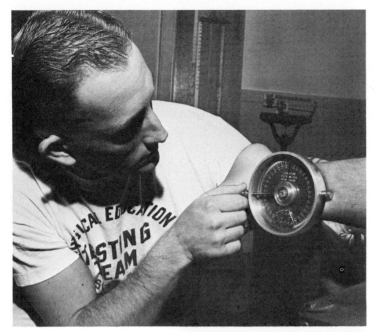

Knee-joint extension.

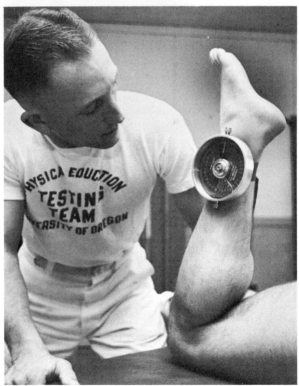

Knee joint flexion.

Fig 11.   The Leighton Flexometer.

99

ance, self-control, loyalty, extroversion and the like. The activities and methods of physical education have also been utilized by physical educators in the treatment of neuropsychiatric conditions, ranging from mild manifestations of "combat fatigue" to the more organic disturbances encountered in mental hospitals.

If physical education is to deal effectively with social, emotional, and personality problems of boys and girls, those with specific needs must be identified. Such identification, as has largely been the case, may be merely the recognition of atypical modes of conduct, such as bullying, "grand standing," "hogging the ball," quarreling, insubordination, cowardice, withdrawing, and the like. However, physical education would be of much greater service to the individual if these personal problems could be systematically discovered—and discovered when such behavior was in an early stage rather than after its culmination in overt misconduct. The utilization of tests, therefore, would be helpful in identifying boys and girls with social, emotional, and psychological problems.

PHYSICAL EDUCATION TESTS

Unfortunately, physical education tests related to personal-social adjustments are meager. Blanchard's Behavior Rating Scale[45] contains 24 trait actions, grouped under the following nine classifications: leadership, positive active qualities, positive mental qualities, self-control, co-operation, social action standards, ethical social qualities, qualities of efficiency, and sociability.

After studying factors which differentiate junior high school boys who tend to participate wholeheartedly in physical education and those who are reticent to so participate, Cowell[46] developed ten pairs of behavior "trends" representing good and poor adjustments. A pupil's social adjustment score is the total of the ratings of three teachers. Cowell has also prepared a "Personal Distance Ballot," which may be used to represent boys' attitudes toward accepting boys; each boy in the group checks on a seven-point scale how near to his family he would like to have each of the others in the group. Percentile scales are available for each of these tests and may be found in the reference and in Clarke's measurement text.

EDUCATIONAL PSYCHOLOGY TESTS

Many tests evaluating various personality traits have been developed in educational psychology. Certain of these are of the inventory type,

---

[45] B. E. Blanchard, "A Behavior Frequency Rating Scale for the Measurement of Character and Personality in Physical Education Classroom Situations," *Research Quarterly*, VII, No. 2 (May, 1936), p. 56.

[46] Charles C. Cowell and Hilda M. Schwehn, *Modern Principles and Methods in High School Physical Education* (Boston: Allyn and Bacon, Inc., 1958), pp. 234-238.

and may be used by the teacher with some training in psychology and an acquaintance with counseling procedures. In utilizing these tests, the physical educator should realize he is not a trained psychologist; therefore, he should understand the importance of referring problems beyond his competence in this area to guidance personnel, in much the same way he refers students needing medical consultation or nutritional guidance. If a guidance department exists in the school, such testing could well be done by this department and programs of developmental and adapted physical education worked out jointly to meet the individual needs of those with atypical social, emotional, and psychological tendencies.

Among the personality tests which may be considered for evaluating phases of social, emotional, and psychological adjustment of students are the following.

Mental Health Analysis.[47] The Mental Health Analysis is divided into two sections of five categories each. Section I is designed to measure the presence of mental health liabilities, using the following categories: behavorial immaturity, emotional instability, feelings of inadequacy, physical defects, and nervous manifestations. Section II is intended to test the presence of mental health assets, with these categories: close personal relationships, inter-personal skills, social participations, satisfying work and recreation, and adequate outlook and goals. The selection of test items in this analysis was made from the literature and researches in the field and from the reactions of students, teachers, principals, and employees.

Washburne Social Adjustment Inventory (Thaspic Edition).[48] This inventory is intended for all ages above the eighth grade, and is designed to determine the student's degree of social and emotional development. The eight traits evaluated are truthfulness, happiness, alienation, sympathy, purpose, impulse-judgment, control, and wishes. Reliability coefficients are satisfactory.

Bell Adjustment Inventory.[49] There are two forms of this test, the *Student Form* for high school and college students and the *Adult Form.* The student inventory provides four separate measures of personal and social adjustment: home, health, social, and emotional; for the adult inventory, occupational adjustment is added. The reliability of this test is satisfactory, equaling .90 for the total score.

SRA Junior and Youth Inventories.[50] Two inventories have been devised, the SRA Junior Inventory, grades 4-8, and the SRA Youth In-

---

[47] Louis P. Thorpe, Willis W. Clark, and Ernest W. Tiegs, *Manual of Directions: Mental Health Analysis* (Los Angeles: California Test Bureau, 1946).

[48] World Book Company, Yonkers-on-Hudson, New York.

[49] Stanford University Press, Stanford, California.

[50] Science Research Associates, 57 West Grand Avenue, Chicago, Illinois.

ventory, grades 7-12. The subjects in both inventories are questioned about their health, getting along with others and their home and family; in addition, the youth inventory has questions related to "boy meets girl," things in general, and looking ahead. The reliability co-efficients are satisfactory in most instances; the intercorrelations of the eight area scores composing the youth inventory are between .20 and .67, with a median of .46. The authors caution that use of scores by themselves to indicate maladjustment is not warranted and that scores on the test merely indicate the relative frequency, not the intensity or severity of problems.

Mooney Problem Check List, 1950 Rev.[51] The Mooney Problem Check List is not a test, but a list of problems encountered by different age groups. The Check List is designed as an aid in counseling—to identify personal problems which may be considered and to help the student in reviewing his own problems. Four forms of the test are available: junior high school, high school, college, and adult. The junior high school form contains 30 items in each of seven problem areas: health and physical development; home and family; money, work, and the future; boy and girl relations; relations to people in general; and self-centered concerns. The high school and college forms are expanded, each including 330 items in eleven problem areas.

Bernreuter Personality Inventory.[52] This inventory is for high school and college students and adults. It consists of 125 questions designed to measure the following personality traits: neurotic tendency, self-sufficiency, introversion-extroversion, and dominance-submission.

Winnetka Scale for Rating School Behavior and Attitudes.[53] One of the most usable instruments for evaluating personality traits of younger children is the Winnetka scale. This tests is designed to rate the following five factors: co-operation, social consciousness, emotional adjustment, leadership, and responsibility. The scale was constructed by analysis of actual incidents occurring in the classroom, the data being classified into situations and response levels, the final scale consisting of 13 situations.

SUMMARY

In this chapter, various tests of value for developmental and adapted physical education have been considered. Included are tests of organic soundness, nutrition, physique types, muscular and circulatory fitness,

---

[51] Psychological Corporation, 522 Fifth Avenue, New York, N. Y.
[52] Stanford University Press, Stanford, California.
[53] Winnetka Educational Press, Winnetka, Illinois.

cable-tension strength, flexibility and range of joint movement, posture and body mechanics, and social, emotional, and psychological adjustment.

SELECTED REFERENCES

Astrand, P. O., "Human Fitness with Special Reference to Sex and Age," *Physiological Reviews*, 36, No. 3 (July, 1956), p. 325.

Bovard, John F., Frederick W. Cozens, and E. Patricia Hagman, *Tests and Measurements in Physical Education*, 3rd ed. Philadelphia: W. B. Saunders Company, 1949.

Clarke, H. Harrison, *Application of Measurement to Health and Physical Education*, 3rd ed. Englewood Cliffs, N. J.: Prentice-Hall, Inc., 1959.

McCloy, C. H., and Norma D. Young, *Tests and Measurements in Health and Physical Education*, 3rd ed. New York: Appleton-Century-Crofts, Inc., 1954.

Mathews, Donald K., *Measurement in Physical Education*. Philadelphia: W. B. Saunders Company, 1958.

Willgoose, Carl E., *Evaluation in Health Education and Physical Education*. New York: McGraw-Hill Book Co., Inc., 1961.

5

Values and Effects of
Physical Activities

F ITNESS FOR LIVING, BE IT IN THE HOME, ON THE FARM, IN the factory, or at the front, implies freedom from disease or significant deviations from normal structure and function; enough strength, speed, agility, endurance, and skill to accomplish the maximum tasks that the day may bring; and mental and emotional adjustments appropriate to the age of the individual. Physical fitness (really physical aspects of fitness) is only a phase of total fitness. The limitations of fitness are determined and modified by inheritance, but within these limitations daily practices may develop and otherwise limit fitness." The statement in which this quotation appears was prepared by the Joint Committee on Health Problems in Education of the National Education Association and the American Medical Association. The full statement indicates the role of exercise in a program seeking greater physical fitness of the American people.[1] The purpose of this chapter is to support the above assertion by showing the value of exercise for total fitness and the effects of exercise upon the organism.

---

[1] National War Fitness Council, *The Role of Exercise in Physical Fitness* (Washington: American Association for Health, Physical Education, and Recreation, 1943).

FITNESS VALUES OF PHYSICAL ACTIVITIES

No doubt exists that the right kind and amount of exercise will develop muscular strength and endurance, body flexibility, and circulatory-respiratory endurance. In fact, properly directed exercise is the only known means for acquiring the ability to engage in tasks demanding sustained physical effort. For this reason, physical education is indispensable in schools and colleges in order to develop strong and enduring bodies.

Physical education has a special responsibility for boys and girls who are below satisfactory levels of physical fitness. Such individuals, although not ordinarily so considered, are, nevertheless, handicapped physically, many seriously so, with accompanying defections of mental power and social adjustment. Thus, physically unfit boys and girls are incapable of prolonged physical effort, are unable readily to learn and apply skills, and are awkward and lacking in poise; at all levels of intelligence, they have greater difficulty in maintaining mental effort and alertness; the sub-fit experience difficulty in day by day personal adjustments with others and in developing active social habits and attitudes.

Extensive studies over a period of years by many investigators in a number of fields have shown the basic relationships of adequate physical fitness and exercise to sound organic functions, to stamina for sustained activity, to proper mental alertness, to good social adjustment; in fact, they have a relationship to almost every desirable phase of mental health, physical well-being, and social efficiency. Very briefly, some evidence of these assertions follows. Other reviews by one of the authors[2] and others[3] have summarized the research pertaining to physical-mental-social relationships. Those mentioned here are representative of the studies found in this area.

Organic soundness. While Kraus coined the phrase earlier, Kraus and Raab[4] extensively developed the concept of hypokinetic disease, defined as the "whole spectrum of inactivity-induced somatic and mental derangements." They developed the thesis that a minimum of physical activity is a prerequisite for healthful living, that lack of it is in part responsible for disease, and that lack of exercise constitutes a cause for a deficiency state comparable to avitaminosis. As in every deficiency

---

[2] H. Harrison Clarke, "Physical Fitness Benefits: A Summary of Research," *Education*, 78, No. 8 (April, 1958), p. 460; *Application of Measurement to Health and Physical Education,* 3rd ed. (Englewood Cliffs, N.J.: Prentice-Hall, Inc., 1959), chap. 3.

[3] "The Contributions of Physical Activity to Human Well-Being," *Research Quarterly*, 31, No. 2, Pt. II (May, 1960).

[4] Hans Kraus and Wilhelm Raab, *Hypokinetic Disease* (Springfield, Ill.: Charles C. Thomas, 1961).

state, its results are most telling on the growing boy and girl. A number of investigations have shown that physically active people are much less prone to such chronic and disabling diseases as coronary heart attacks, duodenal ulcers, and other internal conditions.

After reviewing reports of medical studies published in the United States, Canada, England, Scandinavia, and Austria, Kraus and Raab[5] conclude, ". . . *the overwhelming majority of published reports, based on statistical criteria and techniques, seems to lend strong support to the concept that a relationship between exercise habits and the susceptibility to functional and degenerative diseases of the myocardium does indeed exist.*" In agreement with this observation, Hein and Ryan[6] of the American Medical Association, after evaluating evidence in this area state: "A high level of physical activity throughout life appears to be one of those factors that act to inhibit the vascular degeneration characteristic of coronary heart disease, the most common cause of death among cardiovascular disorders."

Low back pain is much more prevalent in the sedentary than in the physically active. Kraus[7] reported that 80 per cent of his patients with this trouble were unable to pass his test of minimum muscular fitness. Physically active individuals, in general, age more slowly, have better weight control, and maintain a lower blood pressure level.

Mental alertness. A number of researches support the belief that physical fitness is related to mental accomplishments, especially as affecting mental alertness. Thus, it may be contended that a person's general learning potential, *for a given level of intelligence,* is increased or decreased in accordance with his degree of physical fitness. Some studies have shown little or no relationship between physical measures and mental achievement. These investigations, however, have been correlational in nature and have ignored the intelligence of the subjects. By contrast, in the studies showing physical-mental relationships, either the subjects were limited to those who were physically unfit, or subjects with high and low fitness scores were contrasted, or the subjects were equated by intelligence quotients but separated into high and low groups on physical tests. These studies indicate that the individual is more prone to be mentally alert, to be vigorous in his applications, and to suffer less from efficiency-destroying fatigue when he is fit than when he is unfit.

Social adjustment. Among boys, especially, a positive relationship of

---

[5] *Ibid.,* p. 98.

[6] Fred V. Hein and Allan J. Ryan, "The Contributions of Physical Activity to Physical Health," *Research Quarterly,* 31, No. 2, Pt. II (May, 1960), p. 279.

[7] Hans Kraus, *et al., Hypokinetic Disease* (New York: Institute for Physical Medicine and Rehabilitation, New York University-Bellevue Medical Center).

strength to "prestige" traits has been demonstrated. Jones[8] found that boys high in strength tend to be well adjusted socially and psychologically; boys low in strength show a tendency toward social difficulties, feelings of inferiority, and other personal maladjustments. Popp[9] reported that five teachers and administrators generally selected boys with high relative (to age and weight) strength scores as most nearly like sons they would like to have; the reverse was true for boys with low relative strength.

FITNESS STATUS OF U. S. YOUTH

Despite the beliefs and assertions discussed above, too many boys and girls in our schools and colleges show clear indications of inadequate organic power, as reflected in early fatigue under a normal demand of muscular effort and muscular inefficiency reflected in poor motor skills, low strength indices, and lack of endurance. If proof is needed, consider the following summary made from many studies available.

Kraus[10] reported that 57.9 per cent of eastern seaboard school children failed to meet even a minimum standard of muscular fitness. These children were far below similar accomplishments of children in Switzerland, Austria, and Italy, only 8.7 per cent of whom failed to meet this standard. He indicated further that this situation is not being alleviated, since American boys and girls leave their schools in much the same condition as when they enter. High failure rates on this test by American children have also been found by other investigators from many parts of the country. Kraus also produced clinical evidence to show that adult patients with failures on two or more of his simple strength and flexibility tests were prone to lower back pain and manifested constant strain and, frequently, emotional stress. These symptoms disappeared when patients performed prescribed exercises to strengthen the muscles of the abdomen and back and to stretch the muscles of the back and legs.

The AAHPER Youth Fitness Tests have been used to contrast the fitness of American children with their counterparts in other countries.[11] In all instances, the American children were revealed with much lower typical performances on most of the items composing this test battery. For example, the American boys and girls exceeded the means of the

---

[8] Harold E. Jones, *Motor Performance and Growth* (Berkeley: University of California Press, 1949).

[9] James Popp, "Case Studies of Junior and Senior High School Boys with High and Low Physical Fitness Indices," Microcarded Master's thesis, University of Oregon, 1959.

[10] Hans Kraus and Ruth P. Hirschland, "Minimum Muscular Fitness Tests· in School Children," *Research Quarterly*, 25, No. 2 (May, 1954), p. 178.

[11] H. Harrison Clarke, "British, Japanese, Danes Top U.S. Youth," *Physical Fitness News Letter*, University of Oregon, Series VII, No. 5 (January, 1961), p. 1. (This report contains a summary of the three studies involved.)

Japanese only on the test involving abdominal endurance; in the 600-yard run-walk, 98 per cent of the Danish boys and 99 per cent of the Danish girls exceeded the American averages for boys and girls; and British boys on the average for all tests and for all ages were at the 64th percentile for United States performance scores.

Utilizing Rogers' Physical Fitness Index, Clarke[12] reported that male students entering the University of Oregon with four years of high school physical education had a considerably higher average than did those with two years or less. Typically, large numbers of students enter college with low Physical Fitness Indices, not only in Oregon, but generally throughout the country. Whittle[13] found that 12-year-old boys in elementary schools with good physical education programs had much higher scores on fitness and motor ability tests than did boys of the same age who had little or no physical education.

After administering physical fitness tests, Karpovich and Weiss[14] concluded that personnel entered the Army Air Forces during World War II in fairly poor physical condition. Despite relatively high acceptance standards, these men were deficient in running speed, endurance of the abdominal muscles, and arm and shoulder strength. Other branches of the armed forces had and continue to have similar experiences.

Cureton[15] studied the fitness of 1000 young men upon entrance to the University of Illinois shortly before World War II with these negative results: 64 per cent could not swim 50 yards, 26 per cent could not chin four times, and 24 per cent could not jump an obstacle waist high. Similar results were obtained one year later with a larger sample of 3099 Illinois freshmen.

PHYSIOLOGICAL EFFECTS OF EXERCISE: MUSCULAR STRENGTH AND ENDURANCE

Brains without muscles would not get animals very far or the human body out of an armchair. The capacity to move is a dominant factor in biology. In order to understand and to evaluate the effects of movement and exercise, *per se,* upon the human organism, a knowledge of the related physiological processes is needed. The proper selection of the types of exercise to achieve physical fitness results should be based upon the insight which this knowledge should provide. Consequently,

---

[12] H. Harrison Clarke, "Physical Fitness of University of Oregon Male Freshmen," *Physical Fitness News Letter,* University of Oregon, Series II, No. 4 (March, 1955).

[13] H. Douglas Whittle, "Effects of Elementary School Physical Education upon Some Aspects of Physical, Motor, and Personality Development," Microcarded Doctor's dissertation, University of Oregon, 1956.

[14] Peter V. Karpovich and Raymond A. Weiss, "Physical Fitness of Men Entering the Armed Forces," *Research Quarterly,* 17, No. 3 (October, 1946), p. 184.

[15] Thomas K. Cureton, "The Unfitness of Young Men in Motor Fitness," *Journal of the American Medical Association,* 123 (September 11, 1943), p. 69.

a brief discussion of the physiology of exercise is presented. The physiology of muscular strength and endurance will be considered in this section; and the physiology of circulatory-respiratory endurance, in the section immediately following.

MUSCLE FIBERS

The process of developing muscular strength through exercise is physiological; muscle fibers cannot reproduce, although they can increase in size. This growth is due to a number of factors, which include toughening and thickening of the sarcolemma (wall) of the muscle fiber, increasing the amount of connective tissue within the muscle, enlarging individual muscle fibers, and increasing circulatory and respiratory activities during repeated contractions. Individual muscle fibers do hypertrophy as a result of certain types of exercise. Furthermore, latent and normally unused fibers and fibers that are small from lack of use are developed in response to demands made upon them.

Increase in a muscle's size is related to the amount of work it performs. Seibert[16] exercised rats on a treadmill at various speeds and found that those running at higher speeds developed larger muscles. The muscles reached an optimum size for a given speed and remained at this level no matter how long the speed was continued; the size enlarged further when the speed was definitely increased.

The gain in the endurance of a muscle as a result of exercise, however, is out of all proportion to its gain in size. Therefore, the quality of contractions must be improved through such factors as the following: fuel is made more available and in greater amount; oxygen is more abundant, owing to improved circulation of the blood through the muscle; and better co-ordination of the individual muscle fibers and more complete use of all fibers are realized. Systematic exercise facilitates the transmission of nerve impulses across motor end-plates, which, in turn, leads to a more complete use of all muscle fibers. Also, improved co-ordination of agonists and antagonists and of the timing of impulses which reach the individual muscles are significant contributors to the amount of strength and power that is possible.[17]

The condition of muscles is reflected somewhat by their tone, a muscle condition manifested by a quality of firmness, which may be noted by palpation when the muscle is at rest. Muscle tone results partly from sustained contractions when the muscles are at rest. Such action is reflex in nature with the sensory stimulation provided by the proprioceptors located in the muscles and by the tendinous attachments to

---

16 Reported by Arthur H. Steinhaus, "Physiology at the Service of the Physical Educator," *Journal of Health and Physical Education*, 3, No. 6 (June, 1932), p. 36.
17 Charles R. Brassfield, "Some Physiological Aspects of Physical Fitness," *Research Quarterly*, 14, No. 1 (March, 1943), p. 106.

bones. From a review of electromyographic studies, Ralston and Libet [18] stressed that no action potential is obtained when a muscle is completely relaxed. As a consequence, factors other than contractile fibers must account for muscle tone, in part at least. After reviewing research on this subject, Pantin [19] proposed that muscle tone might conceivably be due to connective tissue as well. At any rate, the stretch reflex is a fundamental factor in muscle tone and is usually well developed in the antigravity (extensor) muscles; and it is mainly responsible for maintenance of body posture.

CONNECTIVE TISSUE

Ingelmark [20] reported the following changes in fibrous, cartilaginous, and osseous tissues. Functional strain on connective tissue increases the thickness of ligaments, tendons, and other connective tissue in muscles; the hypertrophy of a tendon under training conditions is as great as that of its muscle. The hyaline cartilage, which covers the articulating surfaces of bones in joints, shows similar changes in training. Conversely, the thickness of joint cartilage reduces very rapidly when joints are immobilized. These rapid changes appear to be due to changes in the fluid content of cartilage. The functional adaptation of cartilage brought on by exercise is confined to those parts of the surface which are normally load bearing; other parts are much less capable of such adaptation, probably because their nutrition is poorer. Normal cartilage surfaces are always rough and scratched and the synovial fluid contains particles abraded from the cartilage. The amount of abraded particles in exercised joints varies with the kind and degree of exercise. Bones show marked changes in the amounts of calcium phosphate and calcium carbonate as related to the degree of training.

Steinhaus [21] suggests several applications of Ingelmark's findings to conditioning situations. The rapid functional adaptation of the cartilage to exercise has the same value as the long term training effects and may be a hitherto unrecognized reason for "warming up" before strenuous athletic participation. The presence of abraded cartilaginous substance in the synovial fluid may support the inference that long-continued pounding in joints, as experienced in boxers' elbows and the knees of football players, could cause permanent damage to cartilage.

---

[18] H. J. Ralston and B. Libet, "The Question of Tonus in Skeletal Muscle," *American Journal of Physical Medicine*, 32, No.2 (April, 1953), 85.

[19] C. F. A. Pantin, "Comparative Physiology of Muscle," *British Medical Bulletin*, 12, No. 3 (1956), p. 199.

[20] B. E. Ingelmark, "Morpho-Physiological Aspects of Gymnastic Exercises," *FIEP Bulletin*, 27 (1957), p. 37.

[21] Arthur H. Steinhaus, "Some Effects of Exercise on the Locomotor Apparatus," *Contributions No. 6, American Academy of Physical Education* (Washington: American Association for Health, Physical Education, and Recreation, 1958), p. 74.

CAPILLARIES

Either new blood capillaries or the opening of unused ones result from the continued use of muscles. Upon comparing one side of the body with the corresponding inactive muscle on the other side, Krogh[22] found that the number of capillaries in the active muscle ranged from 40 to 100 times the number in the inactive muscle. An increase of 45 per cent in the number of capillaries in guinea pig muscles during exercise was obtained as compared with no capillary increase in those muscles not exercised. This increase in capillarization provides a more generous circulation of blood to the muscles, resulting in a better supply of fuel and oxygen and the more effective removal of waste substances.[23] Maison and Broeker[24] demonstrated that the endurance of muscles with adequate blood supply increased more rapidly and reached a higher level than those without an adequate supply.

MUSCLE HEMOGLOBIN

There are two types of skeletal muscles, known in general by their color, red and pale. The color of muscle is dependent upon the amount of hemoglobin present. The red muscles control more muscle hemoglobin, which has the property of combining with oxygen more rapidly than does blood hemoglobin. Thus, these are the muscles located where long continued contractions are required. The pale muscles, which are rapid-acting, contain high concentrates of cytochome oxidase, which are primarily concerned with the activation of molecular oxygen and its utilization in oxidative processes. It is believed that flabby muscles become pale because of the rapid loss of myohemoglobin.[25] Whipple[26] found two to three times as much hemoglobin in the muscles of active dogs than in inactive ones. A consequence of exercise, therefore, is to maintain and improve the amount of this compound in the muscles.

CHEMICAL ACTIONS

It has generally been thought that lactic acid production from glycogen was a fundamental chemical process in providing energy for

---

[22] Reported by Philip J. Rasch and Richard V. Freeman, "The Physiology of Progressive Resistance Exercise: A Resume," *Journal of the Association for Physical and Mental Rehabilitation*, 8, No. 2 (March-April 1954), p. 35.

[23] Khalil G. Wakim, "The Physiological Aspects of Therapeutic Exercise," *Journal of the American Medical Association*, 142 (January 14, 1950), p. 100.

[24] G. L. Maison and A. G. Broeker, "Training in Human Muscles Working With and Without Blood Supply," *American Journal of Physiology*, 132 (March, 1941), p. 404.

[25] Earl C. Elkins and Khalil G. Wakim, "The Physiological Basis for Therapeutic Exercise," *Archives of Physical Medicine*, XXVIII, No. 9 (September, 1947), p. 555.

[26] G. H. Whipple, "The Hemoglobin of Striated Muscle," *American Journal of Physiology*, 76 (May, 1926), p. 693.

muscular contraction. Lactic acid accumulates in the absence of oxygen. Thus, at the beginning of exercise, some lactic acid may be deposited in the muscles due to the circulatory-respiratory lag, but is removed when the oxygen supply becomes adequate to meet the energy requirements of the activity. During fatigue states, lactic acid is again produced and becomes a limiting factor in the ability of the organism to sustain exercise. Severe fatigue results when the amount of lactic acid reaches about 0.3 per cent. After exercise, the accumulation of oxygen debt permits continued removal of lactate and the refilling of oxygen stores. Lactic acid is rapidly diffusible and is uniformly distributed throughout the body, so that concentration of lactic acid in the blood is proportional to the amount of lactic acid in the body at a given time.

Based on Szent-Gyorgyi's theory of muscle contraction,[27] Henry[28] has described the process of muscle shortening, as follows. When the muscles are in their resting state, the actomyosin-ATP complex is in delicate balance; this is a high-energy state that contains its own potential energy for reaction. Actin globules are held together in the form of fibrous F-actin by the presence of ATP molecules. In the resting state, the balance between myosin-ATP and F-actin is very delicate. By means of a slight change in ionic concentration caused by the nerve impulse, probably involving the release of potassium, the balance is upset and the filaments come together. With this union, an electric charge, dehydration, and folding up of the fibers occur, which consists of the contraction. As a result of the contraction, F-actin breaks up the globular G-actin, which separates from myosin. The myosin enzymatically splits ATP, releasing its Nph which furnishes the energy required to dissociate the actomyosin-ATP complex. Once dissociated, the G-actin molecules spontaneously unite to again form the fibrous F-actin. Myocine attaches to a new molecule of ATP, hydrates, and stretches out again to line up close to, but separate from, the F-actin fibers in the actomyosin-ATP complex.

In summarizing this research, Henry[29] indicated that oxygen does not participate directly in energy release; the only function of oxygen, whether at rest, during exercise, or during recovery from exercise is to remove and convert into water the hydrogen atom that the enzymes have abstracted from foodstuffs. The energy for muscular work comes from the enzymatic removal of oxygen from the food. All levels of muscular work necessarily produce oxygen debt, since the continuation of energy production and physical activity would be impossible if oxygen

---

[27] A. Szent-Gyorgyi, "Attacks on Muscle," *Science*, 110, No. 2860 (October 21, 1949), p. 411.

[28] Franklin M. Henry, *Physiology of Work: The Physiological Basis of Muscular Exercise* (Berkeley: Associated Students' Store, University of California, 1950), p. 30.

[29] Franklin M. Henry, "Recent Research in Exercise Physiology," undated mimeographed paper.

did not dispose of the hydrogen molecules. Pyruvic acid assists oxygen in removing hydrogen from the energy-releasing enzymes, being converted into lactic acid as it does so.

Chemically, both the phosphocreatine content and the amount of glycogen in the muscles definitely increases as a result of training; the quantity of non-nitrogenous substances is also increased. The color of the trained muscle, as indicated before, is darker than that of the untrained muscle, indicating a more favorable state for the transport and utilization of oxygen. Inasmuch as phosphocreatine may be directly resynthesized without lactic acid accumulation, it is probable that the highly perfected oxygen transport of the trained individual provides the conditions necessary for more of this direct resynthesis, thus reducing the need for the indirect process involving the formation of lactic acid. The finding of an increased glycogen content in an intermediate state of training and its subsequent disappearance in highly trained dogs lends support to this hypothesis.

MUSCLE FATIGUE

When fatigued, the ability of the muscle to contract is greatly reduced. The site of this fatigue has been variously proposed as being in the synapses of the central nervous system, in the motor end-plate, and in the muscle itself. Evidence cited to refute the muscle as the site purports to show that fatigued muscles will continue to contract when stimulated by electrical charges. Merton,[30] however, demonstrated that a muscle does not contract by electrical stimulation after it has become actually fatigued by voluntary effort. Experimenting with the thumb adductor of the hand, voluntary strength was compared with maximal tetani and the two were found to be equal. When strength failed, electrical stimulation of the motor nerve did not restore it, thus suggesting that fatigue is peripheral. To further substantiate this position, action potentials evoked by nerve stimulation were not significantly reduced even in extreme fatigue; and recovery from fatigue did not take place if circulation to the muscle was arrested.

Loss of strength application is a common phenomenon of muscle fatigue, but recovery rate is not so well understood. Clarke and associates[31] isotonicly exercised the elbow flexor muscles to a point where voluntary movement was not manifested, utilizing the Kelso-Hellebrandt ergograph with a load equal to three-eighths the strength of each subject's exercised muscles. The loss in strength 30 seconds after

[30] P. A. Merton, "Voluntary Strength and Fatigue," Journal of Physiology, 123, No. 3 (1954), p. 553.

[31] H. Harrison Clarke, Clayton T. Shay, and Donald K. Mathews, "Strength Decrements of Elbow Flexor Muscles Following Exhaustive Exercise," Archives of Physical Medicine and Rehabilitation, 35, No. 9 (September, 1954), p. 560.

exercise was approximately one-third; a rapid gain in strength occurred, to about one-half the loss, during the next twelve minutes. Strength recovery was still not complete for most subjects two hours after the cessation of exercise. In a study by D. H. Clarke,[32] strength decrements of equal amounts were obtained immediately following prescribed isotonic and isometric exercises.

Training increases the endurance, or retards the fatigue of muscles. Training also improves their strength recovery rate after exhaustive efforts. In the ergograph study mentioned above, the recovery of trained muscles was much faster than that of untrained muscles. Furthermore, the strength recovery of trained muscles was quicker when the subjects moved about, thus increasing general body circulation, than when they were required to lie quietly during the recovery period.

MUSCULAR STRENGTH-ENDURANCE RELATIONSHIPS

The absolute strength of a set of muscles does not necessarily indicate the degree of their endurance, or resistance to fatigue. The following eight relationships between these two factors are proposed by Clarke,[33] largely supported from his own research. (1) The amount of resistance required to induce muscular exhaustion in a relatively short time varies among individuals, depending on the strength of the muscles primarily involved. (2) The work output of muscles in exhaustion performances is greater when they are in position to apply greatest tension at the point of greatest stress. (3) The speed of muscular contraction affects muscular endurance performance; there appears to be a specific combination of load and cadence which produces maximal work output of each muscle group. (4) Individuals with greatest muscular strength have greatest absolute endurance; however, stronger muscles tend to maintain a smaller proportion of maximum strength than do weaker muscles. (5) An immediate effect of fatiguing muscles is to reduce their ability to apply tension; the amount of this decrement is an indicator of the degree of muscular fatigue. (6) Strength recovery rates resulting from muscular fatigue are increased by muscular condition and by general body movement following exercise. (7) Muscular fatigue patterns from total-body activity can be revealed by the strength decrements of individual muscle groups. (8) The strength decrement of all involved muscle groups may be used to determine total-body muscular fatigue resulting from strenuous activity, and may serve as a criterion for evaluating the muscular fatigue effects of such activity on the body as a whole.

---

[32] David H. Clarke. "Strength Recovery from Static and Dynamic Muscular Fatigue," *Research Quarterly,* 33, No. 3 (October, 1962), p. 349.

[33] H. Harrison Clarke, "Muscular Strength-Endurance Relationships," *Archives of Physical Medicine and Rehabilitation,* 38, No. 9 (September, 1957), p. 584.

MUSCLE SKILL

Volitional contractions are involved in the development of motor skills. In the initial phases, before real skill is attained, greater attention is devoted to the component movements in a skilled act. The motor apparatus controls these, although visual and proprioceptive mechanisms aid in the necessary adjustments of strength and the extent of movements. With practice, the proper sequence of the various components of skilled movements are learned and complete attention is no longer as necessary. Finally, the act may be performed entirely by proprioceptive guidance. The elements that contribute to neuromuscular skill are principally strength, power, speed, agility, accuracy, form, rhythm, and balance.

Where heavy muscular work is involved, the condition of the muscles as reflected in their fatigue is obviously a factor in neuromuscular skill. Whether failure of the muscles involved has much to do with fatigue observed in light but highly skilled tasks is not clear. However, Merton[34] reported that handwriting may be continued without difficulty for one minute 30 seconds with circulation to the writing arm occluded; in the following 30 seconds, it was extremely hard to write at all. In another experiment, the subject wrote for two minutes with free circulation, after which it was arrested; whether he continued writing at once or took a two-minute rest first, he was able to continue for only 30 seconds without severe difficulty. Very similar results were obtained with an expert violinist and with a pianist.

Royce[35] verified these findings in part when studying fatigue curves for the forearm muscles during sustained isometric contraction. He found no difference between the curves obtained with or without artificial occlusion of the circulation down to a point where the exerted force became less than approximately 60 per cent of the maximum strength. Below this critical level, the amount of exerted force continued to diminish under the occluded condition, but leveled off when there was no occlusion.

Clarke[36] examined the rate and pattern of muscular fatigue and recovery from both isometric and isotonic exercises. The isotonic exercise consisted of maximum grip and release once every two seconds for six minutes; the isometric exercise consisted of maintaining a single maximum effort for two minutes. The rate of recovery was much faster following static fatigue, although the two recovery curves were nearly identical 250 seconds after the cessation of exercise and thereafter. The investiga-

---

[34] P. A. Merton, "Problems of Muscular Fatigue," *British Medical Bulletin,* 12, No. 3 (1956), p. 219.

[35] Joseph Royce, "Isometric Fatigue Curves in Human Muscle with Normal and Occluded Circulation," *Research Quarterly,* 29, No. 2 (May, 1958), p. 204.

[36] David H. Clarke, *op. cit.*

tor suggested that the difference in recovery curves may be due to (a) the work being carried on over a longer period of time by the isotonic group, thus slowing its recovery rate, and (b) the sudden release of circulation which had been occluded by the static fatiguing exercise of the isometric group, thus hastening its recovery.

Merton concluded from such studies that muscular fatigue is likely to cause a sudden breakdown in performance when work approaches reserve limits. This will not always be the case because of the excellence of the muscle's proprioceptive servo-control, which compensates automatically for fatigue. It is difficult to know at present, however, which tasks strain the reserves of the muscles they use, for, until the reserves are gone, there is little or no subjective sense of fatigue.

CIRCULATORY-RESPIRATORY ENDURANCE

Contrasted with muscular endurance, which is the lasting power of a single muscle or group of muscles, circulatory-respiratory endurance involves the continued activity of the entire organism, during which major adjustments of the circulatory and respiratory systems are necessary, as in running, swimming, climbing, and the like. "Perfect endurance" may be defined as the ability to maintain top speed of movement indefinitely. Obviously, this is impossible of attainment. Instead, maximum efforts can be maintained only for brief periods at best. Thus, most athletes cannot run 15 seconds at capacity speed. Lesser efforts can be sustained longer. Moderate activity for some and mild activity for many can be long continued. The physiological factors involved in such endurance are considered below.

RESPIRATORY FACTORS

Chest expansion is enlarged as a result of exercise; the rate of breathing is reduced and its depth is increased. Large areas of the lungs are seldom utilized in the respiratory function of sedentary individuals, but with training the entire volume is most readily reached. Thus, the blood is exposed to oxygen over a much greater lung surface. The trained individual breathes less air and absorbs a greater proportion of oxygen than does the untrained individual in the same accomplishment. The increased aeration of the lungs makes this possible.

An adequate supply of oxygen is a fundamental requirement for maintaining the activity of any cell in the body. The resting body consumes approximately 250 cc. of oxygen per minute. This amount may increase 1600 per cent (four liters per minute) when the individual is engaged in continued vigorous exercise. In championship performances, the oxygen consumption has reached 5000 cc. per minute and more. When work demands continuous effort over a considerable period of time, the individual works comfortably as long as he maintains an approximate equilibrium between the oxygen required by the muscles and that which is absorbed. Bannister[37] reported the performance of four subjects on a severe standard exercise on a treadmill while breathing controlled mixtures of air and oxygen. In atmospheric air, exhaustion forced the subjects to stop exercising after eight minutes. When breathing 33 per cent oxygen, their performance was much improved; while, with 66 per cent oxygen, they could continue running for a greatly increased length of time.

The percentage of carbon dioxide in expired air for a work period was employed by Briggs[38] to determine the amount of work which constitutes the *crest-load*. With exertions of increasing magnitude, the percentage of expired carbon dioxide rises at first and then falls. So long as this percentage rises proportionately with each added increment of work the loads are considered normal; when the percentage does not rise proportionately, or begins to decrease, an overload has been reached. The crest-load is that load for which the percentage of exhaled carbon dioxide is the largest.

Oxygen debt is the amount of oxygen taken during recovery from physical exertion which is in excess of resting oxygen consumption. This excess is necessarily accompanied by a greater circulation rate, in order that oxygen may be transported from the lungs and distributed to the muscles. The length of the recovery period depends on the duration and severity of the exercise and on the physical condition of the individual. Because of this phenomenon, the rate of recovery of the heart rate after exercise has been proposed as a measure of the individual's fitness.

With a "normal" load of exercise, the oxygen supply is adequate to meet the needs of the muscles, while with an overload, it is inadequate. Schneider[39] defined a crest load as one in which the oxygen-supplying mechanism, working at full speed, is just able to supply the oxygen needs and thus maintain an even balance between the call and use of oxygen. The body, however, can incur an oxygen debt during a short period of violent exertion by postponing the oxygen intake equivalent to the excess work until the period of recovery from exercise.

DeMoor[40] reported that when speed of movement is kept constant, an increase in work load causes a reduction in mechanical efficiency, probably due to a larger proportion of lactate debt present in the total oxygen

---

[37] R. G. Bannister, "The Control of Breathing during Exercise," *FIEP Bulletin*, 2 (1954), p. 47.

[38] Edward C. Schneider, "A Respiratory Study of the Influence of a Moderate Amount of Physical Training," *Research Quarterly*, 1, No. 1 (March, 1930), p. 1.

[39] *Ibid.*

[40] Janice C. DeMoor, "Individual Differences in Oxygen Debt Curves Related to Mechanical Efficiency and Sex," *Journal of Applied Physiology*, 6, No. 8 (February, 1954), p. 460.

debt caused by the heavier work load. Similar conclusions have been reached by other investigators. Henry[41] demonstrated by an empirical analysis that the lactate component is responsible in large measure for the increasing loss in efficiency as running speed is increased. Thus, the question is posed as to whether or not individual differences in mechanical efficiency are related to individual differences in relative amount of inefficient lactate in total oxygen cost.

CIRCULATORY FACTORS

Certain forms of sport, particularly those in which endurance running occurs, lead to physiological cardiac hypertrophy; this makes the heart more efficient in performing its task. Such hearts are not pathological and are not injured by strenuous exercise, unless first damaged by infection or other disease entities. Hypertrophy of the heart from exercise tends to regress with the cessation of training.

The heart rates of trained athletes are 10, 20, or even 30 beats slower per minute than the heart rates of sedentary individuals. An effect of training is to reduce the resting pulse rate. A fundamental difference between conditioned and unconditioned persons is that the conditioned heart pumps more blood per minute with fewer strokes than does the unconditioned heart. The heart muscle undergoes changes similar to those of skeletal muscle. Thus, capillaries in the heart muscle increase in number; greater vascularization takes place; intracellular hemin increases and provides for improved carriage and storage of oxygen. The increase in respiratory products insures protection against oxygen deficiency during exercise.

Blood pressure is the result of the interaction of heart rate, stroke volume, arterial elasticity, and vascular resistance. An adequate response of the circulation to exercise is associated with a considerable increase in heart rate and in arterial blood pressure. The resting systolic pressure in normal individuals ranges from 110 to 135 mm. Hg.; the range for diastolic pressure, 60 to 90 mm. Hg.; for pulse pressure, 30 to 35 mm. Hg. The increase in systolic pressure is greater for static muscular contractions, as in lifting weights, than for running activities.[42] No appreciable difference has been found in the resting blood pressure measurements of conditioned and unconditioned individuals. However, training does diminish the height to which blood pressure rises as a result of a given performance; the recovery rate after exercise is also shortened.

In order to transport four liters of oxygen from the lungs to the

---

41 Franklin M. Henry, "Influence of Athletic Training on the Resting Cardiovascular System," *Research Quarterly*, 25, No. 1 (March, 1954), p. 28.

42 Peter V. Karpovich, *Physiology of Muscular Activity*, 5th ed. (Philadelphia: W. B. Saunders Company, 1959), p. 219.

muscles, 34 liters of blood are required; inasmuch as the volume of blood in the body is approximately five liters, the blood must circulate seven times a minute in order to meet this requirement. Severe exercise involves an enormous output of the heart, so any impairment in cardiac function is revealed by the inability of the subject to tolerate exercise of such severity. If the circulatory response to the demands of the muscles for oxygen during muscular exertion fails, the blood will be severely deoxygenated and cyanosis can develop.[43]

The blood vessels to the viscera are constricted and those of the exercising muscles are dilated, at least at the beginning of exercise. This factor, combined with the effects of increased blood pressure and greater minute volume of blood pumped from the heart, results in practically no change in the quantity of blood going to the viscera, but permits a much greater quantity to go to active muscles.[44]

Red blood corpuscles are developed in the bone marrow. Before leaving the marrow, each cell loses its nucleus and, as a dead cell, enters the circulation. The red blood cell serves primarily as a carrier of oxygen, but of almost equal importance are its abilities to carry carbon dioxide and to serve as a buffer against acids and alkalies. The number of these cells and the percentage of hemoglobin in each unit of blood are increased by exercise training. Thus, the functioning of the bone marrow in the production of red corpuscles is facilitated by exercise. Destroyed red blood cells are quickly replaced in the trained person as a consequence of strenuous exercise. Just as a disused muscle becomes weakened and atrophied, so presumably may bone marrow lessen its functional capacity when not working constantly to replace worn out cells. In the sedentary person, some anemia may result following prolonged strenuous muscular effort.[45]

Muscular exercise also effects the morphological composition of the blood, which includes definite changes in white blood corpuscles. A lymphocytic phase is characterized by an increase in lymphocytes up to 55 per cent, appearing after exercise of short duration. A neutrophilic phase is distinguished by an increase in neutrophils, sometimes as much as 78 per cent; this may develop during exercise requiring a considerable amount of energy. Regenerative intoxication is a higher degree of the neutrophilic phase, during which neutrophites rise to 90 per cent with lymphocytes dropping to 5 per cent; this type may develop during exercise of great duration, as in marathon running. In this latter condition, a marked drop in the total number of white blood corpuscles also occurs; it resembles the blood picture in some serious diseases where prognosis is unfavorable. The degenerative type is most apt to develop

---

[43] Wakim, *op. cit.*
[44] Elkins and Wakim, *op. cit.*
[45] Wakim, *op. cit.*

after strenuous exercise undertaken by persons in poor physical condition.[46]

Karpovich[47] studied the effect of basketball, wrestling, and swimming upon the white blood corpuscles. Basketball games of eight to 20 minutes produced a neutrophilic reaction and monocytes were usually increased. Short periods of wrestling resulted in the lymphocytic phase; long periods produced the neutrophilic phase. Swimming from 60 to 220 yards caused a lymphocytic phase with a tendency toward neutrophily; longer distances gave a markedly neutrophilic reaction. The increase in the number of white blood cells is largely due to a redistribution of the blood and release of the corpuscles from their "storage" places in the body. Also, exercise probably stimulates the release of the younger forms by the red bone marrow. Anderson[48] reported a tendency for the amounts of leucocytes, lymphocytes, and monocytes to increase concomitantly with increased running time. A peak in leucocytosis was reached 15 minutes after termination of the run; the return to preexercise level was reached in 30 to 60 seconds.

METABOLISM

Basal metabolism is the amount of energy expended by the body at rest. It is quite constant in the same person from day to day, but may vary over longer periods with varying conditions of life. While the heat production of the body is the measure of metabolism, actually the metabolic rate is calculated from oxygen consumed and carbon dioxide expired.

Two metabolic phases occur during exertion, an initial rise and a steady state. The initial rise is delayed a bit to permit the circulatory-respiratory adjustment at the beginning of exercise. Normally, oxygen is not used in the initial process of muscular contraction (anaerobic process); the energy requirements are met by adenosine triphosphate and phosphocreatine. However, glycosis and ovidation accelerate rapidly to meet the energy demands of the exercise. In the steady state, equilibrium is established between the processes of breakdown and recovery, when the oxygen intake meets the needs of the muscles (aerobic process). When exercise is sufficiently severe, the equilibrium cannot be maintained, as lactic acid and other waste products accumulate beyond the power of the blood to remove them.

The oxygen consumption and carbon dioxide recovery curves are exponential—an initial rapid component lasting a few minutes and a

---

[46] Peter V. Karpovich, "The Effect of Basketball, Wrestling, and Swimming upon the White Blood Corpuscles," *Supplement to the Research Quarterly*, 6, No. 2 (May, 1935), p. 42.

[47] *Ibid.* p. 42.

[48] Lange K. Anderson, "Leucocyte Response to Brief Severe Exercise," *Journal of Applied Physiology*, 7, No. 6 (1955), p. 671.

longer component with its length depending upon the exercise intensity and the physical condition of the individual. Berg[49] found that the rate of payment of the oxygen debt is more rapid than the elimination of the corresponding carbon dioxide excess. The oxygen and carbon dioxide constants, however, are not independently variable, as the correlation obtained between them was .84. In any age group, the more physically fit persons tended to have longer lower recovery constants; in addition, the vigorous training of one subject brought about a 16 per cent reduction in oxygen and carbon dioxide constants.

BODY TEMPERATURE

The resting muscle under constant conditions liberates heat at a constant temperature. The temperature is substantially increased by keeping a muscle under tension. During shortening, a muscle does mechanical work, according to the load lifted; in addition, heat is given out. Heat is produced in the contraction, not in the relaxation, of the muscle. The rate of heat production depends on the natural speed of the muscle. A rapid muscle produces a large amount and a slow muscle produces a small amount of heat. The slowest muscles can maintain contraction for a long time with little expenditure of energy; the faster ones fatigue very quickly.

Inasmuch as the mechanical efficiency of a muscle (considering the whole cycle of contraction and recovery) is only about 25 per cent, a relatively small amount of the chemical energy from oxidation is effectively applied to exercise. The balance is converted into heat, most of which is lost from the skin and lungs. The heat remaining in the body raises its temperature. Some of the factors which determine the magnitude of this rise are severity of exercise, clothing worn, amount of adipose tissue on the body, humidity of the atmosphere, and the like. This increase in temperature from exercise speeds metabolic and other bodily processes.[50]

BLOOD VISCOSITY

The viscosity (specific gravity) of the blood varies from 1.041 to 1.067, with an average for males of 1.055, according to early studies by McCurdy and McKenzie.[51] Benson[52] found that adults with known dis-

---

[49] W. E. Berg, "Individual Differences in Respiratory Gas Exchange during Recovery from Moderate Exercise," *American Journal of Physiology,* 149, No. 3 (1947), p. 597.

[50] A. V. Hill, "The Thermodynamics of Muscle," *British Medical Journal,* 12, No. 3 (1956), p. 174.

[51] James H. McCurdy and R. Tait McKenzie, *The Physiology of Exercise,* 2nd ed. (Philadelphia: Lea & Febiger, 1928).

[52] Louis Benson, "Plasma Viscosity," *Journal of Laboratory and Clinical Medicine,* 35, (May, 1950), p. 667.

ease processes had relative viscosity readings of 1.6 to 2.2; associated with an increase in viscosity, he noted peripheral resistance, a capillary blood flow decrease, and cardiac work increase. The degree of viscosity, however, is apparently unaffected by athletic training. Bannister[53] includes it among the factors which are innate properties of muscle; thus, it may be considered one of those factors which limit athletic performance.

URINE ANALYSES

Alyea and Boone[54] were unable to separate the effects of exercise on the kidneys from the effects of physical renal trauma in the contact sports of boxing and football. Consequently, they studied the albumin changes in crew men, since rowing can normally be considered a form of non-traumatic exercise. None of the subjects had albumin in the urine before exercise, but a large proportion showed it following exercise; the more severe the exercise, the higher were the abnormal findings. Hyoline, granular casts, and red blood cells were also found in the urine following exercise.

In a second study, Alyea and Parish[55] reported that the findings of red blood cells in the urine of participants in swimming, lacrosse, and track were about 80 per cent, and approximately 55 per cent in football and rowing. The 1500-meter swimmers and long-distance runners showed the greatest number of atypical urinary conditions. The duration of the event played a major part in this situation; and, in the 1500-meter race especially, the urine was often loaded with red blood cells and casts; these usually disappeared within 24 hours.

The actual cause of the urinary changes mentioned is unknown. Alyea and his associates suggest, however, that the glomeruli in the kidneys may cease to function during vigorous exercise, since the albumin appears in the filtrates of damaged glomeruli when the flow and filtration are reestablished after exercise. As a consequence of their findings, also, these investigators question whether kidneys handicapped by previous infections can go through strenuous, protracted athletics without cumulative damage.

Strenuous muscular exercise ordinarily introduces a transient protein-uria whose extent is related to the intensity of the exercise. Those unaccustomed to exercise and most tired by it tend to excrete the most protein. Cantone and Cerretelli[56] suggest that the increase in serum pro-

[53] Bannister, op. cit.

[54] Edwin P. Alyea and Alex W. Boone, "Urinary Findings Resulting from Non-traumatic Exercise," Southern Medical Journal, 50 (July, 1957), p. 905.

[55] Edwin P. Alyea and Harner H. Parish, "Renal Response to Exercise: Urinary Findings," Journal of American Medical Association, 167 (June 14, 1958), p. 807.

[56] A. Cantone and P. Cerretelli, "Effect of Training upon Protein-uria Following Muscular Exercise," Internationale Zeitschrift Fur Angewandt Physiologie Einschiesslich Arbeitsphysiologie, 18 (July, 1960), p. 324.

tein level is connected with haemoconcentration due to water flow from blood to muscles consequent to increase of the osmotic pressure in muscles during strenuous anaerobic exercise.

STRESS ADAPTATION

Selye[57] described the general adaptation syndrome (GAS) as the response of the organism to non-specific stress. The whole syndrome evolves in time through three stages: the alarm reaction, the stage of resistance, and the stage of exhaustion. The GAS comprises depression of the nervous system, adrenal stimulation, shrinkage of lymphatic organs, gastrointestinal ulcers, loss of body weight, and alterations in the chemical composition of the body. All of these changes form a syndrome, a set of manifestations which appear together.

Assuming that Selye's GAS is basically concerned with the adrenal cortex and a "learning" process against future exposures to the same stress, Michael[58] reviewed studies related to the effects of exercise upon the adrenal glands and the autonomic nervous system. The evidence thus produced supported the contention that repeated exercise conditions the stress adaptation mechanism in the following ways. Adrenocortical activity along with the autonomic nervous system is involved in adjusting to stress. Adjustment to stress is enhanced by reducing the time necessary to elicit a response to stress and thereby lessening the duration of the adjustment phase of the body's reaction to stress. Adaptation to exercise produces a degree of protection against emotional stress. Increased adrenal activity resulting from repeated exercise seems to cause an increased reserve of steroids available to consider stress. A lack of activity reduces ability to withstand stress, as if the reaction to a shock were a learned process.

AGE AND SEX DIFFERENCES

Several studies have provided evidence of the differences in physiological processes between boys and girls. Astrand[59] reported that, before puberty, considerable similarity exists between boys and girls in respect to rest and work values for different functions. With puberty, however, he found a decrease in the capacity of girls for hard work. Their capacities for oxygen transport and certain other functions were 25 to 30 per cent lower than for boys; when comparisons were made relative to body weight, girls were still 15 to 20 per cent below boys. Astrand contended

---

[57] Hans Selye, The Stress of Life (New York: McGraw-Hill Book Co., Inc., 1956).
[58] Ernest D. Michael, "Stress Adaptation through Exercise," Research Quarterly, 28, No. 1 (March, 1957), p. 50.
[59] P. O. Astrand, "Human Physical Fitness with Special Reference to Sex and Age," Physiological Reviews, 36, No. 3 (1956), p. 307.

that these differences are due to the lessened amount of active muscle mass in the female in relation to weight; this was true even for girl athletes who were in no sense overweight. In this investigation, also, the child who was older than seven years had as much oxygen transport, relative to body weight, as the adult.

Mugrage and Andresen[60] compared the quantity of hemoglobin, the number of red blood cells, and the volume of packed cells in samples of venous blood from 80 boys and 80 girls, 13 to 21 years of age. The values obtained were compared with similar determinations on the blood of infants, children, and adults. The following conclusions were drawn. The averages for boys and girls are nearly identical at 13 years of age; these means gradually increase for boys until the adult level for men is reached at 17 years. Averages for girls show little variation during the adolescent period from the adult level for women. In the adolescent as well as in the adult, the mean volume of the individual red blood cell of the male is smaller than that of the female; the volumes for adolescents of both sexes are slightly higher than those for adults. The corpuscle hemoglobin concentration does not change level throughout adolescence.

DeMoor[61] found that men have a faster alactic velocity constant than women. She found no differences in the lactic debt constant.

HARMFUL EFFECTS OF PHYSICAL INACTIVITY

Use by physicians of early ambulation and bed and ambulatory exercises in the treatment of medical and surgical patients is now well established in medical practice. Extensive physical reconditioning activities, extending from hospital bed to return to duty, were employed in hospitals and convalescent centers by the armed forces during World War II. These practices now constitute essential therapy prescribed for patients in Veterans Administration hospitals and are found, but to a lesser extent, in private hospitals and rehabilitation centers. Unnecessary bed rest is considered debilitating; thus, there should be lessons for physical education in a consideration of its harmful effects.

According to Dock,[62] the hazards of phlebothrombosis in the veins of the lower extremity and pelvis and of pulmonary embolism are increased as a result of bed rest. The hazard is greater in obese than in thin patients, in the elderly than in the young, and in lethargic as contrasted with restless patients. Thrombosis was found to be the most frequent sequel to complete bed rest and a common cause of serious pulmonary complications.

---

[60] Edward R. Mugrage and Marjory I. Andresen, "Red Blood Cell Values in Adolescence," *American Journal of Diseases of Children*, 56 (November, 1938), p. 997.

[61] DeMoor, *op. cit.*

[62] William Dock, "The Undesirable Effects of Bed Rest," *The Surgical Clinics of North America*, New York Number (April, 1945), p. 437.

Dock further pointed out that cardiac output and work of the heart is increased by changing from the sitting to the lying position; this change is considerable since it consists from one-eight to one-third of the sitting-level flow. There is evidence that edema in the tissues above the diaphragm is formed at a much greater rate when recumbent as compared with an erect or sitting posture. Thus, when lying, the heart is carrying a definitely greater load; further, the rate of edema accumulation in the lungs, the brain, and in other tissues of the thorax and head is greater. Pulmonary edema due to latent heart disease, to anesthetics, or to low plasma protein, is most rapid in onset and most serious in extent, if the patient is kept flat in bed; it will be minimal while he is sitting up.

Experiments carried out on healthy individuals have shown that complete bed rest causes a marked decrease in bowel activity, with constipation and fecal impaction. Wasting also occurs, with loss of nitrogen, potassium, and phosphorus from the body tissues. Even with a high protein intake, the nitrogen balance is negative as long as recumbency continues. Loss of calcium with atrophy of bone is another common effect of bed rest over long periods, but it is more prevalent in sick patients than in healthy subjects. Usually, there is a loss of vasomoter tone and in blood volume, which causes postural hypotension and tachycardia.

Taylor and associates[63] studied the effects of bed rest for a three- to four-week period on cardiovascular functions and work performances of healthy young men. Bed rest produced a 17 per cent decrease in heart volume and an 8 per cent decrease in the transverse diameter of the heart. The average resting pulse increased one-half beat per minute for each day in bed. The pulse rate at the end of a half-hour treadmill walk of 3.5 miles per hour at a 10 per cent grade increased 40 beats per minute after the bed rest. The oxygen intake during a 90-second run at seven miles per hour up a 15 per cent grade was reduced by 730 cc. of oxygen, or 16 per cent; this was accompanied by increases in oxygen debt and blood lactate. After bed rest, the rate of recovery of the various functions was roughly proportional to the extent of deterioration during bed rest. Grip strength was not influenced by this amount of bed rest and back strength showed only a slight deterioration.

Leithauser[64] observed that surgical illness is produced by powerful stimuli, resulting from trauma, which tend to inhibit function and thereby produce a sluggish circulation. Circulatory insufficiency, which is prolonged and intensified by confinement to bed, is the primary factor in the development of adverse biologic changes after surgery. Walking institutes substitution reflexes, which stimulate pulmonary ventilation and general circulation. Voluntary contraction of the large leg muscles forces the sluggish venous blood into the arterial system.

---

[63] Henry L. Taylor, et al., "Effects of Bed Rest on Cardiovascular Function and Work Performance," Journal of Applied Physiology, 2, No. 5 (1949), p. 223.
[64] Daniel J. Leithauser, "A Survey of Early Ambulation After Surgery," Surgery, Gynecology, and Obstetrics, 106 (January, 1958), p. 100.

In another report, Leithauser[65] stated that, in some instances, vital capacity is reduced over 60 per cent on the first postoperative day, and seven to 14 days are usually required for it to return to normal. Pulmonary complications increase in direct proportion to the reduction in vital capacity. The curve of postoperative vital capacity was also found to be an index of the stage of convalescence. Limiting bed confinement to 24 hours after surgery relieves postoperative distress and rapidly restores the patient to health.

Abramson[66] analyzed atrophy resulting from disuse and presented the following definition: "Disuse atrophy is the decrease in size of tissues, due to the inability of these tissues to develop full function." The optimum stimulus for the prevention of atrophy in muscle is the production of tension by contraction of the muscle itself. Contraction through a full range of joint motion and against a load is considered most effective; this is also true for the prevention of bone atrophy.

STRUCTURE AS RELATED TO FUNCTION

It is not startling to contend that the nature of an individual's physical structure is an essential factor in his motor performance. Evidence of this assertion may be supported by common observation; witness the well-proportioned physiques of boxers and gymnasts, the superstructure of great basketball competitors, the solidarity of top-flight football players, the wiriness of champion distance runners, and the powerful builds of wrestlers, shot putters, and discus throwers.

From studies with nine anthropometric tests, Clarke[67] reported that four measures were particularly significant as structural indicators and were found to be significantly related to various strength tests; these are tensed-flexed upper arm girth, body weight, chest girth, and lung capacity. A summary of his report follows.

1. The intercorrelations of the anthropometric variables were much higher for junior high school boys than for upper elementary and senior high school boys. Reasons for this phenomenon may be related to the accelerated growth peculiarities of boys of junior high school age.

2. Very high correlations were obtained between McCloy's pull-up and push-up scores [Arm Strength = 1.77 (Wgt.) + 3.42 (Pull-ups or Push-ups) — 46] and body weight, chest girth, and arm girth. These high relationships were due to the heavy weighting given to body weight

---

[65] D. J. Leithauser, "Confinement to Bed for Only Twenty-four Hours after Operation," *Archives of Surgery*, 47 (August, 1943), p. 203.

[66] Arthur S. Abramson, "Atrophy of Disuse," *Archives of Physical Medicine*, 29, No. 9 (November, 1948), p. 562.

[67] H. Harrison Clarke, "Relation of Physical Structure to Motor Performance of Males," *Contributions No. 6, American Academy of Physical Education* (Washington: American Association for Health, Physical Education, and Recreation, 1958), pp. 63-73.

in the McCloy formula, combined with the fact that the three anthropo-metric measures have very high correlations with each other.

3. The highest correlations of anthropometric with strength tests were with lung capacity. The highest of these correlations were .86 with composite of 12 cable-tension strength tests, .84 with McCloy's Athletic Strength Index [ASI = R. Grip + L. Grip + 2 (Pull-up + Push-up Strength) — 3 (Wgt.)], .81 with elbow flexion strength, and .80 with Rogers' Strength Index.

4. Such correlations as the following were obtained between arm girth and strength measures with junior high school boys as subjects: .78 with McCloy's Athletic Strength Index, .74 with sum of seven arm and shoulder cable-tension tests, and .67 with the Strength Index.

5. Again for junior high school boys, body weight correlated .82 with McCloy's Athletic Strength, Index, .75 with composite of 12 cable-tension strength tests, and .70 with back lift.

Clarke and Petersen[68] found that outstanding junior high school ath-letes had higher means on anthropometric tests of body size than did boys at other levels of athletic ability; the order, by size, was outstand-ing athletes, regular players, substitutes, and non-participants. Also, a much greater proportion of mesomorphic physiques was found among the outstanding athletes and regular players than among the substitutes and non-participants. While strength and explosive muscular power were more consistent and significant differentiators of athletic ability, as shown in inter-school competition, body size and physique type have fundamental importance for both junior high and elementary school boys.

For boys 9 through 15 years of age, Clarke, Irving, and Heath[69] re-ported the following differentiating characteristics between five somato-type categories. Endomorphs and endo-mesomorphs had large physical bulk and inferior strength; mesomorphs were superior on such tests as the Strength Index, Physical Fitness Index, and arm strength tests; a significantly greater proportion of endo-mesomorphs was advanced and a significantly greater proportion of mid-types was retarded in maturity, as indicated by skeletal age; and the ectomorphs exceeded the mid-types in height.

Nearly all studies of the relationships between structural and strength or motor performances have been conducted with boys as the subjects. However, Rarick and Thompson[70] correlated the muscle size of the

---

[68] H. Harrison Clarke and Kay H. Petersen, "Contrast of Maturational, Structural, and Strength Characteristics of Athletes and Non-Athletes Ten to Fifteen Years of Age," *Research Quarterly*, 32, No. 2 (May, 1961), pp. 163-176.

[69] H. Harrison Clarke, Robert N. Irving, and Barbara H. Heath, "Relation of Maturation, Structure, and Strength Measures of the Somatotypes of Boys Nine through Fifteen Years of Age," *Research Quarterly*, 32, Vol. 4 (December, 1961).

[70] Lawrence Rarick and Jo Ann J. Thompson, "Roentgenographic Measure of Leg Muscle Size and Ankle Extensor Strength of Seven-Year-Old Children," *Research Quarterly*, 27, No. 3 (October, 1956), p. 321.

lower leg by X-ray measurements and the strength of the ankle extensors by cable-tension test with seven-year-old boys and girls as subjects. For the boys, the correlation between muscle area, anterior-posterior view, and ankle extensor strength was .63; for girls, this correlation was .46. The boys were substantially stronger than the girls on the strength test and possessed on the average greater muscle size. When boys and girls were paired on the basis of muscle size, the superiority of the boys in strength was no longer significant.

SUMMARY

In this chapter, research related to the values and effects of participation in physical activities was presented. Evidence of physical fitness values justified the assumption that physically active people are less likely to suffer from chronic disabling conditions, are more prone to be physically and mentally alert, and are inclined toward satisfactory social and personal adjustments. Surveys of American children have shown that too many of them are physically unfit. Physical education programs in schools and colleges designed to improve physical fitness are needed.

An account of the physiological effects of exercise reveals an amazing intricacy of interrelated factors, in which all organs of the body, the lungs, heart, bones, glands, nerves, and muscles, are involved. Man was made for movement, responds to movement, and develops the strength, stamina, and skill of the organism through movement. Lack of movement, disuse of the body to the point of prolonged bed rest, actually creates a hazard to the body, which can only be alleviated by the production of tension in muscles through their contraction.

To a significant degree, the individual's capacity for activity is dependent upon his body structure and form. Various anthropometric measures correlate well with tests of strength and motor ability; a mesomorphic physique is a great asset to the boy who wishes to excel in many forms of athletics.

SELECTED REFERENCES

Abramson, Arthur S., "Atrophy of Disuse," *Archives of Physical Medicine,* 29, No. 9 (September, 1948), 562.

Brassfield, Charles R., "Some Physiological Aspects of Physical Fitness," *Research Quarterly,* 14, No. 1 (March, 1943), 106.

Clarke, H. Harrison, "Muscular Strength-Endurance Relationships," *Archives of Physical Medicine and Rehabilitation,* 28, No. 9 (September, 1957), 584.

———, "Physical Fitness Benefits: A Summary of Research," *Education,* 78, No. 8 (April, 1958), 460.

———, "Relation of Physical Structure to Motor Performance of Males," *Contributions No. 6, American Academy of Physical Education,* Washington:

American Association for Health, Physical Education, and Recreation, 1958, 63-73.

Elkins, Earl C., and Khalil G. Wakim, "The Physiological Basis for Therapeutic Exercise," *Archives of Physical Medicine*, 28, No. 9 (September, 1947), 555.

Henry, Franklin M., *Physiology of Work: The Physiological Basis of Muscular Exercise*. Berkeley: Associated Students' Store, University of California, 1950.

Karpovich, Peter V., *Physiology of Muscular Activity*, 5th ed. Philadelphia: W. B. Saunders Company, 1959.

"The Contributions of Physical Activity to Human Well-Being," *Research Quarterly*, 31, No. 2,P. II (May, 1960).

Wakim, Khalil G., "The Physiological Aspects of Therapeutic Exercise," *Journal of the American Medical Association*, 142 (January 14, 1950), 100.

6

The Case Study
Approach

THIS CHAPTER WILL PRESENT PROCEDURES FOR MEETING
the needs of individual boys and girls who are subpar
in basic physical fitness elements, to be known herein as the *unfit*.
Scores on physical fitness tests provide generalized indices; they are not
essentially diagnostic. In this respect they are comparable to clinical
thermometer readings by physicians. Thus, a high thermometer reading
indicates that the individual has an abnormal condition; this tells the
physician that *something* is wrong, not *what* that something is. In like
manner, an unfit score indicates a deficient condition, not what is causing that deficiency. As the patient with a fever requires medical diagnosis and prescription, so the person with a subfit score should be
studied in order to determine the cause of his condition before appropriate treatment can be planned. The causes of an unfit condition are many.
Certainly the assumption that exercise is all that is needed is short-
sighted and can be positively erroneous in some instances.

Thus, the identification of causes must be a prime concern of the
physical educator in meeting the individual needs of unfit boys and
girls. Once causes are discovered, appropriate follow-up procedures for
each unfit subject can be determined. The case study approach is proposed as the best method to be used for this purpose.

TEN ESSENTIAL STEPS

The procedures presented here for improving the fitness status of boys and girls who are below accepted standards are more than just theories. They have evolved through use over a third of a century in school and college physical education. While these can be variously stated, the ten essential steps are presented.

1. Discover boys and girls with special deficiencies revealed by medical, sensory, nutritional, and psychological tests and examinations. An adequate health appraisal by a physician is the starting point of any physical fitness program.

2. Select those who are below pre-determined standards of strength, stamina, and other basic physical fitness elements through the administration of valid tests available to the physical educator.

3. For the subfit group, conduct physical activities selected to improve their condition. These activities should be presented progressively within each individual's exercise tolerance and by application of proper principles of exercise. The type of exercise to be used for this purpose and the exercise principles will be considered in Chapter 7.

4. After about six weeks, re-test the subfit group in order to determine progress and to identify those who do not respond favorably to exercise, e.g., those whose test scores decrease or do not increase appreciably. For boys and girls who improve at a satisfactory rate, the exercise program should continue with progressive increase in dosage until minimum standards are reached, or, preferably, exceeded.

5. Identify the cause or causes of the subfit condition for those who do not improve scores satisfactorily on retests. These causes may be located by use of case-study procedures, living-habit surveys, personal interviews, and supplementary tests. Details of this process are considered later in this chapter.

6. Refer to other specialists, such as the physician, guidance officer, home economist, school nurse and the like, when physical defects, organic lesions, personality maladjustments, or nutritional disturbances are *suspected* as a result of the case-study process. Actually, case study procedures should be instituted after initial physical fitness tests in some instances, as in the case of obese boys or girls or other easily recognized atypical conditions.

7. Provide individually planned physical fitness programs utilizing the following as appropriate in each case: proper kind and amount of exercise, health guidance, relaxation procedures, methods and activities applied to improve social and personal adjustment, and medical attention.

8. Relate all factors accumulated in the case study to the individual's

somatotype, mental aptitude, and scholastic success. Frequently, these are related, so an understanding of the configuration of the total personality is desirable.

9. Repeat physical fitness tests at intervals of about six weeks, in order to continue checking on the progress made by each subfit boy and girl.

10. Re-direct programs in individual cases as found desirable in the light of retest and restudy results.

This approach to the improvement of subfit boys and girls does not preclude their participation in the regular activities of physical education. If their physical condition warrants it, a decision to be reached after case studies, unfit students should participate in the full physical education program, as they need to learn the skills and to benefit from the social opportunities of these regular classes. For them, however, emphasis on their fitness needs should be primary until such time as they reach the physical standards adopted.

CASE STUDY PROCEDURES

The fifth of the "Ten Essential Steps" proposed above is that the underlying or basic or originating cause or causes of unfitness should be found for each boy or girl thus identified. Preferably, this process should be applied to all unfit individuals at the start, but, in order to save time for those with the greatest need, it may be reserved for those who do not respond favorably to the initial exercise program.

When the unfit person does not improve his score upon retest after an exercise regimen, three reasons may logically be proposed: (a) the physical activity program may not have been properly conceived to develop basic physical fitness elements; (b) the student may not have participated energetically in the exercise plan designed for him; (c) the underlying cause of unfitness may not have been detected, or, if detected, may not have been removed. Assuming the physical educator and the student have worked out proper and co-operative arrangements on the first two of these, the third still remains. It is vital for the present and future well-being of those boys and girls who remain weak and lacking in stamina that action be taken to deal with the causative problem.

A formal device which provides for the systematic accumulation of essential information related to the individual's unfitness is convenient for use in conducting case studies. One such instrument is Clarke's *Case-Study Form and Health-Habit Questionnaire,*[1] as reproduced in Figures 12 and 13. These forms were developed over a period of years through use in school and college developmental programs. They are used in conjunction with Rogers' Physical Fitness Index[2] as the test for

---

[1] H. Harrison Clarke, *Case-Study Form and Health-Habit Questionnaire,* (Cedar Rapids, Iowa: Nissen Medart Corporation, 930 27th Ave., S.W.).
[2] See pages 65-66.

selecting unfit boys and girls. For those who use other tests for this purpose, it is simple enough to make the substitution of tests on the forms, as the case-study process remains the same.

The *Case-Study Form and Health-Habit Questionnaire* are printed separately so that the Questionnaire may be given to a student without showing him the rest of his record, and so that additional Questionnaires may be administered if it seems desirable to check on changes in his habits. The Case-Study Form is in the shape of an 11 x 8½ inch folder; the Questionnaire is of such size that it will fit conveniently into the Form, thus permitting all information pertaining to the student to be kept together and readily available for use.

Three essential stages in conducting case studies may be recognized; these are data gathering, synthesis and interview, and action proposals. In this section, each of these stages will be described; in the following section, their use and integration will be illustrated from actual case studies of unfit boys and girls.

DATA GATHERING

The Case-Study Form provides spaces for the following types of information pertaining to unfit students.

Physical Objective Test Data. Spaces are provided for ten physical fitness test scores, so that retests may be entered. If the Physical Fitness Index is used as the test, space is available for the Strength Index, the norm, and the PFI. If another test is used, this section of the Form would, of course, need to be redesigned.

Somatotype. It is helpful to know the individual's somatotype[3] in interpreting physical fitness scores. Briefly, the dominance of mesomorphy is an asset and the dominance of endomorphy is a hindrance in taking physical fitness and motor performance tests.

Academic Status. In making a case study, records of the student's academic status may be interesting and helpful. Occasionally, his level of scholastic work may fluctuate with his physical condition.

Synthesis. A brief statement relative to the relationships between fitness test scores, somatotype, intelligence quotient, and scholastic success may be made for each unfitness case.

Weight Record. Inclusion of the weight record on the Case-Study Form is not for the purpose of nutritional determination, although the results may be so related. To know the percentage a student's weight is above or below normal is often helpful in those cases involving some form of malnutrition or glandular malfunction. More complete nutritional test data may be desirable in some instances.[4]

---

[3] See pages 62-64.
[4] See pages 59-62.

Health-Habit Questionnaire
(Second Revision)

Name: ....   Grade: .... Date: ....
                (Print last name first)

Instructions: Please answer as carefully and accurately as you can each of the following questions concerning your health habits. You are asked for this information in order that your physical education teacher
may help you to improve your physical condition. Your answers will be kept confidential.

1. How many hours do you sleep each night?....................... Is your sleep restful?...................................

    Do you sleep with your windows open at night?.......... Are you warm at night (especially in the winter)?.......

2. Are you usually rested and refreshed in the morning?................................. Drowsy?............................

    Are you sleepy during the day?................................. In class?............... When studying?.......................

    Do you take a nap during the day?......................,....... How often?................ For how long?.......................

    Do you work and play without being more than comfortably tired mentally or physically at bed time?.....Fatigued?....

    Do you get to sleep easily at night?.................................... If not, why?..

3. Are your living conditions congenial?.....Depressing?....Do you have a room for yourself?.....Bed for yourself?....

4. Are you often "on edge", nervous, or jittery?........................ Is it difficult for you to relax?...................

    Are you subject to worries?.......... Moods?.......... Usually cheerful?.......... Are you really happy?............

5. How far do you live from school?............................. How do you get to school?....................................

    What time do you leave in the morning?....................... When, home at night?.......................................

    How much time do you usually study at home each school day?..

    How much time do you usually work at outside employment (or chores) each school day?...........................

    What do you do?...

6. Do you have a hobby?.......... What is it?..

    How many hours per day of physical activity do you usually get outside of school hours?.......What do you do?.......

    What organizations do you belong to?..

    What social activities do you participate in with mixed groups (boys and girls)?.............. How often?..........

    What extra-curricular school activities do you take part in?...

    What do you do with your spare time?...

    ....

7. Please check (X) the frequency with which you have the following?

	Never	Seldom	Occasionally	Often
a. Headaches				
b. Colds				
c. Sore throat				
d. Ear ache				
e. Indigestion				
f. Bad breath				
g. Coated tongue (bad taste)				
h. Pimples or skin eruptions				
i. Boils				
j. Twitching face and eyelids				
k. Eye strain				
l. Sinus infections				
m. Foot trouble				
n. Joint pains				

Do you wear glasses?........... If so, when were they last tested?............... Do you hear well?....................

Fig. 12.   The Clarke Health-Habit Questionnaire.

8. Do you eat three meals a day regularly?......Is your appetite good?......Do you eat at the school cafeteria at noon?....

   Carry your lunch?.......... Go home for lunch?.......... What do you usually eat at noon?...........................

   ....

   Do you eat between meals? (Check) Never .... Seldom .... Often .... Usually ....

   What do you eat between meals?..

9. How often do you usually eat each of the following kinds of food (check):

	Very Seldom	Once Each Week	Three Times Each Week	Once Each Day	Twice Each Day	Three Times Each Day
a. Meat (including fish and eggs)						
b. Green vegetables (spinach, cabbage, lettuce, etc.)						
c. Other vegetables (carrots, peas, beans, beets, etc.)						
d. Potatoes						
e. Rice, Macaroni						
f. Pie, cake, pastry						
g. Candy, sweets						
h. Fresh fruit						
i. Salads						
j. Oranges, tomatoes						
k. Dried fruits (prunes, apricots, figs, etc.)						
l. Cereals						
m. Pork						
n. Fried foods						
o. Whole wheat foods						

10. How many glasses of water do you usually drink daily?........How many glasses of milk?......Tea?.....Coffee?..

11. Are you troubled with constipation?......................... What do you do to correct it?...............................

12. Do you smoke?............... If so, how much daily?..

    Do you drink alcoholic beverages? .... If so, what?..................... How often?.......... How much?........

13. How often do you visit the dentist?.................... How often do you usually clean your teeth?...................

14. Have you been vaccinated?........... Immunized for diphtheria?..................... Typhoid?.........................

    What other immunizations?...

15. Are your parents healthy and physically fit?............... If not, what is the reason?................................

    What is the physical stature of your father?   Tall................ Medium................. Short.........................

                                                     Fat................. Average................. Thin.........................

    What is the physical stature of your mother?   Tall................ Medium................. Short.........................

                                                     Fat................. Average................. Thin.........................

16. Do you desire to be strong and physically fit (boys)?......... Do you wish to be attractive (girls)?................

    Are you satisfied with your present physical condition?...

    If your *Physical Fitness Index* is low, can you account for it?............. How?.......................................

    ....

    Summary of Interview: ....

Produced by
Fred Medart Products, Inc.
St. Louis, Mo.

Fig. 12   (cont.)

Case-Study Data Sheet

I. *Physical Objective Test Data*

Date of Test									
Strength Index									
Normal Strength Index									
Physical Fitness Index									
PFI Deviation from proportional									

II. *Somatotype:* ....

III. *Academic Status*

         Intelligence quotient: ....

Scholastic Record:

1. Date: .... Record:...

2. Date: .... Record: ....

3. Date: .... Record: :...

IV. *Individual PFI - Somatotype - I.Q. Synthesis:*

V. *Weight Record*

Date									
Height									
Weight									
Per Cent Above or Below Normal									
Gain or loss in weight									

VI. *Mechanical and Functional Impairment*

VII. *Medical Examination*

	Date	Summary of Findings	Physician
Examination prior to Physical Fitness Test			
Re-Examination			
Re-Examination			

VIII. *Recent Illnesses, Accidents, and Operations*

Date	Condition	Physician's Recommendation

Fig. 13.   The Clarke Case-Study Form.

IX. *Faulty Health Habits*

Date	Faulty Habits	Recommendations	Interviewer

X. *Social Adjustment*

XI. *Posture Appraisal*

XII. *Nurse's Report*
(Indicate economic status of family)

XIII. *Physical Fitness Council*
(Give date and summary of suggestions)

XIV. *Clinical or Other Services*
(Give date and explanation of services)

XV. *Treatment and Results*

XVI. *Summary of Case*

Fig. 13 (cont.)

Mechanical and Functional Impairment. Occasionally, the student has an orthopedic defect or functional impairment which handicaps his test performance. Examples are post-polio limb or an injured hand or ankle. These should be noted on the form.

Health Examination. A summary of defects disclosed by the school physician as a result of his health examination should be entered here.

Recent Illnesses, Accidents, and Operations. Any history of recent illnesses, accidents, or operations should be entered on the Case-Study Form. The physician's recommendation as to the type and intensity of exercise in which each subject may engage until ready for full physical activity should also be included.

Faulty Health Habits. A survey of the unfit individual's living habits may disclose causes or contributory reasons for his low physical fitness score. Each unfit student, therefore, should answer a Health-Habit Questionnaire, unless this information is obtained in some other way. The Questionnaire shown in Figure 5 contains questions pertaining to sleeping habits and fatigue (1-2), living conditions (3), tensions (4), out-of-school activities and hobbies (5-6), frequency of minor ailments (7), dietary practices (8-10), constipation (11), smoking and drinking habits (12), dental care (13), immunizations (14), parental health and physical status (15) and self-analysis (16). Any faulty habits disclosed may be checked with a red pencil for ready reference and a summary may be entered on the Case-Study Form.

Social Adjustment. An analysis of the individual's social-personal adjustment should be included in the case study. Certain questions on the Health-Habit Questionnaire are aimed at this situation. Some physical educators may wish to give standard tests or utilize other evaluative procedures in order to understand more fully the social status of the unfit boy or girl.[5]

Posture Appraisal. An appraisal of the individual's posture may be included in the case study. This appraisal may simply provide over-all A-B-C-D ratings or may provide a detailed analysis based on subjective or objective scoring of the various body segments included in the total posture.[6]

Nurse's Report. An efficient and sympathetic school nurse, with her intimate knowledge of the health problems of the school children and the socio-economic status of their families, gained in visits to the homes in some instances, will be valuable in following up cases of unfitness. Where parental co-operation is needed in order to correct physical defects or to change faulty living habits, the nurse can be of essential help. Her report should be summarized on the Case-Study Form.

Physical Fitness Council. The formation and operation of a Physical Fitness Council will be discussed later in this chapter. Suffice it to say

---

[5] See pages 98-102.
[6] See chapter 8.

here that the findings for each unfit student investigated by the Council should be entered on the Case-Study Form.

Clinical or Other Services. Occasionally, unfit students should be given special examinations or tests, especially when the case study points to conditions not usually found in routine school health appraisals. X-rays, basal metabolisms, etc., may be essential when such conditions as ulcers, tuberculosis, glandular difficulties, or psychological disturbances are suspected from the case study process.

Treatment and Results. Any treatments given the unfit student outside the usual resources of the school or college should be entered on the Form.

Summary of the Case. Space is provided on the Case-Study Form for a summary of the case when completed so that all essential facts may be seen at a glance.

Special note should be made that the above instructions for using the *Case-Study Form and Health-Habit Questionnaire* have dealt entirely with low-fitness students. For those using the Physical Fitness Index, however (and this may apply to other fitness tests), it should be pointed out that an unusually high score may or may not be desirable, as it may indicate the presence of a hypertensive state. Further, scores that drop unexplainably from any established level may be danger signs. Such students as these may well be considered with the unfit group.

At the start of the case study, all of the types of information for which units are provided on the Case-Study Form may not be needed. The essential information will vary from case to case, as will readily be seen as individual studies develop. As a general practice, the data to complete Units I through IX are necessary. The Health-Habit Questionnaire should be given routinely. In doing so, good rapport with the student is vital, as discussed below, if true answers are to be freely given. The Questionnaire can be administered to the unfit group as a whole, or may be answered by each unfit student on the occasion of the interview.

SYNTHESIS AND INTERVIEW

Following the initial data-gathering stage, the physical educator should hold personal interviews with each unfit student. At this point, many of the case findings may be negative. For example, the medical appraisal may not show defects which constitute a drain on the body; the student may not have had a recent illness, accident, or operation; there may be no mechanical or functional impairment; no faulty living habit may be revealed on the Questionnaire. Actually, in some instances, the whole physical fitness picture may appear satisfactory, except for the unfitness score.

In conducting case studies, stress should be placed on the fact that the personal information obtained about and discussed with each unfit student will be kept confidential. In most situations, the confidence of the case study will be restricted to the physical educator only; in some instances, however, it must necessarily be extended to other professional people who are helping with various special phases. Naturally, the confidential nature of the case study extends to all those who participate in it and it is the responsibility of the physical educator to make this clear to all concerned. Only by this practice can a fully co-operative relationship be established with unfit boys and girls. The sensitive student would rightly resent having his fitness problems made common knowledge. Furthermore, the channels for information resulting from the school physician's examinations, from mental testing, psychological testing, and the like. would be closed to the physical educator unless their confidential nature was fully protected.

In initiating an interview with an unfit student, every effort should be made to achieve rapport with him. Once rapport is established, the purposes of the conference should be explained to the student. Thus, if he does not already, he should understand the meaning of his low physical fitness score. An intelligent, discerning student may wish to know about the validity of the test used to evaluate his fitness status, the basis for the norms with which he was compared, and may seek a realistic understanding of his position in this pattern. The need to discover the cause or causes of each student's sub-standard condition is the prime reason for the interview. Other purposes are to determine the best approach to follow in order to improve the student's physical fitness and to enlist his full support in his own physical improvement. Time is well spent in obtaining good rapport with the student and in giving him an adequate understanding of his own physical condition, what he can do about it and what it will mean to him; in fact, this is essential for the full success of the low-fitness program.

The main part of the interview should be devoted to an attempt to determine the cause of the student's unfitness. This phase should be based upon information contained in the Case-study Form and upon replies to the Health-Habit Questionnaire. Special attention might well be given to the answer to question 16 on the Questionnaire, in which the student analyzes his own situation. In each conference, the physical educator should be alert for openings that will lead him to the cause he seeks. Many answers on the Questionnaire merely provide leads to underlying causes, and must be followed up with further questions. For example, if the student indicated he was subject to worries; this answer by itself would not be adequate in revealing causation; additional questions should be asked to determine the cause of the worries. Again, if the student checked that he had colds frequently, additional consideration of this situation by a physician might be desirable.

Interviews with unfit students should be held even if their case-study forms and questionnaires reveal no conditions that might account for their poor physical fitness. In talking with them and in checking over the information obtained about them, the physical educator may uncover significant leads. As the individual's case study develops, additional conferences should be held whenever they might prove helpful.

ACTION PROPOSALS

From the various interviews with unfit boys and girls, a variety of action proposals will result, the nature of each being dependent upon the findings of individual case studies. While the following possibilities are not considered all inclusive, they will encompass most of the situations encountered.

1. An exercise regimen, well balanced to improve basic physical fitness elements, may be devised based on the student's exercise tolerance and arranged to provide progressively more vigorous exercise. The preparation of such exercise programs will be commonplace; in fact, exercise will be regularly prescribed for unfit students unless contraindicated by factors disclosed in the case study. Where no causative factors can be identified in individual cases, exercise routines should be utilized to determine their success or until such time as the case study can be continued through referral, as discussed below.[7]

2. Recommendations for the improvement of living habits may be made frequently. Such recommendations will logically take a variety of directions. They may deal with dietary practices and reducing diets, with problems pertaining to fatigue, rest, and relaxation, with the over-burden of out-of-school activities and, possibly, the reduction of scholastic schedules, with social life and dating, with relationships to others, with many situations underlying worries and moods, with factors related to constipation, with home and school problems, ad infinitum.

3. Overweight will be encountered as a cause of unfitness among boys and girls as well as men and women. Frequently, in today's society, weight reduction is undertaken for aesthetic reasons. However, various studies have shown that overweight (obesity) is associated with serious physical impairment and is accompanied by a shortened life expectancy. These are cogent reasons for dealing with the overweight problem, in addition to the fact that obese individuals usually score low on physical and motor fitness tests.

Mayer[8] has pointed out that, in recent years, the role of exercise in weight control has been minimized, if not ridiculed, by a number of lay health educators and some physicians. As Harvard University Pro-

---

[7] See Chapter 7.

[8] Jean Mayer, "Exercise and Weight Control," *Exercise and Fitness* (Chicago: Athletic Institute, 1960), p. 110.

fessor and a world authority on nutrition, he has successfully refuted this concept. Furthermore, he effectively supported the conviction that physical inactivity is the most important factor explaining the frequency of increasing overweight in modern Western societies. He states, "Natural selection, operating for hundreds of thousands of years, made men physically active, resourceful creatures, well prepared to be hunters, fishermen, and agriculturists. The regulation of food intake was never designed to adapt to the highly mechanized sedentary conditions of modern life, any more than animals were made to be caged."[9] Kraus and Raab[10] also maintain that lack of exercise is the most common cause of overweight and that prescription of exercise is important in its medical treatment.

Thus, the developmental and adapted physical educator needs to be alert to the problems of the overweight individual. Exercise is an essential phase of treatment; the principles of exercise presented in the next chapter should be applied as a matter of course. A proper diet should also be suggested; however, as the physical educator has only limited training in nutrition, the advice of specialists in this area should be sought.

4. All unfit individuals should be observed for signs of fatigue and hypertension. Certain queries on the Questionnaire are intended to explore fatigue-hypertension relationships; the answers should be checked and compared to the student's behavior, as observed in his class and school activities. Hypertensed individuals are prone to exhibit signs of being "on edge," nervous, or jittery; they are apt to be constantly in motion—always "on the go." The causes of this condition should be sought. In addition, physical activities designed and presented to reduce tensions should be prescribed for these individuals.[11]

5. Social maladjustment and personality conflicts are frequently found in unfit boys and girls. Which is cause and which is effect may be difficult to determine; obviously, however, both situations need to be remedied. In meeting individual needs, the usual study of causes should be conducted and the contributing conditions eliminated if satisfactory results are to be obtained. In addition, action proposals may include planning physical education participation designed to improve these situations. For example, boys and girls who avoid physical education, especially if avoidance is prompted by a lack of ability to participate effectively, can be placed in situations where they may enjoy some success experiences. For introverts—provide opportunities and encourage them to participate in group activities and team sports. The potentialities

---

[9] *Ibid.*, p. 120.

[10] Hans Kraus and Wilhelm Raab, *Hypokinetic Disease* (Springfield, Ill.: Charles C. Thomas, 1961), p. 139.

[11] See Chapter 9.

for utilizing physical education activities and methods to improve social relationships and to relieve personality conflicts are almost unlimited.[12]

6. If from the case study process, the advice of other professionals, such as the physician, psychologist, school nurse, guidance counselor, home economist, or others, seems desirable, the student should be strongly encouraged to see the appropriate specialist. Such referral will be advisable when the physical educator *suspects* the presence of physical defects, organic lesions, or personality maladjustments as the cause of unfitness. If dietary problems are found which are beyond his capabilities to handle properly (such as pronounced underweight or overweight), with the possibilities of glandular malfunction and the preparation of specialized diets, the assistance of a specialist will be needed. The results of such referral, together with detailed recommendations, should be confidentially transmitted in writing directly to the physical educator. The physical educator should not draw conclusions from diagnoses only; in each instance, specific treatment recommendations should be provided by the specialist.

7. Those boys and girls, who fail to improve their physical fitness after repeated attempts to provide proper exercise for them and who reveal no basic causative factors through the regular case study approach, should be presented to the Physical Fitness Council, as discussed later in this chapter.

ILLUSTRATED CASE STUDIES

Almost exclusively, published case studies of unfit boys and girls treated through developmental physical education programs have utilized the Rogers' Physical Fitness Index (PFI) as the test for measuring basic fitness elements. As a consequence, extensive reference to this test in the illustration of case studies is unavoidable, until such time as similar experiences develop around other tests and become available. As has been stated repeatedly before, however, the method of the case study is descriptive here, without any attempt to justify a particular test, even though that test has proven successful for this purpose.

Formal Studies

Three master's theses, written under the advisement of one of the authors, have systematically conducted and reported case studies on a total of 128 secondary school boys and college men. References to these three theses with a general summary of each follow.

1. C. Getty Page, "Case Studies of College Men with Low Physical Fitness Indices" (Master's thesis, Syracuse University, 1940).

---

[12] See Chapter 12.

In this thesis, 50 case studies of men at Syracuse University, based upon two years of observation, are presented. After analyzing the 50 case studies, the investigator described the typical unfit college man as follows: 20 per cent or more overweight for his age and height; above average mental aptitude but below average scholastic achievement; below normal social adjustment, as evaluated by a standard test; lives at home and commutes daily to the university; employed part time; had participated little if at all in high school physical education; and has such faulty health habits as smoking, insufficient sleep, and incorrect diet.

2. John R. Coefield and Robert H. McCollum, "A Case Study Report of 78 University Freshmen with Low Physical Fitness Indices" (Microcarded Master's thesis, University of Oregon, 1955).

Seventy-eight case studies of University of Oregon freshman men, based mostly upon one term acquaintances, appear in this thesis. The typical unfit college man in this study was characterized as follows: above average in mental aptitude but doing much poorer scholastic work than his classmates; addicted to frequent colds; conformed reasonably well in weight with the Pryor Width-Weight Tables; has such faulty health habits as smoking, eating between meals, excessive worrying, and insufficient time for leisure; 65 per cent felt that their high school physical education programs were inadequate for the development of physical fitness; and, in general, although socially adjusted according to a standard test, 39 per cent of the subjects indicated difficulty in adjusting to people.

3. James C. Popp, "Comparison of Sophomore High School Boys Who Have High and Low Physical Fitness Indices through Case Study Procedures" (Microcarded Master's thesis, University of Oregon, 1959).

Case studies were conducted on the 20 boys with the highest and the 20 boys with the lowest PFI's in the tenth grade at Marshfield High School, Coos Bay, Oregon. Contrasted with the low-fitness group, the high-fitness group had a higher mean intelligence quotient and a higher mean grade-point average. Only one boy (5 per cent) in the high group failed to graduate from high school; in the low group, 8 failed to graduate (40 per cent). Forty per cent of the high group indicated they wanted to go to college; only 15 per cent of the low group expressed this desire. Ten of the low PFI· boys were 15 per cent or more overweight for their age and height, while none of the high PFI boys were in this category. The boys in the low group checked twice as many fatigue problems on the Health-Habit Questionnaire than did the boys in the high group; these problems pertained to insufficient sleep, being tired in the morning, being sleepy during the day, in class, and from studying, and experiencing undue fatigue after work and play. From an alphabetical list of all 40 of these boys, five teachers and administrators independently chose boys they would most and least like to have for sons; 69 per cent of the boys chosen as sons they would *most* like to have were from the high PFI group and 75 per cent of those they would *least* like to have for sons were chosen from the low PFI group.

INDIVIDUAL CASES

Individual case studies are described below in order to illustrate the problems encountered, the action taken, and the results achieved in each case.

Rapport. Paul was 21 years old, 70 inches tall, and weighed 142 pounds; his first test resulted in a PFI of 68. In his interview a strong dislike for physical education was encountered; in fact, he was quite antagonistic and wanted no part of it. Obviously, rapport had to be established if progress was to be made. The interviewer in a friendly, informal manner talked of many things without striking a responsive chord. Finally, he mentioned guns, the discussion of which quickly became a basis for mutual liking, as both the student and the interviewer were avid hunters.

Then, the story came out. This college freshman had not participated in physical education since elementary school. In a sixth-grade physical education class, exercises on the parallel bars were being taught. Paul was inept and failed to perform one of the stunts. The instructor insisted that he try again, with the result that he had a hard fall. His classmates laughed and made fun of him and the teacher joined in the ridicule; the boys continued to tease him on the way home from school. Consequently, but using poor health as the reason, the family physician gave Paul a written excuse from all future physical education requirements.

Fortunately, rapport was formed between Paul and his university physical education instructor. He became convinced that the exercise regimen planned for him was very much to his benefit, so his participation was wholehearted. There were other factors in this case, including an anemic condition, so his progress was slow. However, his PFI rose 18 points, to 86, before the end of the year, when he left the university to attend a theological seminary.[13]

Lack of exercise. The case studies by Page and by Coefield and McCollum showed definitely that many university men with low PFI's had had no physical education in high school, and those who did have such a program were prone to feel that it was inadequate for the development of physical fitness. A typical case of this type follows.

---

[13] Millard Rogers, "The Case of Paul: A Study of Low Physical Fitness" (mimeographed).

George was an 18-year old university freshman, whose initial PFI was 46. He had high scholastic aptitude, normal social adjustment according to his score on the Washburne Social Adjustment Inventory, and had participated "as little as possible" in high school physical education. He had had no serious illnesses in the past and had no noticeable faulty health habits. George thoroughly disliked physical education in high school, so a first task was to change his attitude. It was over a year before he realized the desirability of good physical education; during this time, his participation in the university developmental program was lethargic and his PFI gain was nil. Chiefly under the patient guidance of a student teacher assigned to his class, George learned to play basketball and handball. With enthusiastic participation in these two activities and in his developmental exercise, he made rapid gains during his second year of physical education. On his last PFI test, his score had risen to 91, approximately double his original score.[14]

Obesity. Obesity is an obvious handicap to physical fitness and results in low scores on fitness (and other physical performance) tests; thus, most, if not all, obese boys and girls will be found in the unfit group. Murray provides an interesting case study with this type of involvement. He was an 18-year-old university freshman with an initial PFI of 41; his weight was 215 pounds, which was 71 per cent in excess of the average for his age and height. This student had average scholastic aptitude, normal social adjustment, and had participated "below average" in high school physical education. Murray was co-operative and participated actively in the university developmental program; during the fall and winter terms, his PFI rose 10 points, but, unfortunately, his weight also increased by 6 pounds.

In the spring of his freshman year, Murray went out for the frosh lacrosse team. While out for lacrosse, he lost much of his excess weight partly through exercise and partly by diet. He continued on a regimen of exercise and diet during the summer and "scrubbed" for soccer in the fall. After the soccer season, he registered voluntarily for a developmental class. Murray's final PFI was 85, an increase of 107 per cent; and, he had reduced his weight by 33 pounds. At this time, instead of being a "rolly-polly" boy, he was a fairly well-built and physically active young man.[15]

Lack of co-ordination and participation. David was a 14-year-old boy of ectomorphic build. According to his medical record, his health and physical condition were satisfactory. In his entrance test to Groton School, his percentile rank on the Junior Scholastic Aptitude Test was 87; his intelligence quotient was 115. He had an even temperament

---

[14] C. Getty Page, "Case Studies of College Men with Low Physical Fitness Indices" (Master's thesis, Syracuse University, 1940), Case Study No. 23.

[15] Page, *op. cit.*, Case Study No. 47.

and appeared fairly mature for his age. David's parents were divorced and each had re-married. His home was in New York City where he lived with his father, a well-known surgeon. He had strong religious convictions and had served as an acolyte in the Episcopal Church. His hobby interests were guns, photography, stamp collecting, and reading history. He was not proficient in athletics, but had been active in dramatics and music.

During the administration of various physical tests at Groton School, it was noted that David's co-ordination was very poor and that he was quite conscious of this fact. His PFI was 67, so he was assigned to a developmental class in the morning and participated in soccer in the afternoon. Before going home for Thanksgiving, he asked to take the PFI test again so that he could tell his father of any improvement. He was delighted to find that his score had increased to 82, a gain of 15 points, or 22 per cent.

David pursued developmental exercise very earnestly during the winter months. In the spring, he played intramural baseball; and, after practice, he would be seen frequently in the special exercise room doing his regular developmental routine. His PFI at the end of the year was 94, an over-all substantial increase of 40 per cent. Furthermore, this boy, being intelligent and coming from a family with a medical background, was able to gain insight into what a developmental program could mean to him. He was able to interpret the significance of the PFI from the standpoint of individual analysis and to have respect for the follow-up work made more meaningful by retest results and procedures followed in his case.[16]

Personal problems. Mark was an 18-year-old university freshman with an initial PFI of 76. He was "low normal" in alienation and in sympathy on the Washburne Social Adjustment Inventory; on the Mooney Problem Check List, he checked ten or more problems in the categories of adjustment to college and in self-confidence. He was plagued by colds, indigestion, constipation, coated tongue, and eye strain. In the interview, he appeared quiet and retiring, although nervous, and indicated awkwardness on social occasions. There was no improvement in PFI during the fall term of developmental physical education. However, during the winter term, his class instructor observed a definite personality improvement and stated that, despite his shyness, Mark was friendly and accepted by his peers. Also, during this term, he raised his PFI 18 points, to 94. And, with this increase, a rise of .26, from 1.80 to 2.06, in grade-point average occurred.[17]

---

[16] J. Stuart Wickens, "A Low PFI Case Study," *Physical Fitness News Letter,* University of Oregon, Series III, No. 7 (1957), p. 3.

[17] John R. Coefield and Robert H. McCollum, "A Case Study Report of 78 University Freshman Men with Low Physical Fitness Indices" (Microcarded Master's thesis, University of Oregon, 1955), Case Study No. 3.

Personal-social-religious. As a high school sophomore, John had an initial PFI of 78. His intelligence quotient was average and he had a good scholastic record. According to the health record, he often had headaches, was drowsy during the day, was often nervous, and had difficulty in relaxing; further, he had lost an eye in an accident when seven years old, and had a plastic substitute for appearance's sake. On the Washburne Social Adjustment Inventory, John was "low normal" in happiness and in control and maladjusted in alienation. On the Mooney Problem check list, he felt that he could not get close enough to God, worried about other people and their souls, did not understand his personal and sex life, and wanted to live a good Christian life in order to show others he had been saved. In the interview, he appeared quite religious and talked about quitting school to attend a Bible Institute; also, he believed his parents did not understand him.

John was acutely interested in PFI testing, particularly in his own score. He believed his initial low index was due to a rapid growth period through which he had been passing. He was a hard worker when doing physical labor, but was not too interested in his school courses. He tried diligently to raise his PFI and was happy to learn that it increased 22 points to an even 100. From observation, he seemed to be somewhat better adjusted, although improvement along this line was still needed.[18]

Emotional stability. Sam was in his junior year at the U. S. Military Academy when he failed the Third Class Physical Efficiency Test (he had nearly failed earlier tests) and was dismissed from the Academy as a consequence. He voluntarily went to Springfield College with the objective of preparing to re-take the test in about six weeks. The PFI test was administered immediately to Sam and a case study was started. His PFI was 90; Strength Index, 2624; weight, 165 pounds; height, 72½ inches; and age, 24 years. Chinning and leg lift scores were relatively low; at West Point, his scores were especially low in dodge run, standing broad jump, and bar vault.

The initial case study revealed the following: weight about right for age and height; amount of sleep inadequate; diet heavy on sugars and starches and light on salads, fruit, and leafy vegetables; occasional facial pimples and skin eruptions; social activities consisting of dancing, card playing, and week-end drinking; very little pre-Academy participation in physical education and athletics; and progressive loss of vision in his left eye, which had gone from 20/15 to 20/60 in four years. In the interview, Sam indicated that he had had a protected childhood, and still felt over-protected. He was not allowed to venture and to try

---

[18] James C. Popp, "Comparison of Sophomore High School Boys Who Have High and Low Physical Fitness Indices through Case Study Procedures" (Micro-carded Master's thesis, University of Oregon, 1959), Case Study No. 38.

out ideas of his own. His father was away from home a great deal when Sam was younger, so he had been mostly in his mother's care; she had moved to the village of West Point while he attended the Academy. Sam indicated further that he reacted unfavorably to difficult assignments, stating that he set up mental blocks when he failed in a situation or did not come up to his expectations or the expectations of others.

In this rather complex pattern, efforts were made to cope with as many of Sam's personal problems as the six weeks available would permit. The treatment included advice on sleep, diet, and drinking habits; encouragement was given relative to his psychological problems, although consultation with a clinical psychologist was probably needed; an eye examination by an opthalmologist was recommended; and an exercise program was prepared designed to develop strength, endurance, and agility; the activities were fundamental gymnastics, weight-lifting, apparatus work, handball, and running.

The PFI increased to 103 by the end of his relatively short training period. Checks were made on a number of the Academy test items and Sam appeared to be safely above the minimum standards he must meet when retaking the test. However, in a letter written about this case at the time, fear was expressed that the "psychological blocks" might defeat him under pressure; and advice was tendered "to check more fully into the psychological factors involved when evaluating his fitness to command troops in tense situations." Subsequently, Sam was re-tested by the Academy and again failed. The "psychological" factor seemed to be the cause, as physically he was able to pass the tests. In the bar vault, his height was sufficient but each time he crashed the bar; in rope climbing, he went part way up on each trial and then slid back down. As a consequence, Sam did not return to the Academy. He was a fine young man, in deportment a credit to the Academy, but apparently he was lacking in physical vigor and emotional stability.[19]

Organic drains. When Robert was first tested as a university freshman, his PFI was 68. The initial case study gave no indication of anything especially wrong. However, he had never participated in a physical education program before so it was thought that lack of exercise was the cause of his unfitness. A program was arranged, but a retest six weeks later showed no gain. He was referred to a physician, who, after examination, gave a satisfactory report. This process was repeated five times—and still no progress and still no apparent reason for his continued low fitness score. Finally, after the sixth retest showed no improvement, Robert was referred to a physician attending the university's athletic teams. In the process of examination, a blood analysis was made, which

---

[19] H. Harrison Clarke, "The Case of Sam," *Physical Fitness News Letter,* University of Oregon, No. 2 (1954), p. 1.

showed a definite low red blood corpuscle count; so, Robert was treated for anemia. Within a short time, his PFI went up 10 points, his face had more color, and he admitted feeling better than he had in over a year.[20]

Joan was a high school girl with a PFI of 84. Her medical record was clear, so she was given a physical activity program designed to improve her strength and endurance. After repeated efforts by the physical educator to improve her fitness without success, Joan's family physician was asked to re-examine her. He found no apparent serious defect, but in removing a wen on her side found a cancerous condition beneath. When she returned to school later, her PFI had risen to 113.[21]

Decrease in strength. Joe was an upperclass university student, 24 years of age, weighed 190 pounds, stood six feet tall, and was a well-built young man. His somatotype was appraised as a 362. This student was a major in physical education and an experienced college wrestler. Throughout the wrestling season, he performed in a superior manner, winning all matches and emerging at the close of the season as the Eastern Intercollegiate 175-pound class champion. At the beginning of the season, his grip strength for each hand was 180 pounds.

After a wrestling match in mid-February, Joe noticed a slight pain in the back of his neck. Believing this was "just a stiff neck," he disregarded it. Around the first of March, he awoke at night with a sharp pain running down his left arm to the fingertips. After a medical check-up, which included an X-ray of the troublesome arm, nothing unusual was found. Joe was given daily heat treatments for the arm and was permitted to continue wrestling. At this time, he was given strength tests again. His right and left grips had dropped to 160 and 120 pounds respectively; these decreases represented 11 per cent for the right hand and 33 per cent for the left hand.

While home during spring vacation, Joe visited his family doctor, due to the development of intermittent numbness in his left arm extending into the thumb and forefinger. Accompanying this trouble was a general lethargic feeling. X-ray pictures revealed that the fifth and sixth cervical vertebrae were out of alignment; the intervertebral disc had a small notch on it which prevented alignment and involved the nerves leading to the arm and hand. Joe was required to wear a Thomas collar while sleeping, and to use the Sayre sling for stretching the neck as a part of each day's exercise. Upon return to the university, he was given grip strength tests again. The right grip had dropped to 140 pounds and the left grip to 90 pounds. Orthopedic exercises were con-

---

[20] Millard L. Rogers, "The Case Study Method," *Journal of Health and Physical Education,* 46, No. 3 (1945), p. 119.

[21] Thomas H. Hines, "A New Emphasis on Health," *Journal of Health and Physical Education,* 10, No. 1 (1939), p. 22.

tinued. When last tested, about six weeks later, the right and left grip strengths were 160 and 130 pounds. Joe was definitely on his way to recovery.[22]

Briefly, there is also the case of Phyllis who had a PFI around 120 when tested while attending an Albany, New York, high school. During her freshman year in college, she began to feel lethargic and found it difficult to study for any length of time. A bright girl, her studies began to fall off. Medical examinations and consultations failed to reveal the cause of the trouble. Finally, she was sent home for rest and recuperation. Her father, who was Chief of the New York State Physical Education Bureau, took her to a school for testing; her FPI had dropped to about 65. The family physician finally diagnosed her condition as thyroid deficiency. With medication, Phyllis was soon on the road to recovery and returned to college to complete her education with distinction.[23]

High PFI's. As indicated earlier, high PFI's may be due either to the presence of hypertension of the organism or to a fine musculature developed through physical activity. An example of the former type of high PFI, although there may still be unexplained factors in the report, is the case of Emanuel, who was an exchange student at Syracuse University from a Central American country. He was an unusually good student and did excellent scholastic work during his first year in college. After registering for physical education, he was tested and his PFI was found to be 128. At the end of his first term, he was re-tested and increased his score to 141; his physical education participation during this period was in soccer and touch football.

During the last week of his sophomore year, Emanuel was re-tested and scored 177. Time prevented a complete case study of this student. However, he failed most of his final examinations, and received such low grades that he was dropped from the university. Since the case presented several unusual aspects, his roommates and close friends were contacted. It was found that when Emanuel had matriculated at the university, his fiancée had also entered the same institution. The couple had quarreled, the engagement was broken, and the young lady returned to Central America. During this period, Emanuel had been under an intense emotional strain, as manifested by extreme nervousness, tenseness, and irritability. His friends had been aware of his problem, but, although they tried, were unable to help him.[24]

Although the following brief report is not a case study, it does

---

[22] Carl E. Willgoose, "The Case of Mr. X," Typewritten report, Syracuse University, 1947.

[23] With apologies to those involved for any inaccuracies in this case study reported from memory.

[24] Rogers, *op. cit.*

indicate that high PFI's may just be due to advanced physical development, certainly a logical deduction. Donna was a high school sophomore in Roseburg, Oregon. She was a petite, 102-pound, 60½-inch girl. Her PFI was 184, an extremely high index, seldom achieved. She had a leg lift of 1200 pounds (with a belt); this score alone surpassed the norm for her age and weight (1179 pounds), a remarkable performance. When questioned about this high score, Donna indicated that she had practiced ballet dancing intensively for several years.

Donna was one of five girls who were found to have very high PFI's in tests conducted in eleven Oregon high schools during a single year by University of Oregon testing teams. In all instances, these girls were very active in either dancing or gymnastics, including work on the trampoline. From brief questioning, their teachers stated they possessed pleasant and relaxed personalities. All of these girls, save one, were most attractive and feminine in appearance. This latter observation gives the lie to the oft expressed concept that strong girls appear masculine and unpresentable.

FITNESS COUNSELING

In the case-study approach described in this chapter, the need to discover the causes of the unfit status of boys and girls was considered essential for improving their physical condition, especially for those who do not respond readily to exercise. Some attention was given to the interview as a phase of this process, including the purposes to be achieved, its confidential nature, the necessity for rapport, and the need for referral to health, guidance, and other school personnel. The utilization of tests and other evaluative instruments in order to better understand the student and his fitness problems was stressed. These procedures, of course, are associated with counseling; however, fitness counseling needs much broader attention, as indicated below.

The purpose of fitness counseling is to help the unfit student to develop self-understanding in relation to the causes of his unfitness and to arrive at the point where he is determined to follow through with appropriate procedures for improving his condition. Interviews may be unscheduled or scheduled. In the unscheduled type, the physical educator may either take advantage of chance meetings with the student or seek him out unobtrusively for a brief visit. Such informal chats can be merely for the purpose of getting better acquainted or just asking him how he is "getting along," or may be utilized to check on some point needed to round out the case study account. In this section, however, suggestions for conducting scheduled interviews will be considered.

1. *Do not use interviews to collect routine information.* Interviews should not be used to collect routine information which is readily avail-

able by other means, as this may make the student restless and reluctant to return for additional counseling.[25] To avoid this danger, the interview should be delayed until after the basic case-study data have been accumulated. The student may answer the Health-Habit Questionnaire and execute other formal tests desired, such as personal-social adjustment tests, prior to the interview. By inspecting such information, the physical educator can gain some understanding of the unfit student and his problems, and, therefore, may begin his interviewing more effectively.

2. *Request preparation of autobiography.* The use of the auto-biography to help the unfit student understand his own condition was mentioned in Chapter 3. This practice will also aid the physical educator to obtain significant facts about a student and his problems which cannot be gotten by other means. Occasionally, personal experiences are too intimate to be revealed in face-to-face situations. Other significant facts cannot be remembered or put in a proper setting by question and answer methods.[26] Thus, the physical educator may well ask each unfit student to prepare a brief written account of his life, including what he considers to be his most significant experiences and their effects upon him. This account should not be limited to the physical aspects of his existence, as it should now be amply clear to the reader that the causes of subpar physical fitness are not so restricted, but can well encompass the total being. Usually, no specific outline of points to be covered should be suggested, since it is the student's expressed insight into and reactions toward his experiences that the counselor desires; however, he may be led to speculate on the reason for his unfit condition. In this sense, the autobiography is a loose form of analysis by the free-association method.

3. *Be prepared for the interview.* The physical educator who has followed the case-study procedures for meeting individual fitness problems described thus far will have acquired the essential materials needed in the interview. Thus, preparation for the interview will be relatively simple, consisting largely of reviewing the available information and noting items which may lead him to the cause of the student's unfitness. In some instances, the cause will not be clear; if such is the case, the initial phase of the interview will need to be exploratory in nature as the physical educator seeks for the reason, in co-operation with the interviewee.

4. *Interviews should be conducted in private.* Except in group therapy, it is almost impossible to provoke a frank discussion with a student in the presence of others; privacy is a necessary condition of the interview. Thus, the confidential nature and integrity of the interview can be

---

[25] E. G. Williamson, *Counseling Adolescents* (New York: McGraw-Hill Book Co., Inc., 1950), p. 139.
[26] *Ibid.*, p. 141.

maintained and rapport may be more easily and completely achieved. There must be co-operation in the interview if action proposals are to be accepted and realized.

5. *Rapport is vital for successful interviews.* The need for rapport between the unfit student and the physical educator was mentioned earlier. It may be reiterated here that very little can be accomplished in improving the fitness of the student without rapport, as it is only through his own efforts that positive results can be achieved. Rapport is "a feeling of understanding, acceptance, and comfort."[27] It can be accomplished in many ways, beginning with a friendly welcome in an attractive environment. The first part of the interview should be spent in just getting acquainted and finding out the interests and activities of the student. Certainly, if an autobiography has been written, many items will be found which can lead to discussions resulting in rapport. Above all, however, rapport is accomplished by the physical educator's warmth, interest, and sincerity. Rapport should not be based on tricks and gimcracks; it must be based on a genuine feeling on the part of both the interviewer and interviewee.

6. *Encourage the unfit person to express true feelings.* The unfit student, especially if he shows indications of social maladjustment, must be encouraged to express his true feelings and thoughts without fear of censure or betrayal of confidence. The physical educator should lead the student toward a better understanding of his own problems and toward ways and means of solving them in order to achieve optimal adjustment.

7. *Listen, provide information, and help.* The physical educator should not monopolize the conversation in an interview. His role is not just to tell the unfit student what is wrong with him and to lecture him on what he should do about it. He should encourage the student to talk about his fitness problems; and he should be willing to listen sympathetically, interjecting occasional questions or comments to keep the conversation going. Silence may sometimes be a good thing, although to some, silences are disturbing; in reality, silence may be part of a good interview, as it provides an opportunity to recapitulate mentally what has been said and to plan the next approach.[28] Questions and statements should be phrased in such a manner as to encourage the student to talk freely. If the interviewer's questions can be answered "Yes" or "No," they may be answered in just that way; such answers tend to stop discussion.[29] In this process, the physical educator can weave into the emerging pattern of thought basic information related to the student's fitness

---

[27] Francis C. Rosecrance and Velma D. Hayden, *School Guidance and Personnel Services* (Boston: Allyn and Bacon, Inc., 1960), p. 66.

[28] Clifford P. Froehlich and John G. Darley, *Studying Students* (Chicago: Science Research Associates, Inc., 1952), p. 135.

[29] *Ibid.*, p. 132.

problem and the action proposal deemed appropriate for him.

8. *Develop a positive outlook.* Occasionally, an unfit student may be on the defensive when first confronted with the fact of his unsatisfactory physical condition. As a consequence, he may be antagonistic in his response to the physical educator. In the interview, it is wise to allow expression of these negative feelings. However, after rapport has been established, the student should be led to take a second look at his problem. "It is by looking at both the negative and positive facts and feelings about a problem, plus the slow development of more objectivity, and the bringing to bear of as much information as possible, that one is ever able to develop insight and to determine more satisfying future action."[30]

9. *Use motivational approaches effectively.* The whole case-study approach is motivational in nature. It contains such elements as the use of objective evaluation in demonstrating fitness status and in determining the results achieved from fitness efforts, the assembly of significant information about the student and utilizing it in his best interest, and participation in a sympathetic and personally helpful interview. Otherwise, the fundamental approach to motivation will vary with age and sex and from individual to individual in accordance with a variety of personal interests. For example: some students will respond to facts showing that adequate fitness is necessary for general well-being, for full effectiveness in performing daily tasks, and in enjoying life fully; some boys want to be strong and would like to emulate athletes; generally, girls wish to improve their appearance and to be able to move gracefully. The physical educator needs to watch the reactions of each unfit student to motivational approaches and should not assume that all students respond alike.

10. *Prepare a written summary following each interview.* Memory can be a most unreliable recorder of conversations and interviews. Therefore, a written summary should be prepared immediately after each interview. This summary should include the significant facts learned in the interview, anecdotal records of the student's reactions and comments, his fundamental interests and aspirations, his responses to motivational approaches, and the like.

PHYSICAL FITNESS COUNCIL

As a general rule, unfit students should be re-tested at intervals of approximately six weeks in order to reveal the progress—or lack of progress or retrogression—made by each. If fair improvement is recorded, the physical educator may feel that the treatment regimen adopted is effective, at least for the moment. However, as indicated

---

[30] Rosecrance and Hayden, *op. cit.,* p. 67.

earlier, it is necessary to initiate case studies, if this has not already been done, for students who fail to make significant gains. Case studies would be proper, also, for any unfit boy or girl who registers an initial gain, but whose subsequent progress toward adopted fitness standards stops short of their realization.

Where progress toward fitness goals does not occur after case studies have been initiated, a more comprehensive approach to the student's fitness problem will be necessary. Rechecks on living habits should be made, additional interviews with the unfit student should be held, supplementary tests may be used to help locate causative factors, and quite generally, the school health service should be consulted. There are several other specialists in the school or college who may aid in the search for causes of unfitness in individual cases. Depending on the school system or institution, help may come from the guidance counselor, psychologist, social worker, home economist, nutritionist, health educator, administrator, and classroom teacher. If not available in the school, the services of certain of these specialists may be obtained in the community through the Public Health Service or other agencies.

The formation of a Physical Fitness Council to assist with the follow-up of difficult unfitness cases is usually desirable. The permanent membership of the council might consist of the school physician, school nurse, guidance counselor, health educator, school administrator, and the physical educator. If the school or college has a psychologist, social worker, or nutritionist, these individuals might also be included. The classroom or home-room teacher should be invited to meet with the council when the case involves one of his or her students.

As a matter of course, the physical educator should thoroughly acquaint the council members with the nature and progress of the program for physically unfit students. Obviously, this orientation is essential for the full co-operation of all members and for maximal effectiveness of the Council's efforts.

The Fitness Council members are likely to be busy people. Therefore, the physical educator should solicit their help only in essential cases. In each instance, a brief of the case study as it is known should be prepared in advance and presented at the meeting. This brief should include an account of the steps taken to improve the student's fitness and the success or failure of these steps. Following this presentation, the council should discuss the case, each member contributing as he can from his knowledge of the student. A recommended action proposal should result.

The student under consideration does not necessarily need to be present at the council session. However, there may be instances when his presence would be desirable in order for him to answer questions and to help find a solution to his difficulty. In such cases, a friendly and helpful attitude toward the student should prevail; and, he should be made to feel as comfortable and relaxed as possible.

The confidential nature of the case study and the interview has been stressed in the case-study approach to meeting the needs of unfit boys and girls. Taking this information to the council, then, could well be construed as a breach of this agreement. Consequently, it should be done only with permission of the student. If rapport has been thoroughly established and if the student understands that this action is in his best interest, such permission will be readily given. However, it must now be stressed that all deliberations of the council on individual case studies must remain confidential within the group—and this confidence must be strictly upheld.

Perhaps it might be well to inject a word of warning. Caution should be exercised to avoid making students so conscious of their physical condition that ill health becomes a phobia with them. A frank discussion of his physical condition should be helpful for any student. But if he is constantly met on every side with reminders of his unfitness he is apt to react with apprehension, which in itself could cause lack of fitness, an "inferiority complex," or an attitude antagonistic to the program. On the other hand, the ignoring of students' unfitness is obviously an even worse expedient. Common sense and propriety must always prevail when the physical educator discusses the problems of unfitness with a student. The physical fitness program presented, however, has a distinct advantage in that progress can be measured and proved to the boy or girl, a fact that will counteract to a great extent unfavorable psychological reactions. The student can see his progress and enjoy the emotional satisfaction of work successfully accomplished. Nevertheless, good judgment should be exercised in the follow-up approach, especially in regard to those few students not responding to treatment.

SUMMARY

In this chapter, the case-study approach to meeting the needs of unfit boys and girls was presented. This approach is based upon the concept that the causes of a subfit condition may be varied; the assumption that only exercise is needed to improve the status of all unfit students was considered untenable. It is true that, in the majority of cases, the treatment of unfit students will be concentrated in the physical activity program and in the modification of living (including health) habits. However, there are a sizeable number of physically subpar individuals who need much more. Most often, in these cases, an understanding of the total personality is necessary. The recognition of the interaction of body, mind, and spirit becomes inevitable for any physical educator dealing fully with the problems of students who are deficient in basic physical fitness elements.

Case-study procedures were described as a means of identifying the causes of unfit conditions in individual students, following which appropriate action proposals for the improvement of fitness can be made. Illustrations were presented from actual cases of physically unfit boys and girls treated in physical education.

Such procedures as those described in this chapter require adaptation to local school and college situations. Moreover, the process is difficult to perform and requires both staff and program time. These are handicaps, to be sure, so practical suggestions should be sought to expedite the necessary steps in inaugurating and conducting such programs. Certainly, the presence of handicaps does not justify ignoring the problem of the unfit individual; universal recognition and support of this approach would greatly advance the effectiveness of physical education in its service to the physical fitness of America's youth.

SELECTED REFERENCES

Froehlich, Clifford P. and John M. Darley, *Studying Students.* Chicago: Science Research Associates, 1952.

Hines, Thomas H., "A New Emphasis on Health," *Journal of Health and Physical Education,* 10, No. 1 (January, 1939), 22.

Rogers, Millard L., "The Case Study Method," *Journal of Heatlh and Physical Education,* 46, No. 3 (March, 1945), 119.

Rosecrance, Francis C. and Velma D. Hayden, *School Guidance and Personnel Services.* Boston: Allyn and Bacon, Inc., 1960.

Williamson, E. G., *Counseling Adolescents.* New York: McGraw-Hill Book Co., Inc., 1950.

7

Exercise for the Physically Unfit

THE WAYS BY WHICH BOYS AND GIRLS WHO ARE DEFICIENT in basic physical fitness elements can be identified were described in Chapter 4; the case-study approach for meeting the individual fitness needs of those who do not respond readily to exercise was presented in Chapter 6. In this chapter, the use of exercise to improve the physical status of the unfit will be considered. Emphasis will be placed on the development of muscular strength and endurance and circulatory-respiratory endurance. Body flexibility improvement will be included in connection with strength development.

PRINCIPLES OF EXERCISE FOR FITNESS

In planning exercise regimens for unfit individuals, the specific physical status of each student should be known. No formulae exist to guide physical educators in determining the specific types and amounts of exercise which should be prescribed at each stage of the unfit individual's progress toward the realization of adequate standards of fitness. The following principles may be used as guides in the preparation of exercise regimens.

1. *Exercise should be adapted to the individual's exercise tolerance.* Exercise tolerance refers to the ability of the individual to execute a given exercise, series of exercises, or activities involving exercise, in

accordance with a specified dosage without undue discomfort or fatigue. An exercise performed as specified which is easy for the individual falls short of his exercise tolerance; on the other hand, an exercise which is either impossible for the individual to perform or leaves him in a distressful state exceeds a reasonable interpretation of exercise tolerance.

For the most part, exercise tolerance must be judged by the physical educator through observation of the student, although some rough estimates are possible from his physical or motor fitness scores; the lower the score, of course, the less his exercise tolerance. Furthermore, the scores on the different items composing the test battery may give information related to the student's exercise tolerance. For example, if the student cannot chin himself, the inclusion of chins in his exercise plan would be useless. Such indicators as the degree of discomfort during exercise and the amount of breathlessness following exercise are helpful in judging the tolerance level. Also, the presence of exhaustion, slow recuperation, and excessively sore muscles would indicate that the exercise assigned was too severe. With unfit groups, exercise tolerance will be low at the start, but should gradually rise as the fitness program continues and is effective.

2. *Overloading should be applied to induce a higher level of performance.* In overloading, the individual's exercise is increased in intensity or extended for a longer time than normally. Thus, overload is a relative term; a slight overload exceeds normal activity to a small degree, while a heavy overload equals the maximal performance of which the individual is capable at the moment.

In order to develop either strength or endurance effectively, therefore, the individual must be pushed beyond his customary performance. Athletic coaches use this principle routinely. In track, work-outs are planned to extend the runner more and more as his exercise tolerance increases until his maximum is reached during the competitive season; in football and basketball, scrimmages and other procedures are utilized to accomplish the same end. For the unfit individual, too, overloading means increased intensity and dosage within his tolerance level.

3. *The exercise plan should provide for progression.* Progression is intimately involved with the first two principles. The exercise plan starts with an understanding of the individual's exercise tolerance, then, within this tolerance level, an exercise regimen is prepared to provide for overloading the muscles to develop strength or for increasing the demands on the circulatory-respiratory systems to improve cardiovascular endurance. If the exercise regimen stopped at this point, some improvement in fitness elements could reasonably be expected, but it would soon cease as the body adjusted to the new requirements in output. Both normal exercise and exercise tolerance levels have risen. Progression must now

be effected by increasing exercise in some logical way, thus keeping its demands ahead of the improvement made.

Progression may be accomplished by increasing either the intensity or the duration of exercise. In strength development, the common method of intensifying exercise is by adding to the resistance against which muscles work, as by increasing the amount of weight in weight training. Greater intensity, however, can be achieved by increasing the cadence (speed) of the lift and leaving the load unchanged. Progression in duration for this form of development is accomplished by requiring more repetitions of the same load. In circulatory-respiratory endurance, intensity is increased by stepping up the speed at which a cardiovascular activity, such as running, is performed; duration is enhanced by prolonging the time the activity is continued at the previous pace. Untrained persons should not be overloaded by increasing both intensity and duration at the same time. It is probably best first to increase duration a bit; later, to increase intensity; then, repeat the pattern as often as desired in keeping with the individual's progress.

4. *The type of body exercised should be considered.* Generally speaking, the dominant endomorph will score low on tests of physical and motor fitness; the dominant mesomorph will excel in tests of strength and power; the dominant ectomorph, if he has at least a moderate amount of mesomorphy, will do well on tests involving running and agility. Although not adequately studied, it may be conjectured that many boys and girls in classes for the physically unfit are either above average in endomorphy and/or below in mesomorphy.[1]

In planning exercise programs, therefore, account should be taken of the fact that the dominant endomorphic boy is seriously handicapped in ability to perform physical activities and the dominant mesomorph is favored in this respect. In support of this view, Clarke, Irving, and Heath[2] found that no boys aged nine through 15 years who were dominant endomorphs could chin themselves. Of 18 boys in this somatotype category, only two could perform a one-half chin. At 14 years of age, dominant mesomorphs averaged eight chins, while dominant ectomorphs and mid-types had mean performances of five and four chins respectively. For all boys in their sample, the mean Physical Fitness Indices for the different somatotype categories were as follows: mesomorphs, 124; ectomorphs, 121; mid-types, 116; endo-mesomorphs, 104; and endomorphs, 88. It should be added that the boys in the entire sample reported here were a superior group physically as compared with national standards.

---

[1] For a description of somatotypes, see pages 62-64.
[2] H. Harrison Clarke, Robert N. Irving, and Barbara H. Heath, "Comparison of Maturity, Structural, and Strength Measures for Five Somatotype Categories of Boys Nine Through Fifteen Years of Age," *Research Quarterly*, 32, No. 4 (December, 1961), p. 449.

5. *Consideration should be given to the individual's relative maturity.* The relative maturity of the unfit student may be a factor in his ability to do well on tests of some physical fitness elements. Clarke and Harrison[3] found this to be true for strength tests but not for motor fitness items. These investigators contrasted various physical and motor performances of boys classified as advanced, normal, and retarded on the basis of skeletal age for each of three age groups, nine, 12, and 15 years. In general at each age, the advanced maturity group had significantly higher means than the normal maturity group and this latter group in turn had significantly higher means than the retarded maturity group on such gross strength tests as the Strength Index and the average of 12 cable-tension tests. However, for pull-ups and push-ups, significant differences between the means were not obtained; at two ages, this was also the case for the standing broad jump.

The determination of relative maturity, i.e., whether the boy or girl is advanced, normal, or retarded for his or her age, has its difficulties. The use of skeletal age, which is based on an assessment of an X-ray of the hand and wrist is now generally confined to the research laboratory. During adolescence, some estimation of maturity can be made by judging pubescent development. For girls, the date of menarche is also a helpful index. Pubescent development, however, is a crude indicator of maturity and has limited use, as shown by Clarke and Degutis[4] in a study of 10, 13, and 16 year old boys. These investigators found that, at these three ages, physical maturation was differentiated by this means most effectively at 13 years, although it was not so sensitive to maturational change as skeletal age. At 16 years of age, maturational differentiation by pubescent assessment was much more limited. At 10 years of age, little or no value was attributed to this method.

6. *Individuals must desire to improve.* The desire of the unfit student, his basic attitude toward his own physical condition, is an essential factor in the attempt to improve his fitness status. Every effort must be made to secure the student's full cooperation, as the effectiveness of his exercise prescription will only be in proportion to the degree of his voluntary participation. Inasmuch as motivation has been presented in Chapter 3, additional development of this topic will not be included here.

7. *Advance the unfit individual's psychological limits of effort.* For unfit students, psychological tolerance for strenuous exercise is usually reached long before their physiological limits are attained. The psycho-

---

[3] H. Harrison Clarke and James C. E. Harrison, "The Relationship Between Selected Physical and Motor Factors and the Skeletal Maturity of Nine, Twelve, and Fifteen Year Old Boys," *Research Quarterly,* 33, No. 1 (March, 1962), p. 13.

[4] H. Harrison Clarke and Ernest W. Degutis, "Relationships Between Selected Physical and Motor Factors and the Pubescent Development of Ten, Thirteen, and Sixteen Year Old Boys," *Research Quarterly,* 33, No. 2 (October, 1961).

logical limit is frequently conditioned by habit, boredom, slight aches, breathlessness, and by such mental factors as anxiety and fear of physical harm. All too frequently, such mildly distressful feelings halt exercise before there has been any real overloading; consequently, no appreciable increase in strength or endurance results. Here, some judgment must be exercised, since certain of the factors related to psychological limits also serve as safeguards, preventing overstrain.

Except for participants in highly competitive athletic events, very few boys and girls have ever been fully extended physiologically. Actually, most live through the years of their youth—and, hence, through life—at a low level of energy expenditure. The stepping up of physical effort in intensity and duration is most desirable. For the unfit student, this process may be a gradual progression, in which he constantly attempts to improve his own former performances. Psychological tolerance for exercise, especially for the unfit, can best be developed in this way.

Thus, there may be considerable difference between a person's physiologic capacity and the output he is able to express through muscular effort at any given time; psychological limits are generally imposed in strength and endurance activities involving "all-out" performances. The "cracking" of this psychologic barrier was demonstrated by Ikai and Steinhaus[5] by use of hypnosis, a loud noise made by a starter's pistol, and a shout produced by the subject himself. Pastor[6] demonstrated the value of simply setting goals, as opposed to urging subjects to exercise to exhaustion on the ergograph, in increasing the amount of work done by college men. After considerable experimentation, Lawther[7] observed that a subject's maximum effort is affected by his degree of motivation, his background of punishing experience, and his willingness to endure the pain of all-out effort.

8. *Physical development should be tested and recorded at set times.* A number of the exercise activities frequently included in unfit programs, such as chinning, sit-ups, dips, weight lifting, and the like, are automatically self-testing. This self-testing may be formalized by use of individual progress charts, upon which the student records his performances on a particular day each week. Individual items on the physical or motor fitness test used to identify unfit students may be included on the progress chart as well, with a repetition of the entire

---

[5]Michio Ikai and Arthur H. Steinhaus, "Some Psychological Factors Modifying the Expression of Human Strength," *Health and Fitness in the Modern World* (Chicago: Athletic Institute, 1961), p. 148.

[6] Paul J. Pastor, "Threshold Muscular Fatigue Level and Strength Recovery of Elbow Flexor Muscles Resulting from Varying Degrees of Muscular Work," *Archives of Physical Medicine and Rehabilitation,* 40, No. 6 (June, 1959), p. 247.

[7] John D. Lawther, "The Pennsylvania State University Studies on Strength Decrement, Maintenance, and Related Aspects," *61st Annual Proceedings of the College Physical Education Association,* 1958, p. 142.

test every five or six weeks. It may also be desirable to record body weight from week to week; some unfit students should increase, some decrease in weight. These charts can be excellent motivational devices. More important, however, they provide constant checks on student progress.

In the light of these eight principles, the question may now be asked: How should an exercise program for any particular unfit student be prepared? This is an individual process to be studied by trial for each student. The first step is to determine his exercise tolerance by trying him out on different activities, including both strengthening and endurance elements. Thus, the unfit individual who cannot chin or dip should not be expected to do apparatus work, but should start on the mats with simple conditioning drills and modified chinning and dipping. If he cannot do sit-ups or leg raisings, modified forms of these exercises must also be used at the start. If "once around the track" leaves him exhausted, the distance must be shortened or the pace lessened. Eventually, the amount of work the individual can do without unreasonable discomfort will be determined. The other principles given can then be applied. The starting point, however, must be a proper evaluation of his exercise tolerance.

STRENGTH DEVELOPMENT

In selecting the right kind and amount of physical activity for any particular unfit boy or girl, the physical educator should consider the place of strength in the total physical fitness pattern. As viewed in this book, strength is a basic element; emphasis upon its development is vital for those who are sub-standard. However, for total-body fitness, exercise should not be limited to strengthening activities, but should be balanced properly by endurance (circulatory-respiratory) activities. Moreover, provisions should be made within the framework of the strength-endurance activity program for other important developments, including skill, agility, flexibility, co-ordination, grace, poise, and so forth.

ISOMETRIC VS. ISOTONIC EXERCISE

In this presentation, *muscular strength* is defined as the maximum contraction that can be voluntarily applied in a single contraction. Two types of muscular endurance are recognized: *isometric*, whereby a maximum static muscular contraction is held; and *isotonic*, whereby the muscle continues to raise and lower a submaximal load.

A great many studies have been conducted to determine the relative effectiveness of isometric and isotonic exercises and of various systems of progressive resistance exercise in the development of muscular strength and muscular endurance. These studies have been summarized by Clarke; the conclusions drawn from his synthesis follow.[8]

1. Both isometric and isotonic forms of exercise improve muscular strength. However, the evidence shows little if any difference in the effectiveness of the two forms in achieving strength increase; the same result was obtained for different systems of progressive resistance exercise. Considerable variation in individual strength improvement exists for both forms of exercise.

2. No study has verified the strength gain of 5 per cent per week for ten weeks (50 per cent for the entire period) from a single six-second daily contraction against resistance consisting of two-thirds of the muscle's strength, as reported by Hettinger and Mueller.[9] Apparently, a more realistic, although perhaps still generous, figure is nearer 2 per cent each week.

3. The effects of isotonic exercise favor the improvement of muscular endurance and the retention of muscular strength following the cessation of exercise for a period of time. Isometric contractions restrict blood circulation to a greater extent than do isotonic contractions. For isometric work, Clarke[10] found that the amount of oxygen, oxygen debt, and total oxygen requirement increase linearly in proportion to the size of the load; this constriction of circulation with attendant effects on the oxygen supply to the muscles logically restricts the development of muscular endurance when training with isometric exercise.

4. Hypotheses have been supported that the amount of tension developed in a muscle is a major factor in determining strength improvement and that the work done per unit of time is the factor essential in the extension of muscular strength and muscular endurance performances.

5. Nearly all studies on the conditioning effects of isometric and isotonic regimens of exercise utilized very limited training sessions. Possibly these brief exercise sessions are insufficient for adequate strength development or for any one method of exercising to achieve superiority over another. It may be contended that a person's rate of strength improvement depends largely upon the degree he overloads and that, in most of these studies, the overload principle has not been adequately applied.

---

[8] H. Harrison Clarke, "Development of Volitional Muscle Strength as Related to Fitness," *Exercise and Fitness* (Chicago: Athletic Institute, 1960), pp. 200-212.

[9] T. Hettinger and E. A. Mueller, "Muskelleistung and Muskeltraining," *Arbeitsphysiologie*, 15, No. 2 (1953), p. 111.

[10] David H. Clarke, "The Energy Cost of Isometric Exercise," *Research Quarterly*, 31, No. 1 (March, 1960), p. 3.

Hellebrandt and Houtz[11] have shed some light on the mechanism of muscle training in an experimental demonstration of the overload principle. In their application, the overload principle implies that the limits of performance must be persistently extended to improve muscle strength; and the rate of improvement depends on the willingness of the subject to overload. Comparisons were made with the manner in which athletes extend themselves in training for and participating in their events. The following conclusions were drawn from their experimentation. (a) The slope gradient of the training curve varies with the magnitude of the stress imposed, the frequency of the practice sessions, and the duration of the overload effort. (b) Mere repetition of contractions which places little stress on the neuromuscular system has little effect on the functional capacity of the skeletal muscles. (c) The amount of work done per unit of time is the critical variable upon which extension of the limits of performance depends. (d) The speed with which functional capacity increases suggests that the central nervous system changes contribute an important component to training. (c) The ability to develop maximal tension appears to be dependent on the proprioceptive facilitation with which overloading is associated. Hellebrandt and Houtz further demonstrated that currently popular systems of progressive resistance exercise, such as the DeLorme and the Oxford techniques, are conducted at a low level of overload.

STRENGTHENING ACTIVITIES [12]

As will be surmised from the above, in choosing physical activities to develop strength, those which offer the greatest resistance to muscles should be selected. In this section, various ways by which resistance may be applied to muscles are presented.

Resistance supplied by parts of the body. In this category, the legs, arms, and trunk may supply the resistance elements, as is the case in "conditioning" drills, football "grass drills," "guerrilla exercises," Danish drills, and the like. Although calisthenics are in disrepute with many physical educators today (largely because of the atrocious manner in which they have been conducted), nevertheless they are valuable in developmental programs, especially when individually arranged. The dosage of exercise can be controlled, especially for convalescents and extreme sub-strength students; the exercise series can be systematically planned to cover all muscle groups of the body with emphasis being

---

11 F. A. Hellebrandt and Sara Jane Houtz, "Mechanism of Muscle Training in Man: Experimental Demonstration of the Overload Principle," *Physical Therapy Review*, 36, No. 6 (June, 1956), p. 371.

12 H. Harrison Clarke, *Development of the Sub-Strength Individual* (St. Louis: Fred Medart Products, Inc., 1951).

placed on areas of greatest need; and progression can be regulated from very mild forms to vigorous and exhaustive efforts. Also, exercises of this type may be performed daily at home as special apparatus and exercise rooms are not required. Excellent systems of mat exercises can be devised which will provide for the development of body control, flexibility, and good posture, as well as increased strength. With good motivation of the unfit individual and with the application of appropriate methods, an enthusiastic response can be obtained and excellent results can be achieved.

Resistance supplied by inanimate objects. Utilizing objects of various types and weights, the amount of exercise can be precisely prescribed through specification of the amount of weight lifted, the number of repetitions, and the cadence of movements. Furthermore, exercises can be designed to include all the large-muscle groups of the body, and exercise concentration can be placed on various muscles as desired. Barbell exercises, use of weighted dumbbells, log drills, drills with iron wands, relays and races carrying weights, and the like, are examples of this type of exercise. These activities, properly applied, are probably the most effective methods of rapidly improving muscular strength and muscular endurance.

Resistance applied by entire body weight. The entire body weight can be used as the resistance medium. Arm strength is developed through chinning the bar, dipping from the parallel bars, use of traveling rings and overhead ladder, some forms of dance, and exercises on the horse, horizontal bar, and parallel bars. Development of leg muscles through vaulting from beatboard or springboard and bouncing on the trampoline, and constant use of abdominal and trunk muscles in lifting the legs and controlling the body are also effective in physical development. Agility, co-ordination, neuromuscular control, flexibility, and poise are other benefits derived from modern dance, apparatus exercises, and tumbling exercises on the mats. The unfit individual, however, especially if he is subpar in strength, will not be able to perform even the simplest exercises on the apparatus. Thus, this form of strength development activity has limited usefulness until strength sufficient to support the body with some facility has been developed by other means.

Resistance applied by another individual. For sub-strength individuals well advanced in development, exercises in which resistance is applied by another person may be used. Thus, wrestling, combatives, tug-of-war, and various pushes and pulls have excellent body-building values. Caution needs to be exercised, however, in utilizing such activities for unfit individuals, until they have been conditioned sufficiently to benefit from them.

ENDURANCE DEVELOPMENT

Circulatory-respiratory endurance is the second basic element in physical fitness as proposed in this book. Activities for the development of this element require moderate contractions of large-muscle groups for relatively long periods of time; circulatory and respiratory systems must be stimulated. In order to provide definite overload for this form of development, the activity should be sufficiently severe and prolonged as to require a definite adjustment of the circulation and respiration to the effort. In other words, it is essential to continue the activity well beyond the stage of "second wind," until a pronounced oxygen debt is incurred.

The basic forms of exercise to develop circulatory-respiratory endurance are those which involve self-propulsion of the body over a distance. Particularly desirable forms are running and swimming, since these exercises can be reasonably well controlled. Thus, distance, speed, and duration can be specified in accordance with the physical fitness status and the exercise tolerance of the individual. Progression in the amount and nature of the exercise can also be planned from day to day. Other activities such as climbing, skiing, and skating have similar values.

Many sports also have a high endurance element. Among those of greatest value in this respect are soccer, basketball, speedball, handball, ice hockey, lacrosse, water sports, and other sports and games requiring sustained running. But, some caution should be employed in recommending these sports for unfit individuals, as the competitive element in these activities may lead to over-exertion. In advanced stages of conditioning, however, such activities, when sustained, are good developers of circulatory-respiratory endurance, provided the student has sufficient skill to permit maximum participation. They also develop fast reactions, quick responses to rapidly and constantly changing situations, agility, and co-ordination. Further, when properly conducted, a host of improved personality and character traits will result from sports engagement.

CONDITIONING EXERCISES

From early times, the physical education literature has abounded with descriptions of conditioning exercises. These have been variously known as calisthenics, free exercises, formal drills, grass drills, guerrilla exercises, and the like. It would be next to impossible to prepare a complete list of exercises of this sort, probably running into the thousands in number, which have been proposed. Furthermore, every qualified physical educator has received instruction in such exercises as a part of his professional preparation, and has, no doubt, developed a series of conditioning exercises which he believes to be effective.

In this book, no effort is made to provide a firm set of conditioning exercises for unfit boys and girls, nor to recommend the number of repetitions for each. Rather, emphasis is placed on the need for a systematic sequence of exercises designed to cover the major muscle groups of the body; and the progression of the exercises presented is indicated, so that the basic principles of exercise discussed earlier in this chapter may be applied. Thus, the exercises which follow should be considered primarily as suggestive, although they may be of immediate, practical value for those who need to plan exercise regimens for the physically unfit for the first time. Necessarily, because of the extensive coverage of this book, the presentation of conditioning exercises will be quite limited.

The primary purpose of conditioning exercises is to develop muscular strength and muscular endurance, although some effect on circulatory-respiratory endurance is sometimes possible. Also, many exercises contribute to the development of other motor fitness elements, such as trunk flexibility, balance, power, body control, and agility. The following exercises are classified according to parts of the body primarily involved; obviously, however, few of them can be so restricted, and most have multiple applications.

WARM-UP EXERCISES

Warm-up exercises should introduce the conditioning series in order to "loosen" the muscles, accelerate the circulation, and get the student into the mood for exercise. Usually, these exercises are of a relatively mild nature, but they can be carried into endurance stages if desired.

Arm swinging. With the feet slightly apart and flat on the floor, rhythmically swing the arms to shoulder height, forward and back for one series and sideward and back for another. *Progression:* (a) swing arms to overhead position; (b) perform exercise with weight in each hand.

Trunk bending with arm swings. With feet well apart, swing arms forward overhead, bending trunk and neck backward; swing arms downward and as far between legs as possible, bending trunk and neck forward and bending knees; the exercise is executed rhythmically. *Progression:* Perform exercise with weight in each hand, increasing amount progressively. Trunk flexibility is involved in this warm-up exercise.

Running in place. Running in place can be performed mildly, simulating a jog, with the feet just clearing the floor and with arms keeping pace in a relaxed manner. *Progression:* Build up tempo to a vigorous movement with knees raised high and arms "pumping" hard. (Running, of course, may also be performed around gymnasium, playing field, or track.)

Bouncing. As with running in place, bouncing can be performed mildly by making low jumps from both feet. *Progression:* (a) increase heights of bounces until maximum height is reached; (b) perform bounces from one foot at a time, then change.

Rope skipping. This is an interesting variation of the warm-up type of exercise.

ARM AND SHOULDER EXTENSOR EXERCISES

While a number of conditioning exercises can be described specifically for the development of the strength and endurance of the arm and shoulder girdle muscles, many exercises and activities intended to develop other parts of the body involve strenuous use of these muscles as well. However, special exercises for conditioning the arm and shoulder extensors are given here.

Push-up or dip. The push-up or dip form of exercise has many variations and can be adapted to the condition of any boy or girl. The *wall push-away* is the simplest and easiest form of this general type of exercise, and is performed as follows: Stand with feet away from wall (distance may be adjusted to the individual's tolerance); place hands on wall at shoulder height; with body straight from heels to head, bend elbows permitting chin to touch wall; push away slowly until arms are straight, and continue. (If a wall is not available, push-aways can be performed against hand resistance supplied by a partner.) *Progression:* The following systematic series of "push-away" progressions is possible.

(a) *Dips from knees.* Lie face-down with knees bent and place hands on floor just outside shoulders; straighten elbows and push shoulders up keeping body straight to a position resting on hands and knees; slowly bend elbows until chest touches floor, still keeping body completely straight; push back to starting position, and continue.

(b) *Dips from bench.* Take position of front-leaning rest with hands on bench, chair, bleachers, or shoulders of a partner on all fours; the fully extended arms and body should form a right angle with weight resting on hands and balls of feet and with body straight from head to heels; lower body slowly by bending elbows until chest touches support, keeping body straight; push back to starting position, and continue. (If dips cannot be done, substitute partial dips.)

(c) *Full dips.* Do the same exercise as bench dips, but with hands resting on floor.

(d) *Dips with feet support.* Do the same exercise as full dips, but with feet raised and resting on a bench, chair, bleachers, or shoulders of a partner on all fours. (Height of feet support can be raised as desired.)

(e) *Partner full dips.* Do the same exercise as full dips, but with a partner straddling legs and leaning his weight on exerciser's shoulders (double full-dip position).

(f) *Parallel bar push-ups.* Grasp ends of parallel bars and jump to free-arm support; lower full body weight until elbows are at less than right angle; raise body without kicking, kipping, or swinging until elbows are straight, and continue.

Stick push. As an isometric exercise for arm and shoulder extensor muscles, place wand, or one-inch dowel, across thighs; push hard and maintain maximum pressure for ten seconds, rest for ten seconds, and continue. Some padding for thighs may be desirable in performing this exercise.

ARM AND SHOULDER FLEXOR EXERCISES

Exercises for the arm and shoulder flexor muscles are not as plentiful or as easy to give as those for the extensor muscles. However, the flexor muscles are in special need of exercise and definite provisions should be made to accomplish this purpose. Many boys cannot chin the bar at all; and others can only perform this feat once or twice. A comparable situation exists for girls.

The use of full chins has not been a common practice in physical education for girls. However, many girls can perform this movement, and, quite probably, many more could if conditioned for it. In a study of 900 girls from seven to seventeen years of age, Ross[13] found that 28 per cent could chin at least once; the range for the different ages was from 19 per cent at eight years to 35 percent at eleven years.

Pull-ups or chins. In performing the well known "chinning the bar" exercise, the choice of grip used, the forward or reverse, should be considered. With the reverse grip (palms rear), the biceps muscle is in a more favorable position to perform; because of the pronation of the forearm in doing chins with forward grip, the biceps is handicapped somewhat in pulling the body up. With the forward grip, however, the pronator teres muscle is placed on stretch and exercised; this is not the case, at least to the same degree, with the reverse grip. The pupil is more prone to lower the body all the way when the forward grip is used, due to better proprioceptive sense; however, the number of chins will be less with this grip than when the reverse grip is used.[14] *Progression:* Progressions for the pull-up type of test are as follows.

(a) *Straddle chins.* Take back-lying position, clasping hands of a partner who stands erect astride the body; chin from this position keeping body straight from heels to head. If this position is·too difficult, perform movement from hips rather than heels.

---

[13] William D. Ross, "The Relationship of Selected Measures to Performance of the Hanging in Arm-Flexed Position Test for Girls," Microcarded Master's thesis, University of Oregon, 1960.

[14] For this analysis, acknowledgment is made to Professor Peter O. Sigerseth, Instructor in Anatomy, School of Health, Physical Education, and Recreation, University of Oregon.

(b) *Modified chins.* Use horizontal bar, or wand held by others, adjusted to height of apex of student's sternum; grasp bar with selected grip; slide feet under bar until body and arms form a right angle, with heels resting on floor; perform chins from this position, keeping body straight from heels to head. By adjusting height of bar, exercise tolerance can be met and progression can be achieved; the higher the bar for this exercise, the easier it is to perform.

(c) *Full chins.* Perform chins grasping horizontal bar high enough so that body hangs free with feet clear of floor (otherwise, bend knees so feet do not touch); perform chins pulling body weight, without kicks, jerks, or kips. If full chins are still too difficult, perform partial chins.

Hanging in arm-flexed position. This is an arm and shoulder flexor exercise which is primarily isometric. Stand on support, grasp horizontal bar with selected grip; flex elbows to permit chin to be at level of bar; after support is removed, hold position for given length of time. *Progression:* Increase time position is held and increase number of times exercise is performed.

Stick pull. As another isometric exercise for the arm and shoulder flexor muscles, the stick pull is useful. For this exercise place wand under buttocks and lift, maintaining contraction for a given length of time. *Progression:* Increase intensity of contraction, increase length of time contraction is held, and increase the number of times this exercise is performed. With the application of some ingenuity, other means for pulling and pushing isometrically can be devised, using ropes or other objects or against resistance supplied by a partner.

Apparatus. A number of pieces of apparatus may be available in the gymnasium or may be improvised and installed outdoors in a special exercise area, which may be used effectively not only for unfit boys and girls but for all pupils, even those at the highest fitness levels. An especially effective use of such apparatus has been made by Le Protti[15] to develop high school boys to a high level of physical fitness. With the necessary apparatus, pupils may climb ropes, travel by hand from one ring to another or across an overhead ladder, and traverse hand-to-hand the length of parallel bars. Once the unfit student has acquired the strength to work out on such apparatus, these exercises are enjoyable, challenging, and self-testing in nature. They can be utilized as part of the regular conditioning class, or can be used to end the physical education period as the class members follow each other through one or more of these devices.

---

[15] Stan Le Protti, "La Sierra's Fitness Program," *Scholastic Coach*, 31, No. 1 (September, 1961), p. 60.

Leg raises. Leg raises can be adapted to nearly any degree of exercise tolerance of the abdominal muscles. A mild form of this exercise is presented first. Lie on back, hands at side, head resting on floor, knees straight; bend right knee, lifting foot off floor and bringing thigh to a vertical position; lower leg to starting position; repeat with opposite leg, and continue. This and the following progressions can be made more strenuous by clasping hands behind head and raising first the head and later the head and shoulders off the floor while performing the exercise. *Progression:* (a) Perform bent-knee leg raises with both legs together, but without arching lumbar spine; (b) Perform same series of leg raises with knees straight; (c) With both legs raised, knees straight, and arms at side, continue leg raise movement on overhead until hips are raised and body weight is on shoulders, reach as far as possible over head with feet (touch the floor, if possible); (d) With the legs raised, weight on shoulders, and hands supporting hips, add scissors or bicycling movements, reaching out each time to stretch the hamstring muscles.

Trunk curl-ups. Trunk curl-ups, or sit-ups, are common exercises in conditioning routines. This exercise should be performed by curling up to a sitting position, as its name implies; this is accomplished first by raising the head, then the shoulders, and finally each vertebra in turn until the erect position of the trunk is reached; the return to the starting position should be in reverse order, a curl-down. Some method of holding down the feet will usually be necessary; this may be done by a partner, by the use of straps firmly secured, or by placing the toes under a heavy object, such as a barbell. For some unfit boys and girls, this type of exercise may be too difficult at first and must be preceded by leg raises or other easier abdominal exercises.

A simple form of this exercise is *partial curl-ups*, performed as follows: Take back-lying position, knees straight, legs together, and arms at side; lift head and, later, lift head and shoulders off floor; hold position briefly, return to floor, and continue. *Progression:* (a) Continue raising shoulders and trunk farther and farther off floor until complete curl-ups are performed; gradually build up to 20 sit-ups from this position. (b) Start with ten curl-ups with hands clasped behind head; build up to 20 curl-ups again, build up further, if desired, by holding weights on chest and later behind head. (c) Perform curl-ups from inclined board with head down, further exercise severity can be achieved by holding weights on chest and then behind head. (d) *Rowing exercise.* Lie on back, legs straight and together, arms over head with thumbs locked; sit-up by swinging arms forward and raising trunk, and, at same time, bend knees and bring heels close to buttocks, reaching as far forward as possible; return to starting position slowly. (e) V *sit-ups*. Same starting position as for rowing, but with arms in front of body; sit-up and raise straight legs simultaneously, keeping weight on hips and reaching toward toes with hands.

Curl-ups can be adjusted easily to provide for hip-trunk flexibility, as follows: (a) With knees straight, reach as far forward toward toes as possible on each sit-up; (b) hook instead of point toes to increase tension on the hamstring and back muscles and ligaments; (c) spread legs and alternately touch right and left elbows (hands behind head) to opposite knees, pulling head well forward with hands each time—this adds a trunk twisting movement to the stretching procedure.

Curl-ups can also be performed with the knees bent, heels close to buttocks. With straight knees, the psoas major muscle, between the femur and the lumbar spine, is used vigorously. When the knees are bent sufficiently, this muscle is shortened to a point where it does little if any pulling; thus, more stress in doing sit-ups is placed on the abdominal muscles. This exercise, consequently, is more difficult to perform than the straight-knee type.

LATERAL TRUNK EXERCISES

The lateral trunk muscles are involved in the various abdominal exercises. However, exercises which more specifically place stress on these muscles may be utilized. These exercises are also useful in increasing lateral trunk flexibility.

Trunk twister. A simple form of this exercise is performed as follows. Lie on back, arms stretched sideward, palms down, knees straight; raise feet one foot from floor and swing them slowly as far as possible to left without touching floor, keeping legs together and knees straight; swing legs, again slowly, back through same arc and as far to right as possible; and continue. *Progression*: (a) Instead of swinging feet back through same arc one foot from floor, swing them through a perpendicular arc; (b) To increase flexibility benefits, hook toes and bring legs as far toward chest as possible without bending knees when performing each right-left arc. (c) *Corkscrew*: Start with back-lying position with hands at sides, gradually raise legs with knees straight until weight is on shoulders and feet are extended as far beyond head as possible; slowly swing legs in corkscrew fashion as far over right arm and to right of body as possible; continue as a controlled swing through an arc one foot from floor until legs are as far to left of body as possible, maintaining the swing over left arm until weight is again on shoulders with feet extended over head as before.

Side bends. Side bends may be used to strengthen the lateral trunk muscles and the shoulder depressors; these exercises should be done on both sides. Side bends may be performed as follows. Take a side-leaning rest position (i.e., resting on one hand with arm fully extended and on side of foot), body straight, free arm along upper side of body; lower hips as far as possible, preferably until side of lower leg touches floor; raise hips to starting position and, if desired, throw free hand over head. *Variation:* Same starting position, except place free hand behind head with upper arm in line with supporting arm, elbow back; instead of bending trunk, raise free leg upward and return. *Progression:* These exercises will be impossible for most unfit boys and girls at first; if so, progression may follow somewhat the same pattern as for the "push-up" series above.

Back Exercises

A number of exercises to condition the back muscles are proposed below.

Leg and arm raises. A number of variations and progressions for leg and arm raises from a front-lying position are as follows. (a) With hands behind neck, raise and lower legs alternately keeping knees straight; progress by raising both legs simultaneously and holding briefly, arms at sides, palms down, to aid in maintaining the position. (b) With arms extended over head, raise and lower arms alternately; progress by raising both arms simultaneously, and, later, by raising chest off floor with hands behind neck. (c) With arms extended, raise both arms and legs simultaneously; as a progression, perform swimming motion with arms and legs.

Arm and leg pulls. The basic back arm-pull movement is as follows. From front-lying position, lock hands behind back; raise chest with head back and force hands away from body vigorously. To progress, perform same movement while simultaneously raising both chest and legs, with knees straight. A variation of this exercise is to grasp feet with hands; pull arms and legs, forcing body into bowed position.

Trunk raises. For this exercise, take kneeling position with buttocks resting on ankles and forehead on floor, arms straight and clasped behind back; pull down on arms and draw shoulder blades together, raising hips, trunk, and head until back is about parallel to floor.

Leg Exercises

In this text, exception will be taken to the use of deep squats, deep knee bends, duck waddles, full squat jumps, and other exercises which require the support of the body weight upon one or both fully bent knees. Klein[16] conducted extensive studies of the deep squat exercise, utilizing anatomical analysis, knee dissection studies (64 cadavers), knee joint instability found in knee injuries resulting from athletics, and the instability of the knees of weight lifters and paratroopers (who used squat jumps extensively in training), as contrasted with control subjects in University of Texas physical education classes. He demonstrated that extensive use of this exercise resulted in frequent knee joint instability; the ligaments especially involved were the lateral and the anterior cruciates.

Klein recommended that the full squat type of exercises, which involve supporting, lifting, or projecting the body with or without weights, should be avoided. The National Federation of State High School Athletic Associations and the Committee on the Medical Aspects of Sports of the American Medical Association are in agreement, as is evidenced by the following statement they issued jointly: "The deep knee bend and 'duck waddle' . . . are now generally disapproved by medical authorities. Both exercises have potential for serious injury to the internal and supporting structures of the knee joint, one of the most vulnerable parts of the athlete's body."[17] Thus, such exercises should be modified so that their use aids strengthening of the leg muscles, but without potential danger of damage to the ligamentous structure of the knee joints.

Knee bends. Knee bends can be conducted so that considerable exercise of upper back and pelvic girdle muscles will also result. Start with feet flat on floor and parallel, hands on hips, back straight, pelvis firm, and head up; rise slightly on toes, slowly flex the knees to half-bend position, contracting buttocks, drawing in abdomen, and keeping back straight. If half knee bends cannot be performed, do quarter movements. *Progression:* (a) Perform half-knee bends with hands behind head; keep elbows well retracted and shoulder blades as close together as possible; keep head up and maintain straight back. (b) Perform exercise with weights on shoulders as described in next section.

Leg push-ups. Leg push-ups are performed as follows. Take back-lying position, arms under hips, and feet stretched up toward partner's shoulders; partner places hands and shoulders on up-raised feet, resting body weight so that subject's legs and partner's body form 45 degree angle; subject then performs leg push-ups by slowly lowering legs to half-knee bends and then slowly pushing them back to starting position. *Progression:* For this exercise, adjustments for exercise tolerance can be made by increasing or decreasing the weight of the partner; and, if half push-ups cannot be done, quarter push-ups may be substituted.

---

[16] Karl K. Klein, "The Deep Squat Exercise as Utilized in Weight Training for Athletics and Its Effect on the Ligaments of the Knee," *Journal of Association for Physical and Mental Rehabilitation*, 15, No. 1 (January-February, 1961), p. 6.

[17] Department of Health Education, American Medical Association.

Squat jumps. As indicated above, squat jumping should be so adapted that the body weight is not supported or projected from the fully bent knee. A simple form of this exercise is as follows. With hands at side, bend knees to quarter squat; extending knees, jump slightly with both feet just clearing the floor, arms swinging upward. *Progression:* (a) Increase number and height of jumps; (b) Perform jump with hands on top of head and progress as before. (c) Execute full squat jumps in the following manner: Take a full squat in stride position, *but* with rear foot far enough back so that knee comes in contact with floor,[18] hands on top of head; straighten knees, jumping slightly off floor; on each squat, permit supporting knee to touch floor lightly.

WEIGHT TRAINING

THE CASE FOR WEIGHT TRAINING

Training with weights in this country was originally largely the province of professional weight lifters and body-beautiful enthusiasts. In addition to commercial and private studies, weight training facilities were frequently found in Y.M.C.A.'s, but seldom in schools and colleges. However, such prominent physical educators as C. H. McCloy, Ellis H. Champlin, and Ralph W. Leighton believed in the fitness value of this activity and practiced it in their daily lives.

During and after World War II, three major influences culminated in an increased respect for and understanding of the value of weight training. The first of these influences came from physical medicine in the use of weights for the physical reconditioning and rehabilitation of patients in the hospitals and convalescent centers of the armed forces; this influence has continued in the medical and psychiatric care of patients in Veterans Administration hospitals and community rehabilitation centers. The second influence was the surprisingly successful use of weights to develop the strength and effectiveness of athletes. The list of modern athletes who stress this form of activity in their conditioning regimens for championship performances is impressive. The third influence is the results of research from many sources, especially physical education and physical medicine. These results have refuted such former concepts that weight lifters are "muscle-bound" and that habitual weight lifting chronically tenses muscles, thus interfering with athletic performance. The findings show that weight training positively improves the individual's fitness.

In this book, weight training is accepted as a valuable modality in the

---

[18] In this way, according to Klein, there is no compression in the knee joint; the forward leg, which is not less than a right angle of flexion, takes the stress of the exercise (footnote 16).

development of muscular strength and muscular endurance, especially for boys, although there appears to be no logical reason why it should not benefit girls equally well. Leighton[19] has reported that Washington State University provided a course in weight training upon the request and insistence of the girls themselves. These university young women had certain definite objectives in mind. They wanted to reapportion body measurements, control weight, firm slack or loose parts of the body, strengthen weak muscles, and improve general body condition.

Weight Training Exercises

Space does not permit a detailed presentation of weight training exercises. Texts by Leighton,[20] Murray and Karpovich,[21] and Peebler[22] are available for those who wish further information. The principles of exercise presented in this chapter can easily be applied to this activity. By trial of several weights, the unfit student's tolerance can be determined accurately; and progression can be provided effectively by increasing the amount of weight, the number of repetitions, or the cadence (pacing, as described and studied by Hellebrandt and Houtz[23]).

The exercises presented in this section are confined to the use of barbells; similar types of exercise may also be performed with weighted dumbbells. The exercise plan proposed is a common one, known as progressive resistance exercise, although variations in the way it is conducted may be found. At the start, each unfit student will need to experiment by trial with several weights in order to determine the amount to be used for a given exercise.

The belief is held by some weight training specialists[24] that relatively heavy loads repeated for fewer repetitions are desirable to develop the strength and endurance of the smaller muscle groups of the arms, shoulders, upper back and chest; and, that the larger muscles of the legs and lower back require more repetitions and can stand greater increases in weight. Until some other method is proven superior, this system is proposed. Some exercises will start with five repetitions; after each third day of exercise, the repetitions will be increased by one until ten repetitions have been completed for three days. Then, the weight should be increased and the process repeated starting again with five repetitions.

---

19 Jack R. Leighton, "Weight Lifting for Girls," *Journal of Health-Physical Education-Recreation,* 31, No. 5 (May-June, 1960), p. 19.

20 Jack R. Leighton, *Progressive Weight Training* (New York: The Ronald Press Company, 1961).

21 Jim Murray and Peter V. Karpovich, *Weight Training in Athletics* (Englewood Cliffs, N. J.: Prentice-Hall, Inc., 1956).

22 J. R. Peebler, *Better Growth and Development of Your Child* (Pullman, Wash.: The Author, Executive Health Club, 1954).

23 F. A. Hellebrandt and S. J. Houtz, "Methods of Muscle Training: The Influence of Pacing," *Physical Therapy Review,* 38, No. 5 (May, 1958), p. 319.

24 Murray and Karpovich, *loc. cit.,* p 72.

For exercises which start with ten repetitions, the number should be increased by two after each third day until 20 repetitions have been completed. In the exercise descriptions below, the number of repetitions will be designated as 5-10 and 10-20 respectively for these two situations.

In this section, ten basic barbell exercises are described, although for three of these, variations are included. The order of presentation starts with the wrists and follows through the elbows, shoulders, back, trunk, hips, knees, and ankles. The developmental and adapted physical educator will need to rearrange these exercises to fit the individual situation and to avoid the fatigue caused by repeated exercising of the same muscle group.

Wrist curls. (a) Take sitting position on bench, knees spread shoulder width apart, forearms resting on thighs with hands extended beyond knees, and grasp barbell palms up; raise and lower bar slowly keeping forearms on thighs. Inhale when lifting weight and exhale when lowering it. Repetitions: 5-10. (b) Execute same exercise, except grasp bar with palms down. In part, different muscles are exercised by each of these hand grasps.

Elbow curls. (a) Stand erect with feet comfortably apart, arms fully extended at side, and grasp barbell in front of body with palms forward; raise and lower bar slowly to the chest, keeping the upper arm at side of body and without bending backward at waist. Inhale when lifting weight and exhale when lowering it. Repetitions: 5-10. (b) Perform same exercise, except grasp bar with palms backward (reverse curls). In part, different muscles are exercised by each of these hand grasps.

Shoulder press. (a) Stand erect with feet comfortably apart, with hands at shoulder width apart, grasp barbell with palms backward, and raise bar to upper chest (palms now facing forward); press bar upward overhead until elbows are fully extended. Inhale when raising weight and exhale when lowering it to chest. Repetitions: 5-10. (b) Perform this exercise from starting position with bar behind neck.

Upright rowing. Stand erect with feet comfortably apart and hold bar in front of thighs, hands shoulder width apart and using palms-backward grasp; bend elbows and pull bar up front of body until it reaches upper chest or neck. During raising of bar, elbows should extend sideward and should be kept higher than wrists. Inhale when raising weight and exhale when lowering it. Repetitions: 5-10.

Floor-overhead pull-ups. Stand close to bar with feet comfortably apart, bend at knees and hips, keeping feet flat on floor and back straight as possible, and grasp bar with hands shoulder width apart, using palms-backward grip; pull the weight upward and continue lifting until it is fully overhead with body straight in erect standing position. Inhale when raising weight and exhale when lowering it to the floor. Repetitions: 10-20.

Sideward trunk bends. Stand erect with feet wide apart and rest barbell across shoulders behind neck; perform sideward bending movement, alternately right and left, keeping knees straight. Pause at upright position with each movement. Exhale as trunk is bent to side and inhale as erect position is regained. Repetitions: 10-20.

Forward trunk bends. Stand erect with feet wide apart and rest barbell across shoulders behind neck; bend trunk forward from hips, keeping knees and back straight, with head up. Exhale on forward bend and inhale as erect position is regained. Repetitions: 10-20.

Back lifts. Stand with feet together and legs straight, bend body forward at hips, and grasp bar resting on floor with hands shoulder width apart using palms-backward grip; raise bar until body is erect, keeping arms and legs straight. Inhale when raising weight and exhale when lowering it. Repetitions: 10-20.

Half squats. Stand erect with feet comfortably apart and rest barbell across shoulders behind neck; lower body until the angle at the knee joint is approximately 90 degrees, keeping heels flat on floor, head up, and back straight, although bend at hips is necessary. Exhale when squatting and inhale when rising to erect position. Repetitions: 10-20.

Heel raises. Stand erect with feet comfortably apart, toes turned in slightly, and rest barbell across shoulders behind neck; with knees locked and body straight, raise heels off floor as high as possible. Inhale when raising heels and exhale when lowering them to floor. Repetitions: 10-20.

CONTESTS FOR STRENGTH DEVELOPMENT

As indicated earlier in this chapter, resistance for strength development may be applied by another person. In the presentation of conditioning exercises, some use was made of such resistance. Moreover, some partner vs. partner contests may also be utilized, as may relays and games selected for this purpose.

For this book, a number of contests have been selected to illustrate the possibilities of strength improvement. These activities should be prescribed with caution to untrained pupils, as the psychological competitive element can lead to disregard of proper exercise tolerance levels. In this type of strength development, dosage is difficult to control and the tendency toward excess is always present. Opposing individuals in these activities should be approximate equals.

For several of these contests, three parallel lines 10 feet apart are needed. The pupils are paired as opponents with the center line between them.

Hand pulls. The partners grasp each other's wrists across the center line. At the starting signal, each pupil attempts to pull his opponent across the center line and on over his 10-foot line.

Hop and pull hands. Each contestant grasps his opponent's right wrist across the center line. Hopping on his right foot, he attempts to pull his opponent over this line. Either contestant automatically loses if he touches his rear foot to the ground.

Back-to-back push. With the center line between, the two contestants stand back to back with elbows locked; each contestant has his right arm inside his opponent's left arm. The object of the contest is, by pushing backward, to force the opponent over his (the opponent's) 10-foot line. The contestants are not allowed to lift and carry their opponents; pushing only is permitted.

Back-to-back tug. Taking the same position as for the back-to-back push, each contestant attempts to tug his opponent across his own 10-foot line. The same contest rules also apply.

Hand wrestle. The contestants stand facing each other; the right feet are forward and based side by side; they grasp right hands. The object of the contest is to force the opponent to move one or both feet from the original position by pulling, pushing, or making other maneuvers. Alternate positions by reversing feet and hands.

Wand wrestle. The two contestants grasp a one-inch wand, or substitute. The contest is to "wrestle" the wand away from the opponent. Complete possession of the wand is necessary to win.

Tug-of-war. Draw a line in the center of the area. Divide contestants into two equal teams and line them up in a single file, on opposite sides of the line, facing each other. Each contestant places his arms around the waist of the teammate in front of him. The two leaders of opposing teams grasp each other around the waist. On signal, each team attempts to pull the entire opponent team over the center line.

Step-on-toes. The contestants are paired off. At the signal to start, each attempts to step on his opponent's toes.

Rooster fight. Each contestant grasps left foot behind body with right hand and grasps right arm with left hand. By hopping on his right foot and butting his opponent, he attempts to force him to release his left foot or right arm. Feinting, evasions, and other maneuvers are permissible.

Horse and rider. The players pair off and one mounts the other's back as a rider. At the signal, the riders attempt to pull each other off their "horses."

CIRCULATORY-RESPIRATORY ENDURANCE

Activities for the development of circulatory-respiratory endurance require moderate contractions of large-muscle groups for relatively long periods of time. Respiratory and circulatory systems must be stimulated; in fact, such stimulation is essential for this form of conditioning, which reduces the importance of speed events when using activities for this purpose.

From long experience attempting to improve circulatory-respiratory fitness in young boys and young men, Cureton[25] has made a number of suggestions for the conduct of such activities, including the following. (a) Several weeks are needed for boys in training to adjust to a fairly vigorous program; some do not fully adjust even in eight weeks but adjustment is usually possible if the endurance program is very gradually increased in dosage and intensity. (b) Every endurance session should be accompanied by an effort to breathe well; deep breathing should be stressed following every work performance. (c) Some competition is needed against one's own times on running tests. (d) Temporary set-backs may be expected if the program is too hard at first. (e) Over-eating should be avoided and the amount of sleep increased for those on intensive (relative to the individual's exercise tolerance) circulatory-respiratory regimens. According to Cureton, endurance work must be hard enough and long enough to increase both capillarization and oxygen transport to the muscles.

Particularly desirable forms of circulatory-respiratory endurance activities for unfit boys and girls are hiking, running, and swimming, since these exercises can be readily controlled. Thus, distance, pace, and duration can be regulated to the specific fitness status of the individual. Progression in the amount and nature of exercise can be planned from day to day. Considerations pertaining to the use of these endurance activities in the developmental program for the physically unfit will be presented in this section.

Walking. Variously known, of course, as marching, hiking, and the like, walking can be used as an activity for the improvement of circulatory-respiratory endurance. Obviously, it is the mildest form of this type of conditioning, when the distance is short and the pace slow. As related to progression, it can be the starting point. Hiking for some distance over rough terrain would be difficult to achieve as a physical education activity. However, walking on the track or around the athletic field is entirely feasible. Distance and pace may be increased as exercise tolerance improves.

Double timing can be added to increase the dosage. Double timing is more of a "jog" or "dog trot" than a run. The feet should skim the surface of the ground; they should be placed flatly on the ground, without running on the toes or permitting the heels to strike first. Double timing may be alternated with walking (or quick timing). From this form of exercise, it is a short step to alternate walking and running.

Walking may be used to develop strength and other components of motor fitness in addition to circulatory-respiratory endurance; this is

25 Thomas K. Cureton, "Scientific Principles of Human Endurance with Suggestions for Its Development," *Journal of Physical Education*, 58, No. 4 (March-April, 1961), p. 81.

accomplished if a pack, weight, or another person is carried. Clarke, Shay, and Mathews[26] reported the following statistically significant gains in mean scores by college men completing one military march of 7.5 miles each week for seven weeks carrying 41-pound packs (61 pounds on last march).

	Means		Difference
	Before First	After Last	
Army Physical Efficiency Test	253	281	28
AAF Physical Fitness Test	56	59	3
Navy Standard Physical Fitness Test	260	275	15
Physical Fitness Index	104	113	9

Running. For a great many unfit boys and girls, running is an effective and the most readily available way of developing circulatory-respiratory endurance. Unless contra-indicated in individual cases, all developmental physical education periods should include sustained running (or swimming) in some form. The run at first should be relatively short and the pace reasonably slow. Initially, too, runs can be interspersed with walking. Keep moving; do not stop and rest. The lengths of the runs should be increased gradually, their tempo should be stepped up, and the interspersed walking eliminated.

Cureton[27] maintains that the best events to develop circulatory-respiratory endurance "so far known" include (a) steeplechase running, (b) continuous muscular endurance exercises done for 30 minutes without stopping, (c) interval training in track running, cycling, swimming, skating, rowing, and taking tests in endurance runs, and (d) circuit training. Ingenuity can be applied to setting up running situations, involving more variety than just "so many times around the track or field." Miller, Bookwalter, and Schlafer[28] suggest that running patterns be laid out which are more interesting than just routine runs; these can be changed as desired. Frequently, it is possible to use the extensive school grounds and, perhaps, nearby areas to establish miniature cross-country courses. Steeplechase running is similar to cross-country running with the addition of various obstacles involving jumping, climbing, crawling, and so forth, to be overcome. When formalized in a school situation, this may become an "obstacle course."

Swimming. When facilities are available, swimming is an excellent activity for the improvement of circulatory-respiratory endurance. The boy or girl, however, needs to be able to swim with some ease before maximum endurance benefit may be acquired from it. The application of

---

[26] H. Harrison Clarke, Clayton T. Shay, and Donald K. Mathews, "Strength Decrements from Carrying Various Army Packs on Military Marches," *Research Quarterly*, 26, No. 3 (October, 1959), p. 253.

[27] Cureton, *op. cit.*

[28] Ben W. Miller, Karl W. Bookwalter, and George E. Schlafer, *Physical Fitness for Boys* (New York: A. S. Barnes and Company, Inc., 1943), p. 218.

swimming to the unfit individual would logically be similar to that of running.

Sports. Many sports have a high circulatory-respiratory endurance element. The endurance contribution of such activities, however, depends on the manner in which they are conducted, especially the amount of sustained running involved. Among those of greatest potential value are soccer, basketball, handball, lacrosse and other running games, and water sports. But, caution should be observed in prescribing these activities to unfit individuals, as the competitive element may easily lead to exceeding proper exercise tolerance levels; it is obviously difficult to control the dosage and to provide systematic progression under competitive circumstances. In advanced states of conditioning, however, some sports are excellent developers of endurance.

SPECIAL EXERCISE SYSTEMS

A number of special exercise systems have been proposed which are designed to develop various physical fitness components by group methods. Typically, these systems permit relatively large numbers to participate during the same time period. The exercises once taught are self-administered, the dosage is adapted reasonably well to the level of each individual's exercise tolerance, and provisions are made for overload and progression. The systems can be arranged for use in conditioning athletes for particular sports and also can be adapted to activities for the physically unfit. Several of these systems will be described below as applied to developmental classes.

CIRCUIT TRAINING

In 1958, Morgan and Adamson[29] in England published a handbook describing a system of circuit training. Circuit training can be used for general fitness purposes or can be adapted as a conditioning medium for various arduous sports. For sports' conditioning, for example, it has been utilized by many professional soccer and rugby teams in England and by Australian-rules football and competitive sailing teams in Australia. According to the originators, circuit training enables large numbers of performers to train together by employing a circuit of consecutive exercises around which each performer progresses, performing an individually derived dosage of exercise and timing his progress. The essential features of circuit training follow.

1. A number of exercise stations, usually from six to ten depending on the time allocated for circuit training and the nature of the exer-

---

[29] R. E. Morgan and G. T. Adamson, *Circuit Training* (London: G. Bell and Sons, Ltd., 1958). (Distributed in the United States by Sportshelf, P. O. Box 634, New Rochelle, N. Y.)

cises, are set up in the gymnasium or outdoor exercise space. The length of time required to perform the exercise at the different stations should be approximately the same, so as to avoid crowding in the circuit. This regulation causes some restriction in the choice of exercises.

2. The specific exercises to be performed in a circuit will depend on the conditioning effects sought; thus, the exercise analysis of the physical educator is vital in devising this sequence. For the development of muscular strength and muscular endurance of unfit individuals, Watt[30] recommends three weight training exercises, three free-standing exercises, and three exercises using some kind of apparatus. The circuit for unfit boys illustrated in Figure 14 effectively combines conditioning exercises to develop muscular strength and endurance, flexibility, and circulatory-respiratory endurance.

3. While the exercises remain the same for all participants, although individual adaptations are possible if desired, the dosage and progression in the circuit is arranged in accordance with each unfit person's exercise tolerance. The dosage for each exercise and the circuit time are determined individually.

4. With unfit individuals, some pre-conditioning should take place before their circuits are established. It is also desirable for each individual to memorize his own circuit, so that he will not waste time checking his card repeatedly.

The circuit described below was proposed for unfit college men by A. W. Willee, Senior Lecturer in Physical Education, University of Melbourne, Australia,[31] after teaching developmental physical education classes at the University of Oregon. This circuit illustrates the total process involved; obviously, adjustments and adaptations will be necessary depending on the age and sex of the participants, the amount of time allowed, and the availability of facilities and equipment.

Circuit exercises. Willee's circuit of ten exercises, with substitutions in some instances, follows. Where exercises listed cannot be performed by unfit individuals, modified forms may be substituted; possible modifications can be chosen from the conditioning exercises described earlier in this chapter. A sample record card for this circuit appears in Figure 14.

1. *General activity.* Select one of the following exercises. (a) Tuck jumps: upward jumps with high knee lift, with or without rebounding. (b) Pike jumps: jumping with leg raising and parting while reaching for toes with hands. (c) Scoring runs: Two lines 15 to 20 feet apart;

---

[30] Norman S. Watt, "Application of Circuit Training to Developmental Physical Education," *Physical Fitness News Letter* (University of Oregon), VI, No. 9 (May, 1960).

[31] Mr. Willee is a leading authority on circuit training in Australia. Not only has he applied this type of training to general conditioning problems, but has successfully utilized it with sports teams of national caliber in his country.

start with right hand on one line; run to touch opposite line and return continuously; scoring each time a line is touched by hand.

2. *Abdominal exercise.* Perform sit-ups or trunk curls: lying on back, hands on front of thighs; sit up until fingers touch edge of knee cap; preferably, for ease of administration, feet are not held.

3. *Dorsal exercise.* Select either of the following exercises. (a) Wrestler's bridge: crook supine lying (knees bent); press on head and feet, raising body to form bridge. (b) Prone lying; raise arms, chest, and legs simultaneously.

4. *Lateral trunk exercise.* Standing astride, back towards and feet a few inches from wall; bend trunk downward to touch hands to floor, if possible; raise trunk and swing arms to left wall as high up and as far behind head as possible; continue alternating right and left wall touches; score each time wall is touched.

5. *General activity.* Choose another general activity from those proposed in No. 1 above, or use step-ups, as follows: step up on bench with four count movement; step up alternately left and right feet.

6. *Abdominal and leg adductor exercise.* Back-lying position with legs raised and separated; leg crossing alternately right and left legs on top; count each time legs are apart.

7. *Arm and shoulder flexor exercise.* Pull-ups on horizontal bar, or modification if subject cannot perform full chins.

8. *Kneel sitting.* Take kneeling position, body erect, arms extended and thumbs joined high over head; sit alternately right and left sides, bending to opposite side, keep hands over head; scoring each time body is raised to kneeling position.

9. *General activity.* Jumping and rebounding with leg parting.

10. *Arm and shoulder extensor exercise.* Floor push-ups, or dips from parallel bars if ability permits.

In the exercise sequence, items should be so arranged that local fatigue from one exercise does not interfere with performance in the next. The last item in the circuit should not be a general activity exercise, since this would place two such exercises together when the circuit is repeated. All items in the circuit must be repeatable and self-testing; thus, balances and skill practices are not applicable. When the number of pupils is large, they can be divided with an equal number starting at each of the general activity stations. If exercises provided in the circuit cannot be done by some, they must be modified; suggested modifications, as well as other possible exercises to include in circuit, may be found under "Conditioning exercises" appearing earlier in this chapter. Good exercises can also be devised and placed in the circuit if medicine balls are available; overhead throws and chest push passes against a wall are excellent when standing close enough to the wall to catch the rebound.

WILLEE'S CIRCUIT TRAINING RECORD CARD FOR LOW FITNESS BOYS												
Name: _____ Age: _____ Weight: _____ Class: _____												
	Date: _____		Date: _____		Date: _____		Date: _____		Date: _____		Date: _____	
	Max. Score	Tng. Amt.	Max. Score	Tng. Amt.	Max. Score	Tng. Amt.	Max. Score	Tng. Amt.	Max. Score	Tng. Amt.	Max. Score	Tng. Amt.
1. Scoring Runs												
2. Sit-Ups												
3. Wrestler's Bridge												
4. Wall Slap												
5. Step Ups												
6. Leg Crossing												
7. Pull-Ups												
8. Side Sitting												
9. Jumping												
10. Floor Push-Ups												
Trail Time	__ Min. __ Sec.		__ Min. __ Sec.		__ Min. __ Sec.		__ Min. __ Sec.		__ Min. __ Sec.		__ Min. __ Sec.	
Target Time	__ Min. __ Sec.		__ Min. __ Sec.		__ Min. __ Sec.		__ Min. __ Sec.		__ Min. __ Sec.		__ Min. __ Sec.	

Fig. 14.

Circuit operation. In establishing and operating the circuit, the following procedures should be followed.

1. Teach all exercises in the circuit, so that each individual is thoroughly familiar with the form of the activity.

2. Test the maximum ability of each person for each exercise. In the interests of controlling the time required for a circuit, time limits should be imposed on some exercises; for others the limits will be self-imposed by the condition of the individual. Willee recommends limits of 60 seconds for boys and 30 seconds for girls; in other instances, all-out performances to exhaustion can be used. For example, in the circuit above, time limits should be used for exercises number 1, 4, 5, 6, 8, and 9. For unfit boys and girls, all-out maximums on the other exercises would probably be feasible; however, if some of these involve too much time to complete, time limits can easily be invoked. Record all test performances on each individual's "circuit-training record card."

3. To establish each person's circuit, take one-half of his test performance. For example, if 32 scoring runs (1–c above) are completed in one minute, 16 runs would be included in this circuit; or, if 11 floor push-ups are completed, 6 of these would be on that individual's circuit. Thus, each participant's initial circuit of ten exercises is established.

4. Practice the circuit exercises. Then, on one day, perform the circuit once for time; and, on the next day, go through the circuit twice consecutively for time. Finally, time each student on the regular circuit, which is a repetition of the circuit three times.

5. From this final timing, the student's target time is set. Usually, this time is two-thirds of the time necessary for the three-repetition

circuit. For example, if the circuit time was 24 minutes, the target time would be 16 minutes.

6. In successive developmental classes, each student trains to bring his circuit time down to his target time. If his target is reached within a short time (three to four weeks), the number of repetitions in some exercises may be increased and the trainee may try again to achieve his target time. If a longer time is needed, the student should be re-tested in the different exercises, or on new ones which may be selected; one-half of the performance amounts should then be taken and his target time again set as a consequence of three repetitions of the circuit.

INTERVAL TRAINING

A German, Woldemar Gershler, is credited with the creation of interval training. Many champion distance runners now use this system or some close variation of it. With this type of training, the track athlete is constantly running shorter distances than the one for which he is training at *faster* speeds than his race pace. Through such a program, he develops speed, endurance, strength, power, and a positive psychological approach to competition. Stein[32] has described a method of interval training for general exercises and calisthenics.

There are four variable situations in interval training: (a) length of time allotted to exercise, (b) number of times a given exercise is accomplished in the given time, (c) number of repetitions for an exercise, and (d) length of rest interval between each repetitive exercise. In interval training for general exercises, work bouts are done in intervals at or nearly at all-out effort, with rest periods intervening. Virtually any conditioning exercise can be adapted to the interval system.

An illustration of the application of the interval system described by Stein deals with the curl-up exercise. At the start, use three all-out curl-up bouts of 10 seconds with 15-second rest intervals between each exercise period. Improvement can be noted from day to day by an increased number of curl-ups in one or more of the three bouts. After one, two, or three weeks, depending on the progress made, add a fourth repetitive bout with the remainder of the timing unchanged. When the group is ready, the process can be changed again: either maintain the four bouts of ten seconds and reduce the rest interval to 10 seconds or require three bouts of 15 seconds duration with the rest interval remaining 15 seconds. Gradually increase to four repetitions of 15 seconds duration with 15 seconds rest; then, reduce the rest intervals to 10 seconds. As the class

---

[32] Julian U. Stein, "Adaptation of the Interval System to General Exercises and Calisthenics," *Physical Educator*, 17, No. 1 (March, 1960), p. 22.

progresses, work into 20-second bouts with intervals of 15 seconds, gradually reducing the rest time to 10 seconds.

With the well-conditioned group, a variety of interval combinations can be used, such as two or three 30-second bouts with 15- or 10-second rest intervals, eight or twelve 5-second bouts with 5-second rests, and combinations of several different bout-times and intervals of rest. The possibilities are extensive, since any of the variable situations in interval training can be changed. Changes can easily be made to adapt the process to the exercise tolerance of the participants.

In events where the performer tends to become exhausted in a short time (e.g. pull-ups), a modified and easier method of performing them is necessary, for obviously when the subject is exhausted he can no longer perform at all. Provide an exercise easy enough to perform repeatedly but require it to be done rapidly to induce overload. Such exercises as the following may be used effectively in interval training: floor push-ups, sitting tucks, curl-ups, leg raises, squat thrusts, squat jumps, side-leg raises, treadmill, bench stepping, half-knee bends, and others included in the circuit-training sequence.

CURETON'S RHYTHMIC CONTINUOUS EXERCISES

In numerous youth and adult fitness classes and clinics in this country and throughout the world, Cureton[33] has popularized a system of rhythmic continuous exercises as a means of over-all physical fitness improvement. This process incorporates features of both circuit and interval training; however, the non-stop exercise session may be from 30 minutes to an hour or more in duration. Muscular endurance exercises are interspersed with walking, jogging, running, hopping, kicking, swinging the arms, deep breathing, and the like, as a type of repetitive work. Cureton refers to this process as repeated "pick-up and rest." Each rhythmic continuous exercise session starts mildly, builds up to an intensity in the middle, and tapers off at the end. He believes that long-continued exercise is needed in order to warm the body and its organs thoroughly; such warming being essential for effective muscular and circulatory endurance.

This system provides for three categories of exercise, designated as Low Gear, Middle Gear, and High Gear, which systematically provide overload.[34] Thus, progression is possible through the three categories. Also, individual adaptations are possible within any of the gears by instructing those who cannot continue with each prescribed muscular endurance exercise to jog, walk, or run in place, but to keep moving. The

---

[33] Cureton, *op. cit.*
[34] Thomas K. Cureton, University of Illinois, Urbana, mimeographed material.

exercise session is conducted with the class following the instructor around the exercise area; pauses are made briefly to perform short bouts of muscular endurance exercises.

La Sierra Fitness Program

A "color system" to develop the physical fitness of boys was developed and conducted successfully by Stan Le Protti, La Sierra High School, Carmichael, California.[35] The program is based on three ability groups, each established on the criterion of a physical fitness testing schedule. These tests are designed to evaluate and motivate individual efforts in the areas of strength, endurance, power, agility, flexibility, and balance. The three ability groups or levels of achievement are designated as beginners, intermediates, and advanced. Each group is identified by the color of its gymnasium trunks. Boys assigned to the beginner's group wear white trunks; the intermediate groups, red trunks; and the advanced group, blue trunks. Boys with unusual ability are a part of the Blue group and wear either purple or gold satin trunks. Gold status represents the highest achievement level possible in the physical fitness category; these individuals may well be identified as physically gifted students and are so recognized in the school and community.

Each color group has a separate battery of conditioning exercises designed for its particular level of physical fitness; these exercises are mass executed by each color group. For example, the Blue group executes daily a nine-minute strenuous strength-endurance routine without rest between exercises. This is followed by Cureton's "endurance-hop" process, which is composed of 200 straddle-hops, 200 stride-hops, 75 hops each toe, 200 toe-hops feet together, and 75 alternating knee-touch hops. For the Whites, the lowest fitness group, the exercise regimen is considerably milder, in keeping with the exercise tolerance of this group.

All color groups are required to run through an outdoor obstacle course daily, rain or shine, at the end of the physical education period. This obstacle course is primarily aimed at providing arm and shoulder development. Furthermore, each day, all boys must do bar dips, pull-ups, hand walking across parallel bars, and hand travels across the overhead horizontal ladder.

SUMMARY

Physical fitness is quite as necessary for girls as for boys. Both sexes need adequate strength and stamina for proper physical development

---

[35] "La Sierra's Physical Fitness Program," *Physical Fitness News Letter,* 7, No. 6 (February, 1961); No. 8 (April, 1961).

and organic soundness. Many great educators have echoed Aristotle in suggesting the complete separation of educational aims and objectives for boys and girls. However, in recent decades, there has been a great increase in the civil, political, and intellectual freedom of women. Aside from definite biological differences, the educational and physiological needs of women are converging with those of men. Women also need strong and healthy bodies to produce robust children and to carry out the arduous tasks of childrearing and homemaking. In addition, the acquisition and maintenance of adequate fitness by all people are vital for national survival. The war experiences of all countries leave no doubt of the basic importance of strength and endurance and the importance of physical education in the complete realization of these goals.

In this chapter, exercise for the physically unfit was considered. Eight principles of exercise were presented as guides in devising any activity program for those who are subpar in basic physical fitness components. Types of exercise for improving these components were discussed. Then, specific conditioning exercises, weight training lifts, individual and group contests, and circulatory-respiratory activities were described; in doing so, the principles of exercise tolerance, overload, and progression were systematically applied. Finally, several special exercise systems were presented.

SELECTED REFERENCES

Clarke, H. Harrison, "Development of Volitional Muscle Strength as Related to Fitness," *Exercise and Fitness*. Chicago: Athletic Institute, 1960, 200-212.

Hellebrandt, F. A., and S. J. Houtz, "Methods of Muscle Training: The Influence of Pacing," *Physical Therapy Review*, 38, No. 5 (May, 1958), 319.

Kiphuth, Robert, *How To Be Fit*. New Haven: Yale University Press, 1942.

Leighton, Jack R., *Progressive Weight Training*. New York: The Ronald Press Company, 1961.

Morgan, R. E., and G. T. Adamson, *Circuit Training*. London: G. Bell and Sons, Ltd., 1958. (New Rochelle, N. Y.: Sportshelf.)

Oermann, Karl C. H., Carl Haven Young, and Mitchell J. Gary, *Conditioning Exercises, Games, Tests*, 3rd ed. Annapolis, Md.: United States Naval Institute, 1960.

Staley, Seward C., *Physical Exercise Programs*. St. Louis: C. V. Mosby Company, 1953.

8

Posture Improvement

Physical education in this country has always been concerned with the correction of posture faults. Since the introduction of Ling's Swedish system of calisthenics in the latter part of the nineteenth century, physical educators have utilized therapeutic exercises for this purpose; this work continues at the present time. In this chapter, attention will be given to the problem of helping people who have deviations from proper body alignment.

VALUES OF GOOD POSTURE

Today, posture is not just related to the standing position, as was generally the case in the past. It encompasses many aspects of a person's stance, involving the correlation of the skeletal, muscular, and nervous systems. This gives a greater scope to posture considerations, including stances required for standing, sitting, walking, lying, and the like. Viewed broadly, three types of values may be advanced for good posture: aesthetic, movement efficiency, and improved fitness.

Aesthetic Values

The advantages of a pleasing appearance are well understood. Good posture contributes positively to such an appearance. No one would judge a person with sagging abdomen, rounded shoulders, and protruding head as being physically attractive. Certainly, all art forms portraying the human body to best advantage show a well-coordinated figure; grace and poise, leading to a pleasing posture, dominate.

Playwrights and actors show personality through body stance. The dynamic leader of a just cause expresses his fervor not only in words; his posture forms an integral part of his dynamic presence. An actor portraying Dr. Jekyll and Mr. Hyde uses radical changes in posture to illustrate vast differences in personality. In the same sense, we can use our bodies, if we will, as expressions of our personalities.

MOVEMENT EFFICIENCY

The athlete is well acquainted with the importance of stance in performing the skills necessary in his event. His coach constantly drills him on form, in the firm belief that he will perform more effectively. Thus, we have the stance of the football lineman, the form of the runner, the grace of the fencer, the beautiful co-ordination of the gymnast. In standing, walking, running, and climbing, it is logical to expect that a person will be more effective, graceful, and co-ordinated if his stance is correct, and his posture is good.

Whenever the body takes an upright position, the antigravity (extensor) muscles must maintain a high degree of tonicity. The so-called postural reflex is essential to maintain a normal standing position. One is in a better position of readiness for movement when this stance is good. However, this good posture is not easy to maintain and requires more energy than a slump, whereby the body weight rests primarily on the joint ligaments rather than being held upright by the muscles. Thus, in many instances, the body musculature must be conditioned to maintain good posture.

IMPROVED FITNESS

One of the authors has discussed the fitness values of posture elsewhere. In so doing, he presented and evaluated available research evidence pertaining to this problem, concluding as follows: "Thus there may be seen in the inability of previous experimenters to measure posture a fundamental reason why attempts to correlate posture with health, scholarship, intelligence, athletic ability, organic condition, and similar criteria have mostly failed. When measures of any one of these are correlated with posture, the result will never be higher than the reliability of the posture tests. Therefore, until the value or lack of value of posture can be definitely established, the conscientious physical educator must decide for himself whether the results derived from good posture are beneficial to the physical well-being of the individual and whether or not he will continue with posture training."[1]

---

[1] H. Harrison Clarke, *Application of Measurement to Health and Physical Education*, 3rd ed. (Englewood Cliffs, N. J.: Prentice-Hall, Inc., 1959), p. 153.

Physical educators who have specialized in corrective exercise generally attribute health values to good posture and to the results of posture training. For example, Stafford and Kelly[2] maintain that blood tends to slow down and "stagnate" in the large veins of the abdomen, if the abdominal muscles are weak and chronically sag, that the excursion of the lungs in breathing is diminished with faulty body mechanics, and that the kidneys, spleen, and abdominal organs are not given proper support in poor posture and, as a consequence, their functions suffer. Lowman and Young[3] also state that faulty posture very directly affects the integrity of the breathing process, due to decreased chest diameter, relaxation of the abdominal wall, and sagging of the large suspensory ligament from the base of the neck which helps hold up the heart and lungs.

NATURE OF GOOD POSTURE

The tendency to describe one pattern of good posture and insist that all individuals should conform precisely to this standard is unfortunate. To generalize is feasible, but allowances should be made for variations in body composition and physique type. The important thing is for posture to show erectness, good body alignment, good balance, and ease of stance; a feeling of alertness, of readiness for movement, of coordination throughout the body segments should be noticeable. It would be much easier to apply a common posture design to all; however, the developmental and adapted physical educator must learn to recognize the postures which are in need of improvement, those which are improvable through guidance and special exercises, those which should be examined by a medical specialist, and those which are merely different because of variations in individual structure.

Balanced alignment provides a body appearance which, when viewed from the side, is vertical rather than zigzag, the various body masses joining smoothly in symmetry and harmony. Generally, the standing stance shows a straight or nearly straight gravitational line starting in front of the ankle joint and passing through the patella, through the middle of the greater trochanter and the acromion, and to the lobe of the ear. Slight deviations from this line may be normal for some, depending on individual differences as shown below.

The posture of individuals with ectmorphic physique types are prone to faults of alignment, largely because of the suppleness of their musculo-ligamentous structures. Moreover, if low in the mesomorphic

---

[2] George T. Stafford and Ellen D. Kelly, *Preventive and Corrective Physical Education*, 3rd ed. (New York: The Ronald Press Company, 1958), pp. 87-88.

[3] Charles L. Lowman and Carl H. Young, *Postural Fitness* (Philadelphia: Lea and Febiger, 1960), p. 154.

component, they are normally weak muscularly, so are more prone to fatigue and thus find it difficult to maintain good posture. Such boys and girls, however, can readily be taught to assume a straight vertical position; with the conditioning of the anti-gravitational muscles, they can show a creditable improvement.

Boys and girls with medium builds, the midtype somatotype, may reflect many of the characteristic of the ectomorph insofar as posture is concerned. They may not be so flexible as the ectomorph but may be better balanced with mesomorphy. Thus, these individuals may encounter more difficulty in assuming correct body alignment but will respond more readily to strengthening exercises.

Mesomorphs are less likely to have serious postural faults. This is because their heavier bone structure provides greater stability; they tend to be less flexible than the other somatotype groups; and they have much greater strength and power with which to maintain a well-balanced stance. For them, however, posture faults once acquired are more difficult to correct because of their greater structural rigidity.

Endomorphic boys and girls are handicapped in making a pleasing postural appearance because of excess fat pads located throughout the body. Thus, the evaluation of their posture presents certain difficulties. For example, the presence of fat deposits around the abdomen creating a rounded contour is unavoidable and does not constitute a posture fault. The gravitational line can be applied to these individuals, if fat is distributed uniformly, but body contours will need to be largely ignored in assessing the posture. Unless endomorphs have a high degree of the mesomorphic component (and even then the endomorphy will be a burden), their posture problems can easily be acute.

In addition, various physical anomalies or irregularities in body structure, when present, will affect the way boys and girls can use their bodies. Thus, an individual with short clavicles will manifest some degree of round shoulders; the mature girl with large bust development will tend to lean backward from the hips; the boy with a post-polio leg will need to realign his gravitational line to compensate for a shortened leg and damaged leg and hip muscles.

The determination of whether or not posture faults are unavoidable adjustments for such conditions as those discussed above or are functional posture faults in need of improvement is not always easy. Stafford and Kelly[4] suggest that in doubtful cases posture exercise should be applied. Then, if no improvement can be achieved or if attempts to convert one fault lead to other faults, the physical educator should suspect that he may be dealing with an atypical body structure or a pathological condition.

---

[4] Stafford and Kelly, *op. cit.*, p. 108.

POSTURE FOR VARIOUS FUNCTIONS

While the emphasis in posture improvement is typically directed toward the standing position, attention should also be given to reclining, sitting, and walking. Standards for judging the correct positions of the body under these conditions of everyday life will be discussed here.

STANDING

The poise of the body should be such as to provide conditions of efficient balance while permitting favorable functioning of the internal organs. Starting from the ground up, the feet should be so placed as to support the body weight with a minimum of strain. Thus, they should be parallel and about two to four inches apart or with one foot slightly in advance of the other; in either instance, the toes should point straight ahead. The weight of the body should be carried toward the outer edges of the feet, so as to place the strain primarily on the outer bony structure rather than on the ligaments of the longitudinal arches. In the more active postures, the body will be forward toward the balls of the feet; such habitual postures correlate .75 with Physical Fitness Indices, so may be indicative of the individual's state of muscular fitness.[5]

With the feet placed as described, the patellas of the knees will point straight ahead. The thighs will be in midposition of inward and outward rotation. The knees should be in easy extension with the quadriceps femoris muscles in slight contraction.

The basic key to proper standing position is the pelvis. A flat lumbar spine and a tucked in or flat abdomen (fat deposits permitting) are desirable. These two conditions are closely associated and are controlled by the position of the pelvis. In order to keep the pelvis from tipping, so that a nearly flat back-abdomen can prevail, the gluteus maximus and the hamstrings pull down on the pelvis from behind and the rectus femoris, psoas, and iliacus muscles pull on the pelvis from in front. The normal angle of inclination is such that the plane of the brim of the pelvis is about 60 degrees with the horizontal.[6]

The thoracic spine should also be shallow, extending through the cervical spine to the head balancing thereon. The head should be held erect with the chin tucked in; this is accomplished by pushing the

---

[5] Thomas K. Cureton and J. Stuart Wickens, "The Center of Gravity Test of the Human Body in the Antero-Posterior Line and Its Relation to Posture, Physical Fitness and Athletic Ability," *Research Quarterly Supplement*, 6, No. 2 (May, 1935), p. 93.

[6] W. M. Phelps, Robert J. H. Kiphuth, and C. W. Goff, *The Diagnosis and Treatment of Postural Defects*, 2nd ed. (Springfield, Ill.: Charles C. Thomas, 1956), p. 94.

back of the head up, so that the acromion is on the straight gravitational line.

SITTING

Sitting for relaxation is typically not a particular problem, as the individual is usually ensconced in a comfortable chair, is free to move easily, and will constantly shift his position at signs of discomfort. However, sitting at work or at study can be quite fatiguing and posture deforming, as the individual is confined to a limited space and has his movement restricted as a consequence of his activity.

An essential feature of good sitting posture for work or study is a properly designed chair and a table surface of correct height. The chair seat should be of such height that the feet can rest on the floor without pressure under the knees which would interfere with circulation; for the same reason, the seat should be shallow enough so that hips can be pushed well back. The seat should also slant slightly toward the rear with a hollow for the buttocks, as an aid in maintaining the hips at the back of the chair.

The back of the chair should be curved backward, or better still should be open at the bottom to allow the hips adequate space; support for the back is needed only below the shoulder blades, at the dorso-lumbar junction. The desk or table surface should be at a height which permits the elbows to rest on it without lifting the shoulders or lowering the chest.

RECLINING

Generally speaking, prescribing the position one should take when sleeping is unnecessary, as the individual is constantly shifting position during the night. The selection of a bed may be more important, as one with yielding springs and a soft mattress permits the body to sag, frequently causing morning backache. On the other hand, an excessively hard bed is apt to be uncomfortable for thin people whose bony structure is subjected to constant contact and pressure from this unyielding surface.

A high pillow is undesirable for those who sleep mostly on their sides, as it permits sagging into a scoliotic position; however, a low pillow is needed to hold the head in line with the rest of the body. Usually, for the young and flexible person, a pillow is unnecessary. When lying prone, a pillow for the head should definitely not be used; if the bed sags, however, one may be placed under the abdomen.

WALKING

Good walks vary within normal limits as expressions of individual structure and personality. Normal limits are judged in relation to the ease, buoyancy, and grace of the stride.. Movements of the arms, legs, and trunk should be in a forward-backward plane; sideward or circular movements should be minimized.

In walking, the legs should swing forward from the hips with the heel striking the ground first; with the toes pointed straight ahead, the body weight should pass over the outer borders and thence to the ball of the foot. The arms should swing freely without rigidity in the shoulder girdle. Stress should be placed upon a fully extended spine, an uplifted abdomen, an erect head, and an expanded chest.

POSTURE FAULTS

"When is a posture fault really a posture fault," is a question frequently asked, although not always in those words. Deviations from the gravitational line may range in degree from slight to marked; some deviations may be due to individual variations in body composition and physique type, and should not be considered posture faults, as discussed above. In posture examinations, perhaps it is best to note all posture faults regardless of degree and whether or not the individual will be subjected to special exercises and guidance for posture improvement. In this section, common posture faults will be presented.

ANTEROPOSTERIOR FAULTS

Forward Head. In this posture fault, the head and neck are held in a forward, downward position; the chin is pulled in toward the neck and the face as a whole is downward at an angle of 30 to 45 degrees from the horizontal.[7] Forward head is frequently associated with a rounded upper back.

Round Upper Back. Round upper back is also known as dorsal or thoracic kyphosis. It consists of an increase in the normal spinal curve in the thoracic region, and may be accompanied by a hollow back. This condition should not be confused with round shoulders which may be found without any spinal variation; however, round shoulders and forward head are usually present with round upper back.

Round Shoulders. In round shoulders, the shoulders are forward with the tip of the acromion anterior of the gravitational line; the sterno-clavicular joint, the only joint support for the shoulders, is depressed. The scapula are separated beyond normal; as they rotate on their long axes, the vertebral borders, protruding backward, become prominent. Flexible as contrasted with rigid round shoulders are distinguished by ability to bring the shoulders to a normal position by either active or passive movement. With forward head, the weight of the arms swings

---

[7] Stafford and Kelly, *op. cit.*, p. 126.

the shoulders toward the front, which, combined with the constant use of the arms in front of the body, results in round shoulders; while not always present, there is a definite tendency to round the upper back. The muscles primarily involved in round shoulders are the rhomboids and trapezius; some stretching of the pectoral muscles will frequently be desirable.

Hollow Back. Hollow back is also known as lumbar lordosis. In this condition, the normal curve of the lumbar spine is exaggerated. The pelvis tips down in front and the abdominal muscles, basic fixators of the trunk anteriorly, become stretched; as a consequence, a faulty position of the visceral organs results. The back muscles and posterior ligaments in the lumbar region are shortened and become tight, holding up the back of the sacrum and rotating the pelvis forward. Lordosis is usually accompanied by a number of other compensatory deviations, such as round upper back, round shoulders, and forward head.

Parenthetically, hollow back decreases the range of motion in the hip joint. When present in a runner, the length of his stride is decreased; thus, reduction of the lordosis can well be a means of improving his competitive time as a consequence of permitting a longer stride. This limitation in range of motion also makes the individual prone to sacroiliac strain and lower back pain.

Flat Back. Flat back, or lumbar kyphosis, decreases the slight normal curve of the lumbar spine until it is eliminated or results in a slight backward bulge. The distinction between individuals with a very erect spine and those with lumbar kyphosis may be difficult to make; as a posture fault, this condition is associated with such other faults as bent knees, protruding abdomen, and rounded upper back.

Overcarriage. Phelps, Kiphuth, and Goff[8] define overcarriage as a stance characterized by a forward tilt of the legs, no increase in the upward roll of the pelvis, and backward inclination of the trunk at the hips. Thus, a plumbline dropped from the seventh cervical vertebra will swing free of the buttocks. In this condition, the iliofemeral ligament is longer than normal, allowing a greater amount of hyperextension at the hip; the lower adbomen and pelvic brim are the parts of the body farthest forward of the gravitational line.

LATERAL FAULTS

Lateral postural faults of the spine are generally grouped under the term, scoliosis, a word derived from the Greek word meaning twisting or bending. While very few spines are absolutely straight laterally, there are some which have well defined bends to one side or the other; usually, these also exhibit some lateral rotary deviation.

---

[8] Phelps, Kiphuth, and Goff, *op. cit.,* p. 127.

A number of scoliotic deviations occur, which may generally be categorized as C and S curves. The commonest scoliosis is the C curve, which consists of a long convexity to one side, usually the left. The S scoliosis consists of reverse curvatures, laterally in one direction in the upper back and in the opposite direction in the lower back. Such a scoliosis might consist of right thoracic and left lumbar curvatures, the direction of the curves being designated by their convexity.

In scoliosis, the shoulders tend to maintain their normal right angle with the upper thoracic spine, so unevenness in the shoulder level results; one shoulder, therefore, will be lower than the other. Some rotation of the spine also occurs, causing the posterior aspect of the attached ribs to become prominent on the side of the curve's convexity and the vertebral border of the corresponding scapula to pull away from the ribs. Unless the legs are of uneven length, the hips will be level; however, the iliac crests on one side will be more prominent than the other, due to the lateral sagging in the lumbar region.

Lateral curvatures have frequently been classified as functional, transitional, and structural. To differentiate these classifications, the functional curve disappears when the effect of gravity on the posture is eliminated. One of the following three tests may be applied: (1) lie flat out in prone position and relaxed; (2) suspend the relaxed trunk by the hands from a horizontal bar; or (3) from a standing position, bend first the head forward, then the shoulders, and on down the back until in a completely relaxed position. If, upon applying one of these tests, the lateral curvature disappears, the fault is functional; if the curvature remains fully in the back, it is structural; if it partly disappears, a transitional state is indicated. Rathbone,[9] however, considers these distinctions false and maintains that a better procedure is to consider scoliosis as progressing from a less fixed to a more fixed condition; she maintains that at every stage there is some disturbance in structure. In the early stages, the disturbance may be in the muscles and soft tissue only; while, in the later stages, the bones will be permanently involved.

POSTURE APPRAISAL

In another book by one of the authors, a chapter was devoted to "Measurement in Remedial Work."[10] In Chapter 4 of this book, evaluation as applied to developmental and adapted physical education is presented. A duplication of posture and body mechanics tests in these

---

[9] Josephine L. Rathbone, *Corrective Physical Education,* 6th ed. (Philadelphia: W. B. Saunders Company, 1959), p. 109.

[10] Clarke, *op. cit.,* chap. 7.

two sources is avoided. In Chapter 4, however, the sections on cable-tension strength and range of joint movement tests may logically have some significance for posture improvement efforts. In connection with strength measures, for example, Klein[11] has provided evidence that differences generally exist between the muscular endurance of right and left quadriceps muscles for individuals whose habitual standing postures were imbalanced (i.e., with body weight being carried habitually on one leg); these differences were not present for those in whose habitual stance weight was evenly distributed on both feet.

The formal-type posture appraisal has usually been made with the subject standing in his "best" position. In addition to any postural faults present, the examiner views the student's concept of what good posture is and his ability to assume this position. This type of information, of course, is valuable. However, knowledge of his habitual posture practices is also helpful. In some instances, the habitual posture can be elicited by asking the subject to stand naturally; in other instances, it will be necessary to obtain this information when the individual is in an informal situation and not aware that he is being appraised.

In the posture examination, of course, the less clothing worn the better. If separate facilities are available for developmental and adapted physical education, the posture evaluation process will be simple enough, especially if the sexes are separated for this type of class work. If such is not the case, perhaps some area can be screened off for privacy. Another suggestion is to use an isolated space in the locker room; the habitual posture appraisal can be made here, too, as the students stand and move about in their dressing and showering.

Considerable time can be saved in giving posture examinations by utilizing screening tests to select those boys and girls who will be given complete posture examinations. In such screenings, each student is quickly inspected from the front, side, and rear by the examiner, who decides whether or not he should be included in the posture improvement program. Those so selected may then be given a careful posture appraisal, in which the various faults are noted and their degrees of deviation recorded.

CAUSES OF POSTURE FAULTS

There are many and diverse causes of posture faults; and, usually, more than one is present in the same situation. Several of the more significant of these causes will be discussed here.

---

[11] Karl K. Klein, "Comparison of Bilateral Quadriceps Strength as Related to Good and Bad Standing Posture," *Journal of Association for Physical and Mental Rehabilitation*, 7, No. 1 (September-October, 1952), p. 16.

Unless boys and girls have been subjected to instruction in proper posture, they do not know what good posture is. Those who have had teachers merely yell at them "suck in your gut," "tuck in your chin," "shoulders back," may have a couple of points in mind, but, more likely than not, they have created other posture faults in their attempt to meet these strident instructions. The starting point of any posture improvement program is to teach pupils proper standing, sitting, and walking stances.

Boys and girls should also be given the kinesthetic feeling of good posture. Preferably, this should be done in front of a full-length mirror, so that they see what they look like as well. Of course, some individuals may not be able to assume good posture, due to lack of co-ordination or the presence of restraining muscles and ligaments. Nevertheless, each should be placed in a position as near the desired one as possible, even though it may be strained or uncomfortable, and impossible of maintenance until later in the posture improvement program.

A simple way to accomplish the correct or nearly correct posture position is as follows. Have the student stand facing the full-length mirror. From the rear, the physical educator manually places the student's head and shoulders into position and asks him to hold them firm. Then, the teacher places the side of his head against the upper back to help stabilize the student's position; with one hand he pulls up on the abdomen in front and with the other he pushes down on the buttocks from behind. This maneuver should tilt the pelvis and flatten the lumbar spine. The student holds this position as the instructor steps away.

Best posture will be practiced habitually only if each boy and girl desires to do so. A student will have such a desire only if he understands thoroughly the aesthetic and fitness advantages which accrue to a well-poised and anatomically well-coordinated body stance. The motivational suggestions made in Chapter 3 may be directed toward this end.

A prevalent associate of posture faults is poor muscular development. Unfit boys and girls are poor-posture prone, since they do not have the muscular strength to maintain good posture for any length of time. Their anti-gravitational muscles lack muscular endurance. The usual "fatigue slump" reveals a relaxation of the whole upright stance, resulting in pelvic tilt, protruding abdomen, lumbar lordosis, thoracic kyphosis, round shoulders, and forward head. A major effort needs to be made with these individuals to improve their general strength and endurance before any posture program *per se* can be effective.

POOR POSTURE HABITS

Poor posture habits, of course, are closely associated with the presence of posture defects. Such habits may involve faulty standing or sitting positions, in which the boy or girl permits the spine to sag, the abdomen to protrude, and the shoulders to round. These defects are most prone to appear and to be accentuated when the student has been standing for any length of time. Poor muscular strength and endurance aggravate this situation, in fact, will make it inevitable.

The practice of some occupations are conducive to poor posture. The student or accountant spends many hours at a desk, where the tendency to round the upper back and permit the body to collapse, so to speak, is ever present. The stance of the violinist or of the boy carrying a heavy bag of papers consistently over the same shoulder promotes lateral deviations of the spine. Even over-specialization in some sports, despite an excellent body development, can lead to postural deviations.

In dealing with posture cases, it is well to investigate the habitual and occupational bodily positions of the subjects; a great variety of situations will be found. Steps to change and/or counteract these influences should be taken.

PHYSICAL DEFECTS

Certain types of physical defects are obvious causes of faulty posture; and provide situations that may or may not be corrected. If one leg is slightly shorter than the other, the hips will be uneven and compensation for this unevenness will take place in the spine, causing a scoliosis. In this instance, the correction may be quite simple, consisting of adding a lift of proper thickness to the heel of the shoe. However, if the short leg is pronounced, or caused by a crippling disease such as poliomyelitis, the individual may need to live with a postural deviation.

All sorts of permanent defects, of course, cause postural faults. These defects may be the results of birth injuries, neurological diseases, nutritional inadequacies, and joint diseases. Individuals with these conditions will typically be under the care of medical specialists and, in some instances, may need to wear braces or other artificial supports.

EXERCISE FOR POSTURE IMPROVEMENT

Good posture depends upon: (1) Knowing what good posture is; (2) Being able to assume good posture; (3) Possessing the strength and fitness to maintain good posture for reasonable lengths of time without fatigue; (4) Having the desire to practice good posture consistently. With these four factors realized, the posture problem will be met.

In posture training, some people will need exercises especially designed to permit the individual to assume proper positions with ease. In order to accomplish this purpose, two types of exercise are generally needed. Where muscles and ligaments have been shortened, thus restricting joint movement, stretching exercises will be necessary; where muscles are weak and lengthened, muscular strength and muscular endurance must be developed in them. These exercises are usually complementary; for example, in lordosis, the lumbar spine is stretched anteriorly and the abdominal muscles are shortened and strengthened.

It should be stressed that the foregoing is true only when the postural fault is functional. Where postural faults have structural involvements, corrective exercise if applied at all should be under the direction of a physician, preferably an orthopedic or physical medicine specialist.

POSTURE IMPROVEMENT EXERCISES

Exercises will not be presented here for separate entities, such as forward head, protruding abdomen, and the like, but, rather as combinations commonly found together. Both stretching and strengthening exercises will be described. Certain of these exercises call for the assistance of a partner; when this is the case partners should be properly instructed and supervised in the part they are to play. Some of the exercises described in Chapter 7 can also be used for posture improvement.

UPPER BACK, NECK, AND SHOULDERS

As explained above, thoracic kyphosis is a round upper back, usually accompanied by round shoulders and forward head. Posture improvement exercises for this general area follow.

1. *Chest stretch:* Supine lying position, sandbag or folded turkish towel under scapulae, knees flexed and abdominal muscles contracted to hold lower trunk in position; extend arms sidewards to stretch chest muscles.

2. *Manual chest stretch:* Sitting position, knees bent and feet flat, hands behind head with elbows out, chin held in, and head held high; partner places knee against upper back and forces elbows backward, stretching chest muscles; subject holds starting position and assists movement, thus contracting upper back muscles.

3. *Neck exercise:* Prone lying position with partially inflated volleyball under chest, arms at sides; raise head against resistance of partner.

4. *Upper back exercise:* Prone lying position, hands behind head; raise head and elbows, holding position briefly.

5. *Overhead wand pull:* Sitting position, chin in, head erect, hands grasping wand (shoulder width) held directly overhead by partner; pull down against resistance applied by partner, keeping shoulders well back, chin in, and elbows back.

6. *Rowing exercise:* Two subjects in sitting position facing each other, legs intertwined alternately to anchor position, both grasping same wand with hands; alternately, each subject pulls against the other's resistance in rowing motion, keeping elbows out and shoulders pulled well back.

LOWER BACK AND ABDOMEN

As considered earlier in this chapter, lumbar lordosis consists of hollow back and is associated with a protruding abdomen and downward tilt of the forward brim of the pelvis. Exercises for the posture improvement of this involved situation are presented here.

Many of the abdominal exercises described in Chapter 7 can be used for strengthening the abdominal muscles and for stretching the lower back. When using them for posture improvement purposes, however, the necessity to keep the back flat at the start and throughout performance should be stressed. Sit-up exercises performed from a hook-lying position are preferable in order to stress contraction of the abdominal muscles and to maintain a flat back. Lower back strengthening exercises will also be found in Chapter 7.

Additional lower back and abdominal exercises which may be used for posture improvement follow.

1. *Sitting back stretch:* Sitting position with knees drawn up and soles of feet together, trunk and head erect and arms passed between and under knees grasping ankles from outside; pull shoulder blades together and force lumbar spine back against resistance supplied by grasp on ankles. (This exercise is especially useful when kypho-lordosis is the posture fault.)

2. *Sitting knee raises:* Sitting position with hands on hips, legs together, and knees straight; holding trunk and head erect and shoulders back, alternately slide heels along floor to position as near buttocks as possible still maintaining specified erect position. *Progression:* (a) Slide both feet together toward buttocks; (b) Perform exercise with hands behind head, elbows back.

3. *Hip raise:* Supine lying position with hands behind head, legs bent, and knees as near chest as possible without raising hips off floor; raise hips bringing knees toward chin, and return to starting position lowering knees only enough for hips to rest on floor.

LATERAL DEVIATIONS

In considering exercises for lateral deviations of the spine, the distinction as to whether a scoliosis is functional or has structural involvements should be made. If structural in nature, the condition should be referred to the student's parents with the recommendation that a physician, preferably an orthopedic specialist, be consulted. If the curvature is functional in nature, the adapted physical educator may proceed with a treatment program.

A first concern in the attempt to eliminate a functional lateral curvature is to locate its cause and either remove it or find a way to counteract its effect. If a person's occupation is such that a lateral twist or bend of the trunk is necessary or desirable, perhaps the position may be alternated so that both sides are equally subjected to the situation, one counterbalancing the other. If this alternation is not possible, occasional brief rest periods during which opposite bending is practiced may help.

Functional lateral curvatures can frequently be traced to poor posture habits. Sometimes, these are fashionable, such as the so-called debutante slouch; at other times, they are simple lapses into a slovenly standing stance, such as slouching on one foot or leaning backwards curving the spine. Proper instructions as to good posture habits with sound reasons for their practice should help in these instances.

Fatigue posture slump due to fatigue and lack of fitness is a common cause of functional lateral deviations of the spine. Obviously, exercises to improve muscular strength and endurance are essential if this type of posture fault is to be improved.

With causes identified and appropriate action instituted for their alleviation, the adapted physical educator may also wish to apply corrective exercises. The exercise procedures used in attempting to improve scoliosis cases are to stretch the side opposite the curve and to strengthen the side having weakened musculature. Most functional scolioses are left total or C curves: this curve can be produced temporarily by standing with a book placed under the right foot. Suggested exercises for this left curve follow; for right curves, reverse the exercise for the opposite side.

1. *Standing trunk bends:* Standing position, feet astride, right arm over head, left hand against lower edge of rib cage; keeping trunk on a strictly lateral plane, flex strongly toward left side using raised arm to stress movement and bracing firmly with hand against ribs.

2. *Kneeling trunk bends:* Kneel on right leg with left leg extended directly to side, both arms parallel and extended over head; with trunk held firmly, no rotation, and arms well extended, elbows straight, bend

trunk sideward toward extended leg. Phelps, Kiphuth, and Goff[12] suggest this exercise and recommend that it be executed on both sides for lateral trunk development.

3. *Side bends:* Side bends with variation and progression are described in Chapter 7.

4. *Creeping exercise:* Position on hands and knees with thighs perpendicular to floor; creep slowly forward against resistance of partner with right arm leading each time. (Resistance is applied by partner holding against thighs from rear.)

5. *Kneeling arm and leg stretch:* Position on hands and knees with thighs perpendicular to floor; stretch right arm forward and right leg backward.

LOW BACK PAIN

Evaluating observations made over a period of years in his physical medicine practice, Kraus[13] concluded that under-exercise was an important factor in low back pain. Based upon his extensive professional experience, as well as that of orthopedic physicians and other physiatrists, he concluded that the most frequently seen orthopedic problem in which weakness of muscles plays as important a part as tension and tightness is the "low back syndrome."[14] The sedentary person rarely uses adequately the large muscle groups needed in the body maneuvers which may be required of him. Typically, the abdominal muscles are kept slack; the back muscles are used in a static rather than a dynamic fashion while keeping the body erect; the hamstring muscles are shortened and the leg muscles weakened. When in this condition, sudden forceful movement may result in acute muscle strain or in more severe damage in the lower back region; and this may lead to further inactivity and increased likelihood of greater incapacity.

The evaluation of low back pain advocated by Kraus[15] includes, in addition to a thorough standard examination of the patient, palpation of the subcutaneous tissues of the back, gluteal, and lateral thigh areas to establish a differential analysis of fibrositis, and palpation of the muscles along the spine and gluteal area for localized or diffused deep tenderness. Following these procedures, however, the patient is given a series of muscle tests. Known popularly as the Kraus-Weber Test of Minimum

---

[12] Phelps, Kiphuth, and Goff, *op. cit.,* p. 153.
[13] Hans Kraus and Wilhelm Raab, *Hypokinetic Disease* (Springfield, Ill.: Charles C. Thomas, 1961), p. 19.
[14] *Ibid.,* p. 10.
[15] Hans Kraus, "Prevention of Low Back Pain," *Journal of Association for Physical and Mental Rehabilitation,* 6, No. 1 (September-October, 1952), pp. 1-4.

Muscular Fitness,[16] this series embodies strength tests of the upper back, lower back, upper abdominals, lower abdominals (with and without action of the psoas muscle), and length (flexibility) of the back and hamstring muscles. Generally speaking, a very strong parallel exists between muscle status on one hand, and pain and disability on the other. Interestingly, the response of functional low back pain cases to exercise varies, depending on the degree of tensions; the strength of the muscles usually progresses in a regular and systematic manner, while flexibility shows a great dependence on tensions, whether caused by psychological problems or outside irritations.[17]

As a consequence of these considerations, it may be deduced that reasonably vigorous physical activity carried on consistently will be a preventive of low back pain for a great many people. Once present, however, it becomes a medical problem until such time as the symptoms disappear. Kraus[18] estimates that the average treatment period is around three months, with two or three treatment sessions per week. The medical treatment depends on the classification of the condition, i.e., fibrositis, acute painful muscle spasm, orthopedic involvement, arthritis, psychosomatic disorder, and the like. In many cases, however, muscular imbalance is the sole cause of the condition.

The exercise regimen for low back pain sufferers advocated by Kraus[19] follows the pattern disclosed by his 6-item test mentioned above. His proposed exercises follow; some supplementation of these may be worked out by the adapted physical educator using exercises presented in Chapter 7.

Abdominal muscles. Abdominal strengthening exercises are used when these muscles are weak. These are all performed from a supine, hook-lying position, with four grades as follows.

1. With arms at sides, raise head and upper shoulders.

2. With arms at sides, bring knees as far toward chest as possible without raising hips.

3. With hands behind head, bring knees toward chest and raise hips and head and shoulders simultaneously.

4. With hands behind head and feet held down by partner, perform sit-ups.

Psoas muscles. For psoas strengthening, abdominal exercises are performed from supine lying position with knees straight.

Upper back muscles. The upper back strengthening exercises are performed from a prone lying position; three grades of exercises are given.

---

[16] See Chapter 4 for testing techniques for this test.

[17] Kraus and Raab, *op. cit.*, p. 18.

[18] Hans Kraus, "Diagnosis and Treatment of Low Back Pain," *GP*, V, No. 4 (April, 1952), p. 59.

[19] *Ibid.*, pp. 58-60.

1. With arms extended forward beyond head, raise arms, head, and upper chest.

2. With pillow under hips, hands behind head, and feet held down, raise upper body to position parallel with floor.

3. Perform same exercise (2), but with arms extended and with hands holding a weight.

Lower back muscles. The following three grades of exercises are presented from a prone lying position to strengthen the lower back muscles.

1. With arms overhead, alternately raise and lower legs.

2. With pillow under hips, hands on floor alongside head, and chest held down, raise both legs off floor.

3. Perform same exercise (2), but with weight attached to ankles.

Flexibility. The following three grades of exercises to stretch the back and hamstring muscles are proposed.

1. From a supine lying position with arms at sides and one knee bent, raise straight leg as far as possible without bending knee. Repeat exercise with other leg.

2. From erect standing position with both arms straight and extended to rear, bend forward from hips while holding position of arms.

3. From erect standing position with arms at sides, bend forward from hips, keeping knees straight, legs as perpendicular to floor as possible, and arms hanging pendulum fashion from shoulders (attempt to touch floor and hold position).

FOOT FAULTS

In the process of man's evolution, changes in the use of the hands and feet began when original homo sapiens adopted ground life as an upright biped and the functions of locomotion were gradually transferred from the arms and hands to the legs and feet.[20] The scope of the hands' activity has expanded tremendously, as evidenced by their extraordinary skill in so many ways; consider the manual dexterity of the surgeon, the artist, the baseball pitcher, the pianist, and the toolmaker for a full realization of this development. In contrast, the use of the feet became restricted to the function of upright weight-bearing and locomotion of the body. As a consequence, the resulting relatively rigidly arched contour of the modern foot distinguishes it from all other types of feet, and, also, from the prehuman model which is now most closely represented in the arboreal grasping foot of the chimpanzee.[21] The feet, however, are capable of supporting and manipulating weights that greatly exceed

---

[20] Dudley J. Morton, *Human Locomotion and Body Form* (Baltimore: Williams & Wilkins Company, 1952), p. 21.

[21] *Ibid.*, p. 22.

the capabilities of even the most powerfully developed adult arms and hands.[22]

Each foot is comprised of twenty-six bones: seven tarsals, five metatarsals, and fourteen phalanges. In weight-bearing, the talus receives the body weight directly from the tibia; the weight is then transferred to the calcaneus (heel bone) behind and to the navicular and cuboid bones in front; finally, the weight comes to rest on the other tarsal bones and the metatarsals. The inner side of the foot forms a longitudinal arch normally held high by ligamentous structure and the action of muscles with origins in the leg. An outer longitudinal arch also exists, although this is usually depressed in weight-bearing so that the body weight rests on the ground. Transverse arches also exist, each foot providing one-half the dome. The transverse arch across the ball of the foot, formed by the heads of the metatarsal bones, is typically called the metatarsal arch; some differences of opinion exist as to whether or not the metatarsal arch is a true arch, but all agree that this area of the foot needs considerable support from the ligaments and muscles.

Six movements of the feet are generally recognized as follows. (1) *Ankle plantar flexion* (or foot extension): pushing the forefoot downward in line with the leg. (2) *Dorsal flexion:* pulling the forefoot upward toward the tibia. (3) *Abduction:* forepart of the foot flays outward while the sole of the foot maintains its normal parallel relation to the floor. (4) *Adduction:* opposite of abduction. (5) *Inversion:* movement within the ankle joint tipping the sole of the foot inward. (6) *Eversion:* opposite of inversion. The medial and lateral movements of the foot may also result from or be co-ordinated with outward and inward rotation of the leg at the hip joint. A foot is considered to be *pronated* when the ankles roll inward, with eversion and abduction of the foot, so that the body weight falls on the inner borders of the longitudinal arch, causing them to be depressed. *Supination* occurs when the ankles roll outward into a position the opposite of pronation.

DEVIATIONS

The foot is in its strongest anatomical position when it is at right angles to the leg and is held in slight supination; in this position, the toes point straight ahead or slightly outward. If this stance can be maintained, many foot faults can be avoided. As for standing posture, individual differences in foot mechanics exist, which may not be considered as foot faults. The desirable height of the longitudinal arch has been a debatable point; the consensus is that considerable variations in this height may well be considered within the normal range. In fact, even flat feet are not always pathological. And, some great athletes have per-

---

[22] *Ibid.*, p. 27.

formed well with low or flat arches; this has been particularly true of some of the great sprinters. Conversely, high arches do not guarantee the functional efficiency of the feet. It appears that the prime consideration should be not the height of the arch but the ability of the feet to withstand strain.

Generally speaking, however, an evaluation of the foot as related to its logical anatomical position should be made. Then, if faults are present, functional criteria of foot efficiency may be applied. Types of foot faults are described below.

Weak longitudinal arch. The weak longitudinal arch may lead to flat feet. This condition denotes a sag in the plantar ligaments and muscles, which permits the keystone bone of the inner arch, the navicular, to drop, eventually to the floor if complete arch flatness results. A weak longitudinal arch is accompanied by foot pronation; a prominence of the bones of the inner border of the foot and a bowing inward of the Achilles tendon are obvious when viewed from the rear. Interference with blood circulation may be involved, resulting in a weak pulse and a cold foot.

Weak metatarsal arch. A weak metatarsal arch may be observed from a depression of the second, third, and fourth metatarsal-phalangeal joints. This condition is usually accompanied by callous formations in the ball of the foot, especially over the heads of the metatarsals. Distress is usual, and may be roughly assessed by manual pressure from below.

Short first metatarsal. The first (inner) metatarsal is the most important bone in the forepart of the foot, both in standing and in locomotion. In his analysis of the function of this bone, Morton[23] has shown that any impairment of the bone's effectiveness induces a corresponding disturbance in the function of the entire foot, although the importance of this disturbance has been challenged by Harris and Beath.[24] The shortness of the first metatarsal can be identified by measuring the distance the most advanced point of metatarsal II extends beyond it. Morton[25] reported that a shortness of two millimeters or more is found in 40 per cent of feet; shortness of about one-half centimeter is relatively frequent; a full centimeter is unusual, and more than that occurs rarely. A short metatarsal I is an inheritable condition running in family strains.

Contracted foot. In contracted foot, or talipes cavus, the arch is very high, the plantar fascia is very tight, and the toes are buckled, so that the tops of the toes rub against the shoe and become calloused. This condition may be due to tight shoes or stockings or the result of residual paralysis within the foot.

---

[23] Morton, *op. cit.*, chap. XX.

[24] R. I. Harris and T. Beath, "The Short First Metatarsal," *Journal of Bone and Joint Surgery,* 31-A (March, 1949), p. 553.

[25] Morton, *op. cit.*, p. 97.

Bunions. Bunions, or hallux valgus, is a condition in which the great toe is deflected toward the other toes. The pressure of shoes upon the exposed metatarsal-phalangeal joint causes irritation; consequent calcium deposits at this site increase the size of the joint.

FUNCTIONAL FOOT EFFICIENCY APPRAISAL

The functional efficiency of the foot may be appraised in several ways. The more common of these ways follow.

Pain. Pain upon weight-bearing is an obvious symptom of foot insufficiency. However, Kelly[26] found that pain on pressure formally applied to the feet differentiated normal from painful and pronated from painful feet. She used the following three pressure points: (1) under the junction of the first and second metatarsals with the first cuneiform bone; (2) under the insertion of the tibialis anterior muscle; and (3) under the posterior of the plantar-calcaneo-navicular ligament into the calcaneus bone. Rathbone[27] suggests five pain centers in the foot: (1) at the metatarsal-phalangeal joints, particularly under the head of the fourth metatarsal; (2) on the sole of the foot close to the heel; (3) under the scaphoid; (4) on the mid-dorsum of the foot; and (5) on the outer surface of the foot. These centers of pain are at points where the ligaments are subjected to stretch or where there is pressure.

Fatigue. A second symptom of foot inefficiency is fatigue, especially after standing for short periods of time. Fatigue may be felt not only in the foot muscles, but may be evident in the calf, thigh, and back muscles as well. When the foot is pronated in a weak position, the strain on the longitudinal arch is pronounced; the accompanying rotation of the leg at the hip joint places additional stress on the knee, hip, and lower back.

Improper foot mechanics. Observation of foot mechanics in standing, walking, and running, as discussed earlier in this chapter, may also disclose functional inefficiency in the use of the feet.

CAUSES AND THEIR ALLEVIATION

While occasional foot faults may be traced to hereditary or congenital causes, the greater number by far are due to abuse of the feet in various ways from infancy throughout life. Certain of these causes and suggestions for their removal or alleviation are presented below.

Shoes and stockings. The main culprits of foot faults are the shoes and stockings worn. Short and tight stockings, worn consistently, com-

---

26 Ellen D. Kelly, "A Comparative Study of Structure and Function of Normal, Pronated, and Painful Feet Among Children." *Research Quarterly,* 18, No. 4 (December, 1947), p. 291.

27 Rathbone, *op. cit.,* p. 24.

press the toes and feet, producing a long-continued, gradual pressure against both ends of the feet. This effect is especially prevalent with children because of the shrinkage of stockings occurring from repeated washings and because of rapidity of foot growth during childhood.

The ill-fitting shoe is a more obvious cause of foot faults. Many shoes are too short or too narrow across the balls of the feet; others are too inflexible, thus retarding the free action, or exercise, of the muscles needed for developing the strength of the arches. Vanity is a factor, as, from adolescence onward, both boys and girls are prone to follow the fashions in footwear; thus, the pointed toe, the high heel, and the short last have all contributed heavily to the presence and severity of foot faults.

Shoes should be selected which will permit the foot to function freely while preserving its natural contour and providing adequate support. Among the characteristics of a satisfactory shoe are the following. (1) The soles should be flat, not of the rocker type. (2) The inner border of the shoe should be straight, extending past the ball of the foot, so as to avoid pressure on the great toe. (3) The heel counter should fit the heel snugly in order to prevent inward rolling of the calcaneus and resultant pronation of the foot; the heel should be low, broad, and made of rubber or a similar material to best absorb jar in walking on hard surfaces. (4) The shank should be narrow enough to fit snugly under the inner side of the arch in passive standing; this shank also should be flexible enough to permit the foot muscles to function effectively in walking. (5) The toe cap should permit freedom of the toes; this should be tested when weight-bearing. (6) The shoes should lace up the front in order to permit some adjustment to individual feet.

Arch supports may be necessary in the treatment of severely weakened feet; their indiscriminate use, however, should be avoided as they inevitably cause additional weakness of the foot muscles by restricting muscle action in walking. If used, they should be prescribed by a specialist after careful orthopedic appraisal. If a person has to stand a great deal, as does a saleslady or a traffic policeman, some artificial arch support during these periods of stress may be advisable.

Occasionally, shoe alterations of various types may be advantageous. For example, the Thomas heel is constructed by using a wedge to raise the inner borders of the heel slightly in order to shift the body weight toward the outside of the heel.

Lack of fitness. As was true for posture faults in general, the condition of the feet suffers from lack of adequate strength and endurance of the muscles involved in foot functions. Physical inactivity as a result of sedentary living inevitably results in such weak musculatures, unless counteracted by proper physical education and athletic participation.

Overweight. For people who are obese, the added weight which must be carried daily may constitute the cause of weak and flat-foot conditions. The effect of gradual weight increase may be met to some extent by the muscles of the feet as they gradually adjust and condition for the additional load. Sudden increases in weight, however, may easily overtax the foot muscles before they are conditioned to meet the new demands. Relief from foot strain from this cause is seldom successful without weight reduction.

Injury. In severe injuries to the foot and lower leg resulting from athletics, industry, and everyday life, immobilization of the part may be necessary for some time. Obviously, this restriction of movement and muscle action may cause muscle weakness to the point of noticeable atrophy. Foot strain should be avoided following the removal of casts by a period of reconditioning those muscles affected. Additional coverage of this situation will be found in Chapter 9.

FOOT CONDITIONING EXERCISES

Before considering foot conditioning exercises, stress should be placed on the obvious fact that the causes of foot faults as presented above should be identified and eliminated in so far as it is possible to do so. Proper foot mechanics should also be taught as a matter of course and should be practiced habitually by the subject. Furthermore, proper exercise regimens should be instituted when general body conditioning is indicated.

In addition, special foot conditioning exercises may be desirable to improve foot faults. The main purposes of such exercises are to improve circulation, increase range of foot motion (flexibility), and strengthen muscles of the foot and leg. The exercises below are presented to achieve these purposes. Usually, they should be performed in bare feet.

Achilles tendon and calf muscle stretching. Stiffness of the Achilles tendon and the calf muscles frequently interferes with normal foot balance and mechanics; this is especially true for girls and women addicted to the constant wearing of high-heel shoes. Stretching exercises for this area are indicated and may be performed in the following ways.

1. Supine lying position with knees straight and legs slightly apart; push down with heel while holding foot inverted.

2. Standing position, facing and about 18 to 24 inches from wall, feet slightly pigeon-toed, hands placed on wall; lean toward wall, keeping body straight and heels on floor until stretch is felt in calf muscles, hold position for 30 seconds.

3. Standing position, feet slightly pigeon-toed, and toes raised one to two inches by resting them on board, book, or similar object; thrust body forward while keeping heels on floor, hold position. This exercise may be changed by bending forward at hips and reaching as far as possible toward toes, keeping knees straight.

Strength development. Exercises for strengthening the muscles involved in the proper use of the feet are as follows.

1. Sitting on floor, legs extended and slightly apart, heels resting on floor, feet inverted with soles facing each other; holding the inverted position, alternately flex and extend the feet.

2. Sit on chair, feet apart and resting on floor, marbles placed in front of but midway between feet; with right-foot toes, pick up marble, invert foot strongly, and place marble in hand resting on left knee. Repeat with left foot.

3. Sit on chair; with foot inverted, grasp pencil with toes and attempt to write own name with large strokes. Alternate writing with right and left feet.

4. Sit on chair with feet parallel, 10 inches apart, and resting on towel; repeatedly grip towel with toes and pull toward heels, inverting feet during process.

5. Standing position at edge of mat with toes reaching over edge; grip edge of mat with toes.

SUMMARY

This chapter was devoted to a consideration of posture improvement through developmental and adapted physical education. The values of good posture were presented from three points of view, aesthetic, movement efficiency, and physical fitness. The nature of good posture was discussed, as well as its application to the functions of standing, sitting, reclining, and walking. Anteroposterior and lateral posture faults and the means of appraising them were described; in so doing, stress was placed on differentiating between functional and structural involvements.

Lack of posture knowledge, poor muscular development, poor posture habits, and physical defects were identified as the general causes of posture faults. Exercises for posture improvement of the upper back, neck, and shoulders, the lower back and abdomen, and lateral deviations were described. Special attention was given to functional low back pain, its characteristics, involvements, and means of alleviation. Finally, foot faults were discussed, considering the structure of the foot, types of deviations, means of appraising functional foot efficiency, causes of foot faults and their removal, and foot conditioning exercises.

SELECTED REFERENCES

Kraus, Hans, and Wilhelm Raab, *Hypokinetic Disease*. Springfield, Ill.: Charles C. Thomas, 1961.

Lowman, Charles L., and Carl H. Young, *Posture Fitness*. Philadelphia: Lea & Febiger, 1960.

Morton, Dudley J., *Human Locomotion and Body Form*. Baltimore: Williams and Wilkins Company, 1952.

Phelps, W. M., Robert J. H. Kiphuth, and C. W. Goff, *The Diagnosis and Treatment of Posture Defects*, 2nd ed. Springfield, Ill.: Charles C. Thomas, 1956.

Rathbone, Josephine L., *Corrective Physical Education*, 6th ed. Philadelphia: W. B. Saunders Company, 1959.

Stafford, George T., and Ellen D. Kelly, *Preventive and Corrective Physical Education*, 3rd ed. New York: The Ronald Press Company, 1958.

9

Orthopedic
Disabilities

T HE TREATMENT OF BONE AND JOINT INJURY AND DISEASE
constitutes a branch of surgery known as orthopedics.
Inasmuch as conditions in this category include minor sprains and strains
as well as more severe and disabling impairments, they constitute the
largest single group of disabilities encountered in schools and colleges.
While it is true that many of the minor injuries will heal completely
with time and rest, others will require extended treatment and even
prolonged rehabilitation. Many students with orthopedic problems can
profit from developmental and adapted physical education, using exercises carefully planned to provide optimum conditioning and strengthening benefits and other long-term goals.

The full potentialities for such programs have rarely been exploited
in physical education in public schools and colleges. The primary concern of this chapter will be to acquaint the developmental and adapted
physical educator with the major disabilities commonly encountered in
the child and young adult population; temporary injuries will be given
only passing attention. Most of these conditions focus on or about the
various joints of the body; as a consequence, they interfere with one's
ability to move. The effect of some of these, such as intervertebral disc
syndrome, will be felt throughout the entire body, while others will
have a more local involvement. The amputee, on the other hand, may
experience both difficulties; the loss of a limb is local in origin, but

217

mechanical problems may restrict his movement in general. In public schools, many students are permanently excused from participation in physical education as a result of such injuries or illnesses. It is hoped that this practice may be eliminated whenever possible, and that the teacher of developmental and adapted physical education will explore the possibilities for meeting the needs of the orthopedically handicapped student.

JOINT INJURIES AND DISABILITIES

The consequence of injury to a limb or joint is usually to restrict the function of that joint, both during the process of healing and later. Preservation of the mobility and function of a joint presents a serious problem not only to the attending physician but to the various medical and paramedical specialists concerned with the physical rehabilitative process. The difficulties encountered in restoring joint function once it has been lost make it clear that preventive procedures are extremely important.

In every injury one or more of the component joint parts may be involved: cartilage, adjacent bone, synovial sheath and capsule, bursa, ligament, tendon, or surrounding soft tissue. In addition, the various muscles attached about the joint may be involved with the pain and disability felt throughout the entire muscle length. Injury to each of the parts involved may require a different treatment. All parts will need special attention and careful protection against further trauma; this will also help prevent the occurrence of secondary complications that often arise from the premature use of manipulation or weight-bearing, from the failure to protect the joint by adequate splinting, or from overly prolonged immobilization.

CLASSIFICATION OF JOINT INJURIES

To facilitate presentation of the joint injuries that occur to the large number of articulations in the body, they have been arranged here in terms of their location, either within the joint, around the joint, or adjacent to the joint.

Intraarticular. The internal structure of a joint is such that injury may cause severe impairment. Some of these conditions are listed as follows:

1. Contusion of the joint cartilages. This is often the result of falling on an extended limb so that the articular surfaces are driven together.

2. Contusion with dislocation or tearing of the articular cartilage or with fracture of the joint margin. This is often found in such sites as the edge of the acetabulum or the glenoid fossa.

3. Rupturing or tearing of the internal ligaments of a joint. Such

an injury is often accompanied by a partial or complete severing of an articular disc or meniscus.

4. Tearing of the internal ligaments with fracture. An example would include tearing off of the tibial spine with consequent rupture of the anterocrucial ligament of the knee.

5. Intraarticular infection following trauma. Such infection may cause destruction of the joint surfaces, a synovitis, or the aggravation of some pre-existing joint disease.

Periarticular. It is more common for the external joint structures to become disrupted; such injuries are well-known. They include the following conditions.

1. *Sprains.* Sprains can be the result of several different causes, including: the incomplete tearing of one or more ligaments; the tearing of a ligament accompanied by the pulling off of a small fragment of periosteum; the tearing off of ligament, periosteum, and a small piece of bone at the site of attachment (a sprain-fracture). All of these conditions are accompanied by a certain amount of excess fluid concentration and hemorrhage into and about the joint.

2. *Dislocations.* These result in the complete tearing of some portion of the joint capsule, with displacement of the head of the bone from its normal position. Dislocations are always accompanied by sprain and the attendant fluid and blood accumulation in the joint and may be accompanied by contusion of the joint surfaces. Often there is synovial sheath and bursa involvement and temporary or even permenent injury to blood vessels and nerves. One of the hazards of dislocations is the tendency for them to recur as a result of permanent joint capsule damage.

3. *Fracture dislocations* resulting in a dislocation accompanied by a fracture in or near the joint. Examples of this type of injury are a fracture through the anatomic or surgical neck of the humerus with dislocation of the head of this bone, or fracture and dislocation of the hip with fracture of the margin of the acetabulum.

Indirect Articular. Indirect involvement of the joint may be the result of injury to the bones, muscles, fascia, skin, nerves, blood vessels, or lymph channels in the same extremity. The following are injuries which might cause such involvement:

1. Fracture in the adjacent shaft or in some bone of the extremity necessitating prolonged fixation and joint immobilization;

2. Tearing off of the tuberosities about the joint by muscle contraction;

3. Injury of the muscles controlling joint movement, the result either of direct trauma or of treatment;

4. Tearing or rupture of tendons;

5. Scars and contraction of the fascia and skin;

6. Loss of muscle control following nerve injuries;

7. Infections spreading to the joint proper or destroying tissues aiding in joint function;

8. Severe crushing or tearing injuries which may involve all of these tissues.

TREATMENT

One of the most important aspects to be considered in the treatment of all joint injuries is the prevention of permanent disability by early diagnosis of all the parts involved and by immediate application of a treatment procedure aimed at the cure and protection of each injured part. Secondly, nonoperative or operative procedures should be employed to restore function when impaired. All of the therapeutic adjuncts should be used to aid in this restoration.

Physically, traction furnishes an excellent means of preventing destruction and proliferation of joint cartilages with resultant ankylosis or immobility. This is especially true if, because of muscle contraction, thickening of the joint capsule, or the excruciating pain accompanying the condition, the extremity has already assumed a position likely to cause deformity. In this case, traction is definitely indicated. However, no method of traction should be applied that prevents the daily assistive or active exercise of the joints that are not immobilized.

When plaster casts are necessary to maintain opposition and fixation of fractured bones, attention should always be paid to the protection of the weaker group of muscles; as early as possible, active movements of adjacent joints should be started. Therefore, traction of the upper extremity is usually applied at the lower end of the humerus leaving the elbow free for daily movement. The same principle holds for the lower extremity.

Prolonged immobilization will invariably result in a certain amount of muscle atrophy and may cause some restricted range of joint motion. However, when mobility returns, these deficiencies can usually be remedied by the use of progressive resistance exercises designed to increase the strength of the involved muscles. Strength return is seen to be rapid and complete in a relatively short time when these exercises are administered.

DEVELOPMENTAL AND ADAPTED PHYSICAL EDUCATION

The teacher of developmental and adapted physical education is not to be considered a therapist in dealing with students who are recovering from joint injuries and disabilities, nor is he dispensing therapy. However, the school or family physician may feel that additional strengthening exercises would be of benefit if the student demonstrates a local muscular weakness of the involved extremity. If the physical educator is to administer these exercises, the instructions given should be followed with great care. Frequent rechecks may be necessary, so close liaison with the medical officials will be imperative. Many of these students are able to attend classes long before their medical treatment has ended, so it may be possible to be of some help to them early in their recovery. In no case, however, should the teacher of developmental and adapted physical education make the decision regarding exercise prescription or administer exercises to the involved extremity without first obtaining appropriate medical clearance. Even then, he must be sensitive to the student's limitations of exercise tolerance, restricted range of motion, or limits of pain. Any change in these factors should immediately be reported to the student's physician. Generally speaking, however, the principles of exercise outlined in Chapter 7 should be followed with any orthopedically handicapped individual.

For the student who has limitations for exercise, it may be possible to provide a program of reconditioning designed to increase strength and circulatory-respiratory endurance without involving extremities that must not be exercised. When this is done, it is found that the general physical fitness can be maintained or increased as the injury is healing. For example, if an arm or shoulder must be immobilized, it is possible to exercise the legs in running or to utilize them in other strengthening activities. Conversely, when restrictions are placed on leg or hip movements, although they often present more difficult problems, there are many upper extremity exercises that can be designed to obtain maximum conditioning benefits. In this respect, the use of adapted sports can often be of help to the teacher of developmental and adapted physical education, although once again, care must be taken to ensure the safe participation of the student in the activities selected.

JOINT INFLAMMATION

By definition, arthritis is synonymous with inflammation of a joint. The inflammation may vary in severity, depending upon the virulence of the causative agent and the resistance of both the individual and the joint. Arthritis is responsible for widespread affliction, involving possibly some five million persons in the United States including large numbers of children.

RHEUMATOID ARTHRITIS

Although the cause of rheumatoid arthritis (atrophic arthritis) is not known, it has been variously linked with traumatic, chemical, or infectious agents. Atrophic arthritis, frequently a disease of children and young adults, may involve many and perhaps all of the joints of the body, with more than one often actively affected at the same time.

Pathologically, there is apt to be bone atrophy about the joint. Rapid deformity occurs, and accompanying muscle spasm leads to contractures and pain, with resultant immobilization that may lead to complete ankylosis. The joint itself presents an enlarged appearance with considerable thickening of the synovial and ligamentous tissues about the articular capsule.

The predominent clinical manifestations in a rheumatoid arthritic joint are the effusion, pain and heat caused by the inflammatory synovitis. Limited range of motion and deformity appear as a consequence of the early symptoms, with the ultimate disintegration of cartilage and subchondral bone noted as later symptoms.

Treatment of rheumatoid arthritis is not curative and does not alter the course of the disease process; however, certain therapeutic benefits have been obtained in relieving symptoms of pain, maintaining normal joint range of motion, retaining normal muscular strength, and protecting the joints from further destructive trauma. Consequently, heat and therapeutic exercise play important roles in the daily lives of such patients. Heat, preferably moist, helps relieve muscular spasm and pain; such application should be followed by range of motion exercise to help maintain the normal joint excursion. Resistive exercises are necessary to maintain strength in muscle groups that may become weak from disuse. Such exercises are dependent not only on the strength of the muscles but vary as to the severity of joint inflammation and limitations of pain. In some cases, the extent of the physical activity may necessarily be very slight, while in others considerable resistance may be applied.

In addition to these rehabilitative procedures, the general treatment of the patient usually includes measures directed toward the removal of infection and building up of body resistance through diet, rest, and a more favorable climate. Certain drugs have been employed with varying degrees of success in relieving the discomfort associated with rheumatoid arthritis. Aspirin, the most common salicylate to be used, has proved to be the most effective and the least dangerous drug of this kind. Other treatments have included injections of gold salts, the use of such steroids as cortisone and hydrocortisone, the hormone corticotropin (ACTH), and the synthetic chemical compound phenylbutazone.

OSTEOARTHRITIS

Osteoarthritis (hypertrophic arthritis) occurs mainly in persons past middle life. This condition generally affects joints which are susceptible to strain and injury, particularly of the knees, hips, hands, and spine. It is characterized by calcium deposits about the joints and an overgrowth of bone. This bony development may limit the range of motion;

in some cases, ankylosis may occur. Hypertrophic arthritis is not considered an acute disease because it is usually not accompanied by any constitutional symptoms. Pain that may appear upon arising in the morning is generally relieved by "warming up."

Certain types of chronic hypertrophic arthritis, e.g., Marie Strümpell's disease, should be given careful consideration if there is involvement of the spine. During certain stages, a round upper back may develop; if not corrected, this posture fault may become solidified and result in complete rigidity.

The involved joints generally show some local enlargement of the synovial membrane and surrounding tissues. X-ray examination usually will show the "spur" of bone that has grown inhibiting the joint motion.

One of the important treatment procedures considered in the care of patients with osteoarthritis is the removal of any mechanical factors that may be affecting postural deviations. Heel lifts, hyperextension, traction, application of braces and plaster casts may be helpful, together with the institution of exercise to the weakened and stretched muscles. Other therapeutic procedures, massage, and heat, are also used to help reduce pain.

BURSITIS

Bursitis (bursal synovitis) is a rather common affliction of the joints of the body and is caused by irritation of certain bony prominences by either outward pressure or by internal friction of tendons, ligaments, or even the skin. Anatomically, these bony protuberances are protected by small sacs called bursae which are filled with a lubricating synovial fluid that is produced from the walls of these sacs. In this manner, the various bony structures may glide over one another without friction.

Inflammation of a bursa may develop, however, either gradually due to continued strain or injury or acutely as a consequence of more severe trauma. The outstanding symptoms include pain, swelling, and marked tenderness. Pain is noticeably increased upon movement.

Treatment of bursitis may include immobilization, oral medication, injection, and even x-ray therapy in extreme cases, as well as the application of heat. Subdeltoid (subacromial) bursitis, one of the most common forms, may in severe cases require an abduction splint and the use of analgesics for the relief of pain. Chronic cases often necessitate joint aspiration and flushing, together with certain therapeutic procedures to restore joint range of motion and strength to the muscles activating the involved joint.

DEVELOPMENTAL AND ADAPTED PHYSICAL EDUCATION

The student afflicted with arthritis or other form of joint inflammation will undoubtedly be receiving medical guidance concerning his disability. In the more severe cases, it may not be possible for him to take part in any formal exercise program, especially during the acute phases of the disease. During this time, perhaps a number of quiet games or activities requiring a minimum of movement may be advisable; these may be very helpful as a form of relaxation and may provide a means of socialization with other students in the developmental and adapted class.

In the less severe cases, mild exercise or moderately active games may be approved by the physician as beneficial. These must be carefully supervised by the teacher so that the student avoids excessive activity. For those individuals who are only moderately handicapped, swimming in a heated pool probably provides the most easily supervised and physically relaxing type of exercise available. The pleasurable effect of the warm water plus the ability to control the amount of activity provides an excellent medium for their participation. As their disability abates, or in very mild cases, more active conditioning may be approved; however, limitations concerning games involving body contact may be imposed.

During the acute stages of bursitis, activity of the involved joint will undoubtedly be contraindicated, and, indeed, the limits of pain as expressed by the student will help to ensure his co-operation. As the inflammation subsides, his participation in games and conditioning activities may be medically approved. Care must be taken to report any increase in pain or tenderness that may be expressed by the student; the exercises themselves should be carefully graded in intensity as he returns to normal fitness levels.

CONGENITAL DEFORMITIES

Each year, thousands of babies are born with some form of physical defect that does not of itself shorten life or interfere with the intellect. These boys and girls, except for the more severely disabled, will attend school, and therefore may be considered candidates for the developmental and adapted physical education program.

Congenital deformities are the result of improper fetal development and may involve any structure of the body; indeed, there is evidence that more than one often occurs in the same individual. The effect of these conditions on the child ranges from one of extreme disability, so as to be actually incompatible with life, to one that is rather insignificant. Many children in the latter class will fully compensate for any inconvenience caused by their deformity and will take their normal place in school activities; they will not require special attention in physical education. Others, however, may be so disabled as to need additional help from the teacher of the developmental and adapted program. As there are a large number of these anomalies, only those most frequently encountered will be discussed.

CLUBFOOT

Although there are many congenital deformities of the foot that come under the general category of clubfoot (talipes), the two types that will be mentioned specifically are the equinovarus and the calcaneovalgus. In the former, the foot is turned downward and inward so that the outer surface, and in severe cases even the dorsum, of the foot becomes the weight-bearing surface. It causes considerable strain on the foot when standing and walking, and as the child grows older further deformity becomes apparent. Talipes calcaneovalgus is often referred to as congenital flat foot, and is the converse of equinovarus. In this deformity, the toe and the top of the foot often lie against the anterior surface of the leg, so that the weight-bearing surface is the inner surface of the foot and ankle. It is a less common anomaly than the equinovarus, but causes rather severe disability unless corrected.

The treatment for clubfoot is most successful when it is begun early. Because these cases can often be recognized at birth, frequently the only treatment necessary is corrective strapping with adhesive, especially in mild cases. However, more severe impairment may warrant the use of corrective casts, with the result that most of the deformity and disability can be prevented. A delay in treatment may necessitate surgical correction; in older children and adults, this may involve the removal of bone with many weeks of immobilization to follow.

CONGENITAL DISLOCATION OF THE HIP

Congenital dislocation of the hip may involve one or both legs; and successful treatment is facilitated by early diagnosis and treatment. Radiographic analysis of the hip generally reveals the upward and backward displacement of the head of the femur as well as the thickening at the base of the acetabulum. There is no pain attendant to this disability, so it may not be noticed until the child begins to walk, at which time he adopts a characteristic waddling gait. The greater trochanter of the femur is prominent in the hip or gluteal region, and there is usually a noticeable sway-back posture. Treatment consists of reducing the dislocation by replacing the head of the femur in the acetabulum. In infancy or early childhood, this can generally be accomplished by manipulation followed by the application of a hip cast to be worn for a number of months. If the congenital dislocation is treated early, a satisfactory function is usually obtained leaving little or no shortening of the extremity. In older patients, excellent results have been obtained with the use of surgical procedures, so that increasing disability is prevented.

WRY NECK

Wry neck (torticollis) is generally the result of overstretching of a sternocleidomastoid muscle during the passage through the birth canal. Consequently, there is a tendency for the baby to hold the head to one side. As a result of muscle tear, the formation of scar tissue causes the muscle to become inelastic and to develop a contracture. As the child grows older, this leads to the development of facial asymmetry, a curvature of the thoracic spine, and an inequality of the height of the shoulders. In most cases of congenital torticollis discovered shortly after birth, treatment is generally successful in a month or two employing the therapeutic modalities of heat, massage, and stretching. In cases where permanent deformity has resulted, surgical intervention may be indicated, to be followed by the application of a plaster of Paris cast to hold the head in an overcorrected position.

ERB'S PALSY

Erb's palsy, injury to the brachial plexus, may occur at birth as a result of a difficult delivery in which traction is exerted on the baby's head without freeing the shoulder. The injury is limited to the roots or trunks of the fifth and sixth cervical nerves; the infant thereby loses the ability to abduct the arm at the shoulder, to rotate the arm externally, and to supinate the forearm. Generally, the strength in the forearm and the hand grasp is preserved, unless the lower part of the brachial plexus is injured. In mild cases, diagnosis may not be made at birth, but if free voluntary movements of the arm are limited, such cases may be suspected.

Prognosis can be made within a few months after birth when the return of muscle power will demonstrate a nerve injury rather than nerve laceration. It is possible for edema and hemorrhage about the nerve fibers to cause paralysis, and in such cases, the strength should return as these conditions subside.

Treatment generally consists in preventing the nonparalyzed muscles from exerting a pull on the paralyzed ones. It is therefore necessary to abduct and externally rotate the arm with the elbow flexed. At a later age, an airplane splint can be used, as well as other therapeutic treatment procedures. In cases where some innervation of muscles exists, exercise carefully prescribed and administered can improve strength and function of the limb.

DEVELOPMENTAL AND ADAPTED PHYSICAL EDUCATION

It is very difficult to generalize when discussing the developmental and adapted physical education program to be employed for students with congenital deformities. The very nature of these anomalies is such that all areas of the body are subject to deformity, with a number of different combinations possible at each site. Certainly each student must be considered on the basis of his physical disability, which must further reflect his incapacity for exercise and activity. Inasmuch as many children do not receive early and adequate medical treatment of their defects, each year large numbers of boys and girls in the public schools present varying needs in the physical education program. It is probably safe to state that a majority of these cases have been routinely excused from participation in such classes in the past.

The student with a congenital handicap may present the teacher with certain emotional problems that are often difficult to deal with. An unsightly appearance, coupled with parental overprotection in some instances, leaves the young child with a difficult adjustment to make. Academically, these students often compensate very successfully by making an extra effort to perform well in the classroom. The physician, however, may feel that it is important for them to adjust more directly to their physical handicaps by learning to perform skills and participate with other students in those activities for which their individual limitations present no obstacle. In fact, a number of such individuals have exceeded national and even world records in certain athletic events.

In the developmental and adapted program for these students, the advice of the physician should be followed very carefully with exercises being given according to his recommendation. Progress can be made toward the development of physical fitness and a number of skills can be learned to the great satisfaction of the student. The person with a lower extremity involvement often does very well in gymnastic activities, especially in the apparatus events. This generally means that added emphasis on improving upper extremity strength must be made; however, individual satisfaction in such performances often brings forth the extra incentive. On the other hand, upper extremity impairment causes different problems, although a number of games and activities are available for such students. Even ball games can be played with reasonable success if only one arm is incapacitated. Insofar as possible, maximum participation should be sought, and every effort should be made to increase both the physical fitness and the emotional adjustment of these students.

BONE DISORDERS

Unlike congenital deformities, which exist in an individual at or before birth, a large number of orthopedic disabilities may develop in a normal person after birth. Some of the more prevalent of these are presented here under the general category of bone disorders. In studying them, it should be kept in mind that the best way to prevent a deformity is to prevent the disease or abnormality which leads to its appearance. Although for some the cause is not known, an understanding of the disease process itself extends the possibilities for a more enlightened approach by the teacher of developmental and adapted physical education. The growing child offers an excellent laboratory for the study of the various bone disorders, as these conditions often alter the rate of growth or distort the various growth centers. Bone adapts to external or internal stresses and generally reacts in a prescribed manner once these stressors become known. The serious nature of such disabilities in children should not be underestimated by any teacher of physical activities.

OSTEOCHONDROSIS

Osteochondrosis is a disease of children, affecting the growth or epiphyseal centers in such a manner as to result successively in a fragmentation and degeneration, which is followed by regeneration with a subsequent return of normal hardness and strength. Various epiphyses may be involved, but certain ones seem to be more commonly affected. These are known by various names, depending upon the site of involvement. For example, Osgood-Schlatter's disease affects the tibial tubercle, Legg-Calvé-Perthes disease (coxa plana) occurs in the femoral capitular epiphysis, and Scheuermann's disease is found in the vertebral epiphyses. It should be noted that osteochondrosis usually begins in childhood between the ages of five and twelve years, and more commonly affects boys than girls.

The etiology for osteochondrosis is largely unknown, although vascular disturbances and mild trauma are possible causative factors. The outstanding clinical symptom is pain in the affected part which causes a voluntary limitation to the range of motion; when the hip or leg is involved, a protective limp may be noticed. In cases of hip disease, pain may be referred to the knee.

X-ray examination reveals irregularities of the epiphysis and eventual fragmentation which may result in a malformation of the growing bone. In Legg-Calvé-Perthes disease, for example, the bone of the epiphyses of the proximal end of the femur becomes softened and if not protected from weight-bearing during this period, the head of the femur may become so flattened that a permanent disability of the hip results. Two years or more may be necessary for this disease to run its course.

Despite a certain amount of bony distortion, the disease generally terminates with good functional results, provided weight-bearing is avoided during the active stage. Therefore, many orthopedic specialists recommend immobilization of the affected joint in a plaster cast to prevent deformity.

SLIPPED FEMORAL EPIPHYSIS

A condition that resembles osteochondrosis is that of a slipped femoral epiphysis. Present among children at about the age of puberty, the condition results in a non-traumatic separation of the femoral head at the epiphysis, and is often associated with individuals who are excessively overweight. Once again, referred pain may be present in the knee, and the child may favor the extremity by developing symptoms of limitation of motion and limping. If there is complete separation, it then becomes a surgical problem; however, care in the early stages will often prevent this occurrence.

SPONDYLOLISTHESIS

A lordotic deformity at the lower end of the lumbar spine sometimes results from a condition known as spondylolisthesis, in which an anterior displacement occurs, usually of the fifth lumbar vertebra. The disability generally manifests itself as the child approaches puberty, often as the result of some minor trauma. Orthopedic and x-ray examinations are essential to the establishment of a diagnosis. If the deformity is accompanied by pain and disability, surgical treatment is indicated.

RICKETS

Rickets is a nutritional disease of infancy which affects the strength and growth of the bones of the body. Etiologically, there is a disturbance of calcium metabolism, apparently due to a deficiency of calcium and vitamin D. In addition, poor eating habits, lack of sunshine, or perhaps some other factor, can be precipitating causes. Rickets often makes its appearance during the first few months of life, but may not become apparent until the end of the first year. Early signs of the disease include failure to sit or to stand. X-ray pictures may reveal the irregularities in the epiphyseal lines of the bones, denoting a disturbance in growth, and gradually the weakened bones may develop certain deformities as a result of muscular and weight-bearing stresses. Knock-knees and bowlegs are frequently seen, as well as deformities of the chest, spinal curvatures, and various other structural deviations of the upper extremity.

Efforts concerning the treatment of rickets are first directed toward preventing its occurrence, for in almost all instances it can be avoided. If the presence of this disease is discovered early, proper diet and an adequate amount of vitamin D and sunshine may help in preventing deformities. However, early correction of structural abnormalities may be necessary by using splints or plaster of Paris casts, or by employing corrective surgery if the disease process itself has first been arrested.

Although other disturbances have been mentioned, the single most important cause of damage to the epiphyseal growth center is trauma. Indeed, specialists in the field of athletic injuries have for years been aware of the hazard presented by competitive athletics to the physical welfare of growing children, inasmuch as it is possible for damage in this area to cause a disturbance of growth that can lead to some later deformity. Inequality of epiphyseal growth may be responsible for such abnormalities as bowlegs, knock-knees, deformity of the arm and wrist, and shortening of limbs. There is no known way to stimulate epiphyseal growth once it has ceased, although it is frequently possible to diminish the growth of the opposite limb through special treatment in order to bring about a better bilateral balance.

Osteomyelitis

Osteomyelitis is an inflammation of the bone caused by a pyogenic (pus producing) bacteria. Although it may remain localized, the disease organisms, especially staphylococcus and streptococcus, generally reach the bone through the blood stream, affecting the bone marrow or such other structures as the cortex, cancellous tissue, and periosteum. Osteomyelitis is seen most frequently among children between the ages of three and ten years, and while any bone in the body may be involved, frequently more than one is affected.

The onset of the disease is characterized by a sense of extreme illness, with a high fever, headache, nausea, and severe pain and tenderness in the region of the affected bone. Localized swelling and tenderness of the area involved usually occurs within a day or two. Pathologically, after the bacteria have entered the bone, their growth may cause pressure and destruction of bone, and if they break through to the surface, their attack on the periosteum may severely impair the blood supply to the bone. New osseous tissue will be formed by the periosteum; the old bone, unless removed surgically, becomes detached and may work its way out of this abscessed area.

Osteomyelitis may also be caused by the direct contamination of the bone by the infecting organism. Very often this is the result of compound fractures or other penetrating wounds into the bone. These localized infections usually do not result in a generalized reaction throughout the length of the entire involved bone, however. Chronic osteomyelitis occurs occasionally in cases in which the resistance of the body has been built up to the infectious organism. The course of this disease in its chronic form is usually long, marked by intermittent exacerbations.

Treatment with sulfonamides is generally considered useful in combatting streptococcus and staphylococcus infections. The child's health should be maintained at a high level, and all sources of infection should be treated promptly. Chronic osteomyelitis is extremely persistent, often recurring throughout the patient's lifetime. Complete removal of all dead bone and adequate drainage are important factors in the treatment of this disease.

SKELETAL TUBERCULOSIS

Tuberculous infection of the bones and joints is still a fairly common disease, in spite of the fact that great medical advances have been made in the prevention of pulmonary tuberculosis. Tuberculosis of the bone, seen more frequently in children than adults, manifests itself in that portion which is near a joint. Occasionally it appears as an irritation of the periosteum and cortical bone, but generally it begins within a joint and then extends to the medullary portions as the result of a secondary infection.

The symptoms of bone and joint tuberculosis vary considerably in individual cases, and may develop gradually over an extended period of time. At the outset, however, there is usually only slight pain and muscle spasm about the joint, but local symptoms may be preceded by poor general health, a weight loss, or a slight fever. An accurate diagnosis requires special tests and laboratory examinations, at which time it is determined if the tubercle bacilli are present, as is true in cases affecting the lungs.

About half of all cases of skeletal tuberculosis occur in the spine, and can be detected clinically by stiffness or lack of flexibility of the back. The characteristic deformity is the development of an abnormal prominence at some level of the back, caused by destructive lesions and fractures in the spine. Treatment of this disease is usually of long duration, frequently lasting several years, and continuing until there has been bony union of the vertebrae above and below the diseased process.

Tuberculosis of the hip constitutes the second most prevalent of these involvements. As would be expected, a common first symptom is limping, and the hip becomes slightly flexed, abducted and rotated externally. As the disease progresses, there is increasing destruction of the head of the femur and often of the acetabulum. Adduction and internal rotation develop and the flexion deformity remains. As is true for spinal tuberculosis, immobility and frequently joint fusion are indicated in the care of these patients.

DEVELOPMENTAL AND ADAPTED PHYSICAL EDUCATION

It should be emphasized that one of the most important features of any treatment of bone disorders is to prevent weight-bearing during the active phases of the disease, a fact so important that many times the child will face long periods of hospitalization. This does not mean, however, that he will be completely inactive during this convalescence. On the contrary, it is essential to provide some means for these patients to exercise that does not interfere with the involved extremity. One is impressed, for example, with the manner in which youngsters with Legg-Calvé-Perthes disease manage to ambulate with crutches while the affected leg is suspended above the floor in a foot sling, or the alacrity with which they manipulate movable litters while lying prone. The factors in the long term hospital rehabilitation of young patients present a number of problems to the orthopedic surgeon as well as to others involved in patient care.

To the teacher of developmental and adapted physical education, the problem seems threefold. On the one hand, he must plan an effective program for those students returning to school after prolonged illness, and yet he must be alert to certain of the symptoms that might reflect an approaching illness. In addition, he may have to adapt activities to the student who retains a handicapping deformity. Keeping in mind that many of these disorders can occur at any age, it is the child who has not attained full growth who is in danger of incurring lasting disability when epiphyseal centers are damaged. It must be stressed, therefore, that any activity program for these students in developmental and adapted physical education must be approved by the physician.

The consequence of prolonged immobilization of extremities is muscle atrophy; following extended confinement in bed, general physical fitness subsides to a low level. Upon the student's return to school, the main objective should be to increase his strength and endurance by means of a progressive exercise program designed to prepare him for regular class participation. The physician may feel that certain specific exercises are indicated, while others must be avoided. This is especially true following such diseases as osteomyelitis and skeletal tuberculosis. Milder participation in activities may be requested for these individuals. Once again, swimming provides a medium for exercise that can readily be adapted to the needs of even the most severely disabled. Therapists in rehabilitation know of its effectiveness as a conditioning medium for patients whose exercise prescription calls for complete abstention from weight-bearing.

All convalescent students should be started on reconditioning programs as soon as possible. For cases involving the juvenile bone disorders, such as osteochondrosis or spondylolisthesis, the elementary school is - the place to begin, although this is the educational level so often neglected in physical education. The number of such individuals in a school district would probably be small, so every effort should be made to include them in the nearest developmental and adapted program. No less emphasis should be placed on those in junior or senior high schools, whose growth needs may be fully as great.

The remaining group of students is composed of those who retain a residual handicap after the disease has abated and the long bones have attained their full growth. In colleges and universities it is not surprising to find a number of such students. In developmental and adapted physical education, a wide variety of exercises is available to the student, exercises that will meet his fitness needs as well as provide new skills for successful participation in a number of activities adapted to his physical limitations.

INTERVERTEBRAL DISC SYNDROME

There seems to be considerable agreement among medical authorities that the symptoms of "backache" are subject to wide misinterpretation. Diagnostically, the challenge is made more severe because disability and pain arising from the back are among the most common of human ailments. Probably none is more pathetic, subject to such misunderstanding, and, in turn, receives such little sympathy. As O'Connell[1] notes, although these symptoms carry little threat to life, they can interfere greatly with living. It would seem apparent that the back and its function should be more generally studied; in this section special investigation will be made of the intervertebral disc, inasmuch as current knowledge suggests that damage to this structure is frequently the cause of back pain. Functional low back pain is discussed in Chapter 8.

TOPOGRAPHY

The spine is an elastic column, the strength and mobility of which is dependent upon the fact that it is made up of a number of vertebrae; the amount of movement between individual bones is slight, but the total range of motion is considerable. The arrangement of these vertebrae is in a series of curves, a condition which strengthens the back by tending to absorb the vertical forces. From a structural standpoint, the spine's weakest point is where the comparatively rigid dorsal spine meets the more mobile lumbar spine. It is this lower back region that is the concern of this discussion.

Each vertebra contains two parts, the body and the spinal arch. The spinal cord passes through the opening formed by the arch, and the muscles and ligaments of the back attach to the five bony finger-like projections which arise from the arch. Between the bodies of each two vertebrae is an intervertebral disc which serves as a buffer to absorb

---

[1] John E. A. O'Connell, "Protrusions of the Lumbar Intervertebral Discs," *Journal of Bone and Joint Surgery*, 33B (February, 1951), p. 8.

the shock of walking or jumping, as well as making bending and stretching more comfortable. These discs have been rather intensely studied in recent years and must be examined here if the nature of low back injury is to be fully understood.

The intervertebral disc is composed of two cartilagenous plates, a semi-gelatinous substance called the nucleus pulposus and a fibrous ring surrounding it, the annulus fibrosus. Coventry and associates[2] compare the disc to a thick rubber ball which is filled with fluid and partially compressed between two rigid discs. Thus, when the force on the disc changes, the position and shape of the ball changes. So, if the annulus fibrosus ruptures, the nucleus pulposus is protruded, often causing pressure on the nerve roots of the spinal cord at that point. The site of this occurrence in approximately 95 per cent of the cases is at the fourth or fifth lumbar interspace,[3] not only because the usual forces are more active here, but there is added the shearing force as the fifth lumbar vertebra tends to ride forward on the first sacral vertebra.

ETIOLOGY

The causes of pain in the lower back are many and varied; in fact, physicians recognize more and more that there may even be multiple factors in any individual case responsible for pain in this region.[4] Although the back may receive referred pain sensations from visceral lesions or from some vascular, metabolic, or neoplastic origin, it must also be kept in mind that it is subject to all the disabilities of other joints, including sprains, strains, fractures, and dislocations. The additional danger inherent in such injuries is the possibiltiy of causing damage to the spinal cord or to the nerve roots that radiate from the central pathway. Each case presents specific problems of treatment, as indeed it reflects a specificity of etiology. However, disturbances of the intervertebral disc offer not only a rather common type of disability, but one in which the problems of management should be of interest to the teacher of developmental and adapted physical education.

Although the function of the intervertebral discs had previously been known, it was not until 1934 that Mixter and Barr[5] discovered that an intraspinal protrusion of a lumbar intervertebral disc was frequently

---

[2] Mark B. Coventry, Ralph K. Ghormley, and James W. Kernohan, "The Intervertebral Disc: Its Microscopic Anatomy and Pathology. Part I. Anatomy, Development and Physiology," *Journal of Bone and Joint Surgery*, 27 (January, 1945), p. 165.

[3] Everett G. Grantham and R. Glen Spurling, "Ruptured Lumbar Intervertebral Disks," *Medical Clinics of North America*, 31 (March, 1953), p. 479.

[4] Joseph S. Barr, "Low Back and Sciatic Pain," *Journal of Bone and Joint Surgery*, 33A (July, 1951), p. 633.

[5] W. J. Mixter and J. S. Barr, "Rupture of the Intervertebral Disk with Involvement of the Spinal Canal," *New England Journal of Medicine*, 211 (1934), p. 210.

the cause of rather acute low back pain. The nature of such lesions would suggest a sudden and rather severe onset; thus, many patients will relate some traumatic incident in the past in explanation of back pain. However, there will be many who will recall only a slight trauma which may have been in the past and was not immediately disabling. To understand how this can be so, one must remember that even small movements can transpose a rather considerable force to the lumbar vertebrae, and bending, lifting, and falling are certainly outstanding causes of ruptured discs. Also, if certain predisposing factors are favorable, the disc may herniate from less severe postural changes which may appear gradually over an extended period of time.

CLINICAL FEATURES

The first and outstanding clinical feature of a ruptured lumbar intervertebral disc is pain, and this usually accompanies the precipitating event. It is further increased by extension and reduced by flexion of the lumbar spine, and is intensified by lifting, sneezing, coughing, or straining. Tenderness will also be elicited upon palpation at the fourth or fifth spinous process.

As a rule, several attacks of low back pain are experienced before the patient develops "sciatica," the symptom so typical of these cases, marked by radiation of pain usually down the posterior or lateral aspect of the leg. This may be delayed for months or years, during which time the recurrences of "lumbago" seem to clear up by themselves.

PATHOLOGY

A rupture of the annulus fibrosus causes the nucleus pulposus to be protruded and press against the surrounding structures, including the nerve roots. It should be recognized, however, that the mere presence of the clinical symptoms does not in itself become diagnostic. Rather, as Policoff[6] says, they suggest that an extra-dural, space-occupying lesion is present with secondary nerve root compression.

Pathologic changes occur in the intervertebral disc with advancing age. As growth slows down, retrogressive changes increase, as is true with all tissues of the body. However, the discs, probably because of the constant wear and tear to which they are subjected, are apparently affected early and retrogress more rapidly and severely than is true with most other tissues.[7] Moreover, the prolapsed disc may degenerate and,

[6] Leonard Policoff, "Diagnostic Challenge of Back Pain," *Archives of Physical Medicine and Rehabilitation*, 41 (October, 1960), p. 441.

[7] Mark B. Coventry, Ralph K. Ghormley, and James Kernohan, "The Intervertebral Disc: Its Microscopic Anatomy and Pathology. Part II. Changes in the Intervertebral Disc Concomitant with Age," *Journal of Bone and Joint Surgery*, 27 (April, 1945), p. 233.

together with the symptoms, disappear, thus accounting for the relief of painful symptoms experienced over the years.[8] That age accounts for certain other disc changes is illustrated by the observation that the water content becomes steadily less, the color changes, and by 40-50 years of age, the nucleus pulposus becomes noticeably less elastic. Lindblom and Hultqvist[9] suggest that the lumbar disc may decrease in volume from approximately 15 cu. cm. to 1 cu. cm. These structural alterations also help explain why low back injuries have a high incidence within the older age groups.

DIAGNOSIS

In addition to determining the clinical symptoms already mentioned, the physical examination includes a number of tests which help the physician to make an accurate diagnosis of the cause of the low back pain. The type of movement of the lumbar spine which elicits pain is quite significant, and observations must be made to determine any muscle weakness. Also, it is important to examine the lower extremities, especially the lower leg and foot, to check any area of sensory loss. A loss of sensation on the medial, anterior, or lateral aspect of the lower leg may indicate a rupture of the third, fourth, or fifth lumbar intervertebral disc respectively. The physician will also include in his examination certain tests of reflexes, notably the knee and ankle jerks.

Roentgen examination of the spine is usually done, and may reveal a subluxation of the nearby articular facets with a certain constriction of the foramina. The intervertebral space is apt to be narrowed, and the vertebra immediately above the involved disc may be displaced posteriorly. In addition to x-ray examination, the myelogram has been recognized as one of the most helpful diagnostic tools for revealing a defect at the level of the involved disc.[10] As a precaution Gurdjian and Webster[11] point out that these are merely implements in the diagnostic arsenal; the results of all tests help make up the total clinical picture. For example, a narrowed intervertebral disc revealed by x-rays does not necessarily indicate a rupture of the disc; Gurdjian and Webster found myelography to be misleading in nearly one-third of the patients they treated.

In making a diagnosis, the physician finds it necessary to rule out other conditions whose symptoms of low back pain suggest a herniated

---

[8] K. Lindblom and G. Hultqvist, "Absorption of Protruded Disc Tissue," *Journal of Bone and Joint Surgery,* 32A (July, 1950), p. 557.

[9] *Ibid.*

[10] Donald Munro, "Lumbar and Sacral Compression Radiculitis (Herniated Lumbar Disk Syndrome)," *New England Journal of Medicine,* 254 (February 9, 1956), p. 243.

[11] E. S. Gurdjian and John E. Webster, "Lumbar Herniations of the Nucleus Pulposus," *American Journal of Surgery,* 76 (September, 1948), p. 235.

nucleus pulposus. Grantham and Spurling[12] group them as follows: rheumatoid spondylitis; trauma; neoplasms; anomalies; and infections.

PROGNOSIS

An exact estimate of prognosis cannot be made, inasmuch as each case of low back pain presents highly specific circumstances, as well as the need for special treatment. The physician will bring relief from painful symptoms in the vast majority of cases in a relatively short time, but, for some, pain may persist despite the best management. Encouraging is the fact that a progressive improvement in results is obtained as the nature of the ruptured disc is studied.[13,14,15]

TREATMENT

Medical specialists generally agree that treatment of a herniated lumbar intervertebral disc centers around two procedures, one conservative, and the other surgical. The difficulty arises, however, in determining how long non-surgical treatment should be given; furthermore, it is often hard to assess in advance the success of operative procedures, sometimes made more complicated by a difficult differential diagnosis.

Conservative Treatment. All patients should be given a fair trial of conservative treatment. If indicated in all new patients, it may play a dominant role in the total picture of the intervertebral disc syndrome. Barr[16] suggests that about 30 per cent of patients with disc lesions will spontaneously recover from a first attack; many of these will be symptom free, perhaps for years. Therefore, everything should be done to permit any possible recovery during this time.

Conservative management consists of rest, sedation, the administration of analgesics, and an exercise program. At the very outset complete bed rest for several days may be considered the most effective treatment, aided by a bed board or an especially firm mattress. Sometimes pelvic traction is indicated, which can be very helpful in relieving painful symptoms, as well as the use of such mechanical supports as corsets, plaster casts, lumbo-sacral braces, or strapping. These latter devices are gradually discarded as the pain subsides. The application of heat and massage, while not curative, also affords temporary relief, and certain

---

12 Grantham and Spurling, *op. cit.*

13 B. M. Skinners and W. B. Hamby, "The Results of Surgical Removal of Protruded Lumbar Intervertebral Discs," *Journal of Neurosurgery*, 1 (1944), p. 117.

14 J. E. A. O'Connell, "The Indications for and Results of the Excision of Lumbar Intervertebral Disc Protrusions: A Review of 500 Cases," *Annual Royal College of Surgeons*, 6 (June, 1950), p. 403.

15 Barr, *op. cit.*

16 *Ibid.*

drugs give considerable comfort to the patient during the acute stage. The use of exercise will be discussed below.

Surgical Treatment. Surgical intervention is considered necessary in a selected number of cases. Grantham and Spurling[17] suggest that the sudden appearance of serious neurologic complications, resulting from protrusions into the spinal canal, is the only absolute requirement for immediate surgery of the intervertebral disc. Severe lower extremity muscle paralysis and bladder or rectal disturbances make this decision imperative. Also, if the radiating sciatic pain makes ambulation impossible, it indicates the need for surgery.

The best surgical technique for protrusion of the intervertebral disc has been the subject for some debate, the issue being whether to fuse the spine in addition to excising the disc. Barr[18] reported excellent results when utilizing the combined procedure, but others have not recommended it.[19,20,21,22] The opinion is expressed rather unequivocally by Munro[23] that a fusion of the spine in the compressed nerve root area has no therapeutic relation to the ruptured disc. Gurdjian and Webster[24] reported limiting the use of this procedure in their series of nearly 200 patients to those cases involving spondylolisthesis, unstable fifth lumbar vertebra, long history of backaches, or to cases where the patient's occupation involved heavy labor.

Therapeutic Exercise. The role of exercise in the treatment of the low back syndrome has been found to be widely endorsed, and one would expect a substantial body of knowledge to exist concerning the treatment and pre- and post-operative care of such patients. However, as Anderson and associates[25] point out, there is a lack of specific information about correction of the mechanical changes which are associated with disc lesions.

---

17 Grantham and Spurling, *op. cit.*, p. 496.

18 Barr, *op. cit.*

19 Guy A. Caldwell and William B. Sheppard, "Criteria for Spine Fusion Following Removal of Protruded Nucleus Pulposus," *Journal of Bone and Joint Surgery*, 30-A (October, 1948), p. 971.

20 I. William Nachlas, "End Result Study of the Treatment of Herniated Nucleus Pulposus by Excision with Fusion and Without Fusion," *Journal of Bone and Joint Surgery*, 34-A (October, 1952), p. 981.

21 Paul Ross and Franklin Jelsma, "Postoperative Analysis of 366 Consecutive Cases of Herniated Lumbar Discs," *American Journal of Surgery*, 84 (December, 1952), p. 657.

22 H. G. Decker and S. W. Shapiro, "Herniated Lumbar Intervertebral Disks," *Archives of Surgery*, 75 (July, 1957), p. 77.

23 Munro, *op. cit.*

24 E. S. Gurdjian and John E. Webster, "Lumbar Herniations of the Nucleus Pulposus," *American Journal of Surgery*, 76 (September, 1948), p. 235.

25 Thomas P. Anderson, Ernest Sachs, Robert G. Fisher, and Robert M. Krout, "Postoperative Care in Lumbar Disc Syndrome," *Archives of Physical Medicine and Rehabilitation*, 42 (March, 1961), p. 152.

Discussing certain extrinsic causes of backache, Rose[26] points out that weak muscles tend to place a greater strain on the joints and ligaments of the back. This causes persistent pain and further reduces physical activity, which in turn may increase the backache, bring about general fatigue, and reduce further the muscle strength. Thus the vicious cycle is complete. While poor posture, of itself, probably does not cause the radiation of sciatic pain, it is undoubtedly true that postural *changes* can sometimes be precipitating factors. In low back pain, the postural deviation of significance is lordosis; the concept in treatment is to reduce the lumbo-sacral angle so as to lift the weight from the posterior structures at this site.[27] The muscles to be strengthened, then, are the abdominal and gluteal muscles primarily, as discussed in Chapter 8.

Undoubtedly, a number of helpful exercises could be fashioned for use by patients with a history of low back pain or a ruptured disc. However, since a few specific ones have been recommended, it seems appropriate to set them forth here, although it is necessary to keep in mind the fact that medical examination and prescription should precede each suspected case of herniated nucleus pulposus. Physiatrists have recognized that no single exercise series can solve all the problems present in such patients, but judicious use of certain of them adapted to individual needs has proven highly successful. The following are commonly employed for these persons, their administration based upon exercise principles previously set forth in Chapter 7.

1. *Partial to full sit-up.* The starting position is supine with the knees flexed and the feet flat on the floor, arms folded over chest. If there is pronounced abdominal muscle weakness or if flexion of the spine is to be avoided, the partial sit-up can be performed by raising the head and shoulders from the floor for three to five counts and return. The full sit-up is used in conjunction with the partial one in many exercise programs, when greater range of joint motion is desired, and when sufficient strength is available.

2. *Back Flattener.* Use the same starting position for this exercise as for the previous one. The task is to contract the gluteals so that the lower back is forced against the floor and the anterior pelvis is tilted upward. As this is a static exercise the intensity is usually varied by holding this position for increasingly longer periods of time, and by performing these bouts with greater daily frequency.

3. *Alternate to double knee tucks.* The starting position is the same as used for the previous exercises, and the alternate knee tuck is performed by slowly drawing one knee to the chest. This is facilitated by pulling on the knee with both hands. The subject then returns to the

---

[26] G. K. Rose, "Backache and the Disc," *Lancet,* 266 (June 5, 1954), p. 1143.

[27] Paul C. Williams, "Examination and Conservative Treatment for Disk Lesions of the Lower Spine," *Clinical Orthopedics,* 5 (1955), p. 28.

starting position and repeats with the other leg. The double knee tuck is performed similarly, except that both knees are drawn to the chest simultaneously. If done slowly, this exercise is helpful in stretching the erector spinae muscles that may have become shortened.

4. *Buttocks raise.* This is similar to exercise 2, except that a positive effort is made to raise the buttocks from the floor by contracting the gluteus maximus and the abdominals. Once again, this static contraction should be held for a few seconds before relaxing and performing the next repetition.

5. *Squat bend.* From a standing position, weight distributed well back on the heels, the gluteals should be contracted and the subject should squat and place his arms between his legs and touch the floor with his hands. Return to starting position and repeat. This exercise is helpful in strengthening the gluteus maximus and the quadriceps muscles, both important in controlling the ease with which one squats and recovers. The importance of this exercise is pointed out by Williams, who says that "the principle involved . . . would avoid most low back disability if rigidly employed in our daily activities."[28]

DEVELOPMENTAL AND ADAPTED PHYSICAL EDUCATION

There is no way of knowing exactly how many people suffer from low back pain, nor can the number of people who have an impairment of the intervertebral disc be determined. Certainly, though, this is a sizable problem, which will frequently come to the attention of the teacher of developmental and adapted physical education. Low back pain is so widespread that physical educators must understand both the problem involved and the manner in which exercise and activities play a part in the non-medical treatment program. This is one disability in which effective preventive measures may be helpful in protecting many students from having future difficulty. Maintaining adequate strength and endurance seems to afford one of the best means of carrying this out, and this is a service that should be of primary concern to physical education.

Another important consideration centers about the issue of posture training. Although this general problem has been dealt with in a previous chapter, it must be reiterated here that physicians familiar with the ruptured disc are in essential agreement that postural changes, even of a long-term nature, may be precipitating causes of many of these symptoms. This is particularly true of lordosis, although sometimes more than one deviation is present causing the ultimate disability. This seems reason enough to be concerned with the teaching of correct posture and trying to interest students in maintaining a body alignment that does not

---

[28] *Ibid.*

place undue stress on any one segment of the back. If additional strength is needed, the administration of appropriate exercises should be accomplished first. Commensurate with this, and its value should not be minimized, is teaching the technique of bending and lifting heavy objects, where safe procedure can prevent painful injury.

Once the pain of the first attack has been partially alleviated and the student is able to attend classes, he may become eligible for the developmental and adapted program. The physician's recommendations should be followed, as the injudicious participation in activities could bring about the onset of acute exacerbation. Generally, extreme flexion or extension of the spine or twisting is contraindicated; exercise may involve heavy reliance on static muscular contractions. If pain is severe, protective bracing may be required, and the more inactive games may be recommended.

The heated pool affords a medium for exercise that has long proven very helpful to these persons. Not only does it help to relax any muscular spasm in the back, but the buoyancy of the water relieves much of the pressure on tender areas caused by the weight of the body. In addition, exercise can be given that will help in conditioning the student and maintaining or increasing his physical fitness. Even walking in the water, both forward and backward, and varying the depth of the water and the intensity with which strides are taken, have proven successful. Upper extremity exercises can be controlled by having him propel himself certain distances by using his arms alone. The stroke used in this instance should be the elementary backstroke because the body position avoids hyperextension of the back and calls for contraction of the abdominal muscles of the trunk, both favorable conditions when there is pain present.

When recovery permits, it may be recommended that more vigorous participation in certain activities be instituted. At this time, consideration should be given to starting a program designed to afford maximum muscular protection against future recurrences. Any contraindications for activity should be discussed with appropriate medical personnel and the progression of conditioning exercises carefully graded. As the subject returns to full participation, individual, dual, and team games may be included in his program, but there may still be some limitations concerning the more severe twisting movements and certain body contact sports.

The student who has undergone surgery for a ruptured intervertebral disc may present certain problems of a slightly different nature than others. The first consideration, of course, is the patient's immediate postoperative care. This is not a matter to be dealt with by the developmental and adapted physical educator; however, it should be understood that maximum benefits may not be fully realized for several months, during which time treatment may involve, among other things, exercises and posture training. The extent of his recovery and the prognosis will dictate the type of exercise program possible for this individual in physical education, but it is anticipated that the majority will experience rapid progress toward more complete participation in a vigorous exercise program.

AMPUTATIONS

The loss of a limb involves an irrevocable anatomical and physiological impairment of major proportions. This is especially true if it interferes with the individual's ability to perform normal activities of living, such as walking or eating; certain emotional difficulties may also be present if the handicap is visually obvious to others. Each year, thousands of men, women, and children suffer an amputation of one sort or another that makes them eligible for consideration in the developmental and adapted physical education program, and for whom a wide range of activities can be made accessible.

The orthopedic surgeon is most intimately concerned with the amputee, although he is not the only one who will perform this type of surgery. The vascular surgeon may do it for various vascular diseases, the general surgeon may amputate as a result of a severe crushing injury, or the internist may amputate because of gangrene that develops in the diabetic patient. All are concerned with the total care of the patient and will be joined by a number of other members of the rehabilitation service. It is contended here that the success of the total treatment program for these persons will largely determine the adjustment in all other phases of their lives. This is certainly true in regard to their acceptance of and subsequent participation in physical education; indeed, it should not be surprising if they experienced a natural reluctance to participate in the types of activities presented in this program. In order to more fully understand this student, it is first necessary to become acquainted with his treatment and the concept employed in his rehabilitation so that a more sucesssful developmental and adapted program can be planned.

SITES OF ELECTION

A great deal of emphasis seems to have been placed upon the election of the particular site on a limb where amputation should be performed. The advance in prosthetic manufacture, especially in the years immediately following the second world war, when great advances were made in their design and fit, was based largely on so-called acceptable areas. More recently, however, this concept has been challenged, as many patients have been fitted with appliances even when their amputations have been performed in what might be termed undesirable locations. Mazet, Taylor and Bechtol,[29] discussing upper-extremity amputations, contend that the surgeon should attempt to save as much of the limb as possible, and should be more concerned with such physical aspects as skin coverage, adequacy of nerve innervation and circulation, and the function of the part to be saved.

Upper extremity. For amputations involving the hand, as much finger area as possible is usually saved, especially of the thumb, with the possible exception of the bulbous distal ends of the phalanges and, in certain circumstances, of the metacarpals. In the past, it was generally believed that the proximal third of the forearm and the distal two inches of the humerus should be sacrificed, again primarily because no adequate prostheses were available. However, this problem has now been surmounted with modern prosthetic equipment; even elbow-disarticulation amputations can be fitted over the flaring condyles of the humerus with new fabrication and fitting techniques.

As much of the humerus as possible in above-elbow amputations should be preserved, for, as Mazet and associates[30] state, "the range of function of every above-the-elbow prosthesis is directly proportional to the length, strength, and range of motion of the humeral lever." Even the short above-elbow stump has a fairly satisfactory range of function if well fitted and harnessed. In addition, shoulder disarticulations and thoracoscapular amputations can also be fitted, although in the case of the former, retention of the head of the humerus, particularly for cosmetic purposes, has been advocated. Fitting thoracoscapular amputees with adequate shoulder cap and harness can restore body symmetry and provide elbow flexion and grasping movement.

Lower extremity. Similarly, in lower-extremity amputations, current thought is that as much functional length of the limb as possible should be preserved. In the foot, the question of providing a weight-bearing stump becomes very important. Amputation through the metatarsal bones gives a fairly satisfactory stump, leaves the patient with a mild handicap, and is fairly functional, but does present some problem of balance. Amputation through the tarsal bones is generally avoided, as little functional value is gained by this procedure. The Syme amputation through the distal ¼ or ½ inch of the tibia and fibula does permit free weight-bearing on the bare stump for short periods, as the skin of the heel is utilized to cover the ends of the bones. The large bulge at the ankle that results is a little difficult to fit with a prosthesis, however, and is somewhat unsightly.

There is general agreement in below-knee (B-K) amputation surgery

---

[29] Robert Mazet, Craig L. Taylor, and Charles O. Bechtol, "Upper-Extremity Amputation Surgery and Prosthetic Prescription," *Journal of Bone and Joint Surgery,* 38-A, No. 6 (December, 1956), p. 1185.

[30] *Ibid.*, p. 1193.

that long tibial stumps should be avoided. The distal third of the tibia has very little soft tissue padding and is relatively avascular, so that these long stumps become very difficult to fit and are also apt to become ulcerated, swollen at the end, and are subject to other vascular complications.[31] The most successful below-knee stump is probably five to six and one-half inches below the knee joint; efforts are usually made to preserve any portion of a below-knee stump, especially when sufficient motion and length is present to control the swing of the prosthetic shank and foot section. Two inches of tibia is considered sufficient for a B-K prosthesis. With the advent of modern prosthetic design, the end-bearing features of the femur now make the knee disarticulation an excellent functional amputation.

For above-knee (A-K) amputations, the Callander or Kirk supracondylar amputation permits an end-bearing stump, but must be performed through or just above the knee. For the standard-type suction socket, the length of femur considered best is about three to four inches above the knee joint. From this level to about four or five inches below the tip of the trochanter, amputations can be fitted with a suction socket prosthesis. Hip disarticulations are usually avoided; every attempt is made to save as much of the head and neck of the femur as possible.

PROSTHETIC APPLIANCES

After the stump has healed, and the use of an artificial limb has been indicated, the actual prescription of a particular prosthesis is next. Lambert and Novotny[32] indicate that the best prosthetists prefer to share this responsibility with the surgeon who performed the amputation. In addition, it is recommended that other personnel concerned with the total rehabilitation of the amputee, such as the physiatrist and social and vocational guidance agencies, enter the picture in order to give the amputee the best possible solution to his many problems.

Proper fit is the most important consideration in selecting an appliance; this should take precedence over other features such as its weight, design, or material. Limb makers have become highly skilled in their trade and are now able to fashion prostheses for nearly all sites of amputation.

Below-knee prostheses. Amputations of the toes generally result in a negligible disability and usually do not require a prosthesis. Even the loss of the first toe seems to offer no real threat to ambulation, although there may be some minor instability on push-off. Careful shoe fitting with a soft toe cap is necessary. The transmetatarsal amputation also

[31] C. L. Compere and R. G. Thompson, "Amputations and Modern Prosthetics," *Surgical Clinics of North America,* 37 (February, 1957), p. 103.

[32] Claude N. Lambert and Albert J. Novotny, "Amputations and Amputees—Adult and Juvenile," *Surgical Clinics of North America,* 37 (February, 1957), p. 120.

results in relatively little disability, as the remaining foot is capable of full weight-bearing. No prosthesis is required, regular shoes can be worn and frequently gait abnormalities appear only during rapid walking or running, thus presenting only a minor disability when considered for the developmental and adapted program. The Syme amputation provides a strong, long stump which requires a relatively simple prosthesis consisting of a plastic or leather leg portion, ankle and foot.

In the case of the lower-leg amputation, normal function is almost certain to be achieved with a prosthesis, so that very little disability is noticed by an observer. The stump at this site is not very satisfactory for weight-bearing, so it is bypassed and the socket is fitted so as to permit the weight to rest on the tibial condyles. An ankle joint must be fashioned, and this will usually provide for plantar flexion and dorsiflexion only, although rubber cushions are installed to permit more normal walking movements to be simulated. More complicated appliances have been designed to provide for other ankle motions, and may eventually become widely used. A prosthetic foot, a leather thigh corset, and a pelvic suspension belt complete the apparatus. The corset is used for suspension as well as some weight-bearing, and the pelvic belt is provided with an anterior support strap which also aids in knee extension.

Because of the normal weight-bearing function of the knee joint, the knee disarticulation amputation provides an excellent weight-bearing stump that is usually quite painless. A prosthesis can be fitted to this site by using outside hinges, although it may present a somewhat wider appearance than the normal knee. The stability achieved is not quite as good as in the below-knee amputation, but is much better than those that employ the above-knee prosthesis.

Above-knee prostheses. Removing the knee joint results in a serious problem to ambulation in addition to causing an imbalance of hip musculature. This imbalance subsequently tends to interfere with prosthetic training because hip contractures may result as a consequence of inadequate post-operative care. These and other problems of stump care will be discussed in a later section.

The suction-suspension socket is most commonly employed for above-knee amputations. A snugly-fitted socket provides an air seal which resists the tendency to pull off by creating a negative pressure within. This appliance can be very satisfactory, and avoids the necessity of having to wear the bulky belt and hip joint that was utilized with the older types of prostheses. However, short stumps may prove inadequate for the suction socket alone, so the Silesian bandage, a leather strap that angles up over the opposite hip may provide the required support. On the other hand, if the suction socket cannot be worn in the usual way, it can be enlarged so the patient can wear a stump sock; in this case, a pelvic band must be attached because there is no longer any supporting negative pressure.

The control of the knee in the above-knee prosthesis actually resides in the hip, for it is the manipulation of the thigh that provides the correct functional alignment of the lower leg. The prosthetic knee joint most frequently employed maintains a constant friction so that more control of the forward swing of the leg is permitted. In the standing position, the body weight must fall slightly behind the knee joint so that it thrusts the knee into extension, because if it is forced into flexion nothing prevents its buckling. In walking, the body passes forward over the prosthetic foot and the stump is flexed at the thigh as the other limb accepts the body weight and is sufficiently balanced. This braking action causes the knee to flex and the movement of the body increases the flexion until the toe leaves the ground and the lower leg swings forward. The hip extensors decelerate this movement until the moment that the heel strikes the ground, and the knee is locked and the body rides onto this foot into the next stepping phase. Occasionally an amputee will have difficulty maintaining balance for some reason, and will require the use of a more complex knee joint which more effectively brakes flexion. This joint also acts as a safety measure against falling and may give the wearer more confidence in his prosthesis.

A hip disarticulation is a more serious amputation of the lower extremities than any of the others previously mentioned, although it is less severe than a hemipelvectomy. The difficulties encountered here present the prosthetist with an engineering problem of vast proportions; he must provide the patient with a hip joint in addition to the rest of the leg capable of both movement and weight-bearing. There are successful wearers of this prosthesis, but it is suspected that it will be limited to use by the younger and well-conditioned individual.

Below-elbow prostheses. The loss of a hand, while small in relation to the total surface area of the body, presents an irrevocable loss, much more vital than its counterpart in the leg, the foot. No prosthesis ever really succeeds in replacing the tactile and functional aspects so important to performance of the thousand daily tasks required of the thumb and fingers. Amputation of the fifth finger does not cause a very severe disability, and the loss of other digits need not be particularly incapacitating—with the exception of the index or middle finger. Loss of the thumb, however, is quite a handicap, and its amputation leaves the individual without the important function served by the thumb of opposing the other fingers. Although finger prostheses can be provided, they have not proved particularly successful. For these amputations as well as for those through the metacarpals, a nonfunctional rubber cosmetic glove can be worn that will largely restore the outward appearance of normalcy.

It is possible to fit the wrist disarticulation amputation with a prosthesis, although the width of the distal portions of the radius and ulna make this task more difficult. Also, it may mean that the prosthesis will be slightly longer than the normal arm because of the long stump. However, saving as much forearm as possible in this way permits the full range of motion of pronation and supination.

The forearm amputation can be fitted easily with a plastic shell over the stump so that the full movement of the elbow joint is preserved, and, depending upon the site of surgery, some pronation and supination of the forearm is possible. A cable controlled by the opposite shoulder operates the terminal device; with sufficient training and practice, the amputee can develop a very efficient movement. With the advent of the APRL (Army Prosthetics Research Laboratory) hand, a very fine substitute for the amputated hand was found, which could be fashioned to simulate both color and appearance, thus making it very acceptable cosmetically. However, once the patient fully accepts his disability and becomes thoroughly trained in the use of the terminal device, many prefer to use the prosthetic hook, which proves to be more quickly operated and more functional.

Above-elbow prostheses. When the elbow joint has been lost, additional problems are superimposed, which makes the handicap more severe. The prosthesis fitted to the upper arm must utilize two cables instead of one, one to operate the terminal device, and the other to manipulate the elbow lock. The co-ordination required to perform these two functions is considerable, and is quite difficult for some to learn.

Retention of the head of the humerus, when a high amputation is necessary, has long been advocated for the sake of appearance in a shoulder disarticulation amputation. It also helps when fitting a prosthesis, for the shoulder cap has a much more secure grip and has less tendency to slide in place than if the essential shoulder structure has been removed.

CINEPLASTIC PROCEDURE

An additional prosthetic technique used with a great deal of success in upper extremity amputations is cineplasty. It has been employed primarily to the biceps and pectoralis major muscles, but only in those cases in which the success of the procedure seems assured. A tunnel is fashioned through the muscle at its distal end, and it is lined with skin; an ivory peg is placed through the aperture thus created. The ends of the peg are connected to an assembly that operates the artificial hand. In order to operate a cineplastic prosthesis efficiently, it is necessary that the muscle begin its pull at or near its resting length, so that it can generate a force sufficiently great to carry out the necessary movements.

Certain factors limit the use of the cineplastic procedure. The principal limiting factor is a range of excursion that is too slight to be completely effective, thus reducing the strength of prehension. Also, care must be taken that the tunnel does not break down, and proper hygienic rules must be followed not only for stump care but for maintenance of the tunnel as well. Inasmuch as this is an elective surgical procedure, these matters can be thoroughly discussed with the patient, and preoperative strengthening exercises can be performed in preparation for future use.[33]

PHANTOM LIMB

The sensation of phantom limb is defined as the persistence of the image of the limb that is no longer present. It is entirely normal for this to occur, and most amputees experience it, some to a greater extent than others. Awareness of the missing member may or may not be described as basically unpleasant, but it is subject to intermittent unpleasant sensations—itching, tingling, or pain. These manifestations may persist for several months, but generally disappear by the end of the first year after amputation. In some cases the pain from the phantom limb is intense, and has been variously described as the feeling of "toes being crushed" or of a "foot burning from a hot wire." In less severe cases the phantom may represent a tingling sensation or may merely be a passive awareness of toes, foot, or ankle.

PRE-PROSTHETIC TREATMENT

The pre-prosthetic treatment of the amputee depends upon the successful administration of exercise and the careful management of stump formation.

Exercise. If at all possible, the patient should begin an exercise regime before surgery so as to hasten the recovery after the operation has been performed. However, this is not always possible, so it should be started as soon after surgery as the surgeon will allow. The use of general conditioning bed exercises to the uninvolved extremities help the patient return to normal strength and prevent muscle atrophy during confinement; at the same time, static exercises can often be started in the involved limb. Also, initial instruction in bed posture and placement of the stump is beneficial to the amputee prior to the more active treatment given when he is ambulatory.

One of the most common problems arising early in the postoperative rehabilitation of the above-knee amputee is that of stump contractures. Since the various adductor muscles of the hip insert along the length of the femur from the lesser trochanter to the medial condyle, these mus-

---

[33] John H. Kuitert and Frederick E. Vultee, "Prosthetic Training for the Upper Extremity Amputee with Cineplasty," *Archives of Physical Medicine and Rehabilitation*, 34, No. 6 (June, 1953), p. 367.

cles are transected during surgery and as a result are weakened. The abductors, on the other hand, arise from the ilium and insert into the greater trochanter and therefore are not disturbed by the thigh amputation. This creates a muscular imbalance which can quickly lead to an abduction contracture of the stump. Extension of the hip is weakened more by division of the hamstrings than is flexion of the hip by division of the rectus femoris; thus flexion contractures can develop quite easily. Stump exercises are usually started as soon as possible after amputation; in so doing, the patient is instructed to maintain the limb in a position of adduction and extension in order to resist the pull of the stronger muscles. Prolonged periods of sitting without placing the hip through a full range of motion often lead to the development of such contractures.

Hip flexion contractures are probably best reduced by causing the hip flexors to be relaxed while the extensors are being actively contracted, thereby helping to strengthen the hip extensor muscles at the same time the hip flexors are being stretched. Childs and Holtzman[34] have pointed out that passive stretching alone may result in a tightening rather than a relaxation of the muscles. Also, placing weights on the stump, a method of stretching the hip flexors commonly seen, more than likely sets off proprioceptive impulses which stimulate the muscles to support the weights and not to relax, thus increasing the contracture.

Stump formation. As soon as the stump is dry, shrinkage is started. Initially, this takes the form of applying a small amount of tension by wrapping with a bandage. After a week or so, the pressure is increased and the stump given a conical shape. In the above-knee stump, this is customarily done from the region of the ischium to its distal end. Another definitive objective is to remove excess fatty tissue before fitting the prosthesis, for additional shrinkage later causes the socket to become too large for the wearer and this may lead to eventual replacement of the prosthetic device.

The suction-socket stump requires less shrinkage; thus, the form of the stump is more cylindrical in shape. Using this type of prosthesis usually causes less shrinkage and frequently the musculature of the stump will develop as a result of the continued use of the limb.

A matter of prime consideration to the amputee is that of maintaining a healthy stump, as an artificial limb cannot be worn as long as there is any ulceration of the skin. Therefore, great care is taken to maintain proper hygienic principles of cleanliness and adequate methods of skin drying.[35] In those stumps that are slow in healing, an intermittent whirlpool bath is frequently included in the hygiene program, a procedure

---

[34] Theodore F. Childs and Milton Holtzman, "Pressure Gauge Device as an Aid in Treating H p Contractures Following Above-Knee Amputation," *Archives of Physical Medicine and Rehabilitation,* 39 (September, 1958), p. 581.

[35] Paul F. Fleer, "A Guide for the Corrective Therapist in the Treatment of Patients with Lower Extremity Amputations," *Journal of the Association for Physical and Mental Rehabilitation,* 5 (July-August, 1952), p. 12.

often helpful in promoting stump circulation and cleaning as well as indoctrinating the patients in total stump care.[36]

PROSTHETIC TRAINING

The fitting of the proper appliance is only one step in the process of equipping the amputee with the tools of proper rehabilitation. Teaching him to use it is a process that can not be taken for granted, for experience has shown that a large percentage of amputees will not learn how to utilize their prostheses by trial and error. One of the frequent causes of prosthetic neglect is the unfamiliarity of the patient with his limb and its use in the activities of daily living. By applying the correct methods and developing proper motor patterns, nearly all amputees can be successful in using their prosthetic appliances.

Learning to walk with an artificial leg or performing co-ordinated maneuvers with a prosthetic arm is accomplished gradually. Teaching these activities should be approached by the instructor in the same way he would teach any athletic skill. Consequently, some individuals will learn at a more rapid rate and will ultimately be better performers than others. In fact, some patients develop rather amazing feats of agility and precision with their appliances that are both fascinating to watch and rewarding to the individual. There is some feeling, however, that the use of such skilled amputees to demonstrate the results of rehabilitation to new amputee patients fosters the mistaken impression that such skills are within the grasp of all patients, when in reality this is not true at all. Actually, only an average amount of skill is needed for successful prosthetic utilization.

In using the lower-extremity prosthesis, the first step is to learn balance. Without this, walking is impossible. Balancing should be practiced until the body weight can be borne by the artificial limb alone for at least thirty seconds, and this done in an erect, relaxed posture. Further training usually involves learning to take steps between parallel bars, with the ultimate aim of doing this correctly without use of the hands for support. It is often advantageous for a full-length mirror to be placed at the end of the parallel bars so that the patient can view his progress and help to make his gait efficient. In order to make the pattern of walking more inconspicuous, Fleer[37] suggests that the amputee walk with his feet close together as well as close to the floor, and with an even, rhythmical gait, striving to take the same length of step with both feet.

After the gait has been learned for walking on a straight and even surface, additional skills of climbing and descending stairs, walking on

---

[36] Harry J. Bugel, William Zilmer, and Jack Grigsby, "Advantages of Intermediate Prosthesis in the Rehabilitation of the Lower Extremity Amputee: Preliminary Report," *Archives of Physical Medicine and Rehabilitation*, 39 (January, 1958), p. 28.
[37] Fleer, *op. cit.*

an inclined surface, rising and sitting, and walking on rough or uneven surfaces must also be mastered. Even falling is practiced, with emphasis placed upon the correct procedure so as to meet emergency situations that can arise for the amputee.

For the upper-extremity amputee, loss of the hand presents a galaxy of special problems. The hundreds of daily tasks performed in perfect co-ordination by the hand and fingers present obstacles for prosthetic designers that are not yet completely overcome by their finished product. However, nearly all of the important activities of daily living can be performed by the upper-extremity amputee; and, with proper training, he can perform intricate co-ordinations with the use of the hook and shoulder harness. As has been mentioned, the cosmetic hands available have limited function, but can be used for dress-up occasions where appearance is considered important to the amputee.

Another problem that must be emphasized for the upper-extremity amputee is to maintain proper posture, as the loss of an arm results in a disturbance in the distribution of weight, frequently causing lateral deviations of the spine. Slight alterations are probably of little consequence, but the more pronounced curvatures often are reflected in muscle spasms as well as in the unsightly appearance of a high or low shoulder. In addition, the amputee who is habitually round shouldered may be limited in the amount of excursion needed for completely successful operation of his terminal device.[38]

CHILDHOOD AMPUTATIONS

Amputations that involve children not only present special problems to the members of the rehabilitation team, but are of particular interest to the teacher of developmental and adapted physical education. Every effort should be made to include these individuals in this program.

Acquired amputations. In general, young children have not grown as accustomed to their normal limbs as have adults, nor have they developed the fine degree of skill that mature persons have achieved. As a consequence, they may react in a slightly different manner to an amputation. A great deal of the difficulty they do have, however, often comes from the unnecessary pressures that the curiosity and ridicule of their classmates in school may bring, both before and after the prosthesis has been fitted.[39] A great deal of careful guidance is needed if the most effective adjustment is to be achieved by these youngsters.

---

[38] Norman Berger and Marshall A. Graham, "Factors Related to Training of the Upper Extremity Amputee," *Journal of the Association for Physical and Mental Rehabilitation,* 5 (January-February, 1952).

[39] Claude N. Lambert and Albert J. Novotny, "Amputations and Amputees: Adult and Juvenile," *Surgical Clinics of North America,* 37 (February, 1957), p. 120.

The juvenile prosthesis is a smaller version of the adult model. The surgeon, however, has to bear in mind that, if the epiphyseal center is saved, growth of bone may be expected to occur; thus, what seemed originally to be a very short stump may turn out to be quite acceptable for prosthetic fitting when the child has experienced his normal gain in stature. This means that refitting of the prosthesis will be necessary periodically and the limb enlarged to keep pace with increased size.

Another consequence of normal growth that is apt to occur is for the bone to grow faster than the surrounding tissues. The tendency will then be for the bone to literally grow out of the end of the stump; this may necessitate a reamputation at this site. This should not prevent the fitting and utilization of a prosthesis, however, as the early training in its use will permit a more lasting and functional adjustment. In fact, the use of some form of lower limb appliance is advocated for children as young as nine or ten months of age. With an early start they will be better able to learn to stand and to walk as soon as the normal child.[40]

Congenital amputations. Frequently neglected is the child with a congenital amputation. Whether it is because the parents wish to hide the disability or because they are in ignorance as to the prosthetic possibilities, or perhaps for some other reason, the proper medical assistance often remains unsolicited for these children. In truth, an artificial limb can nearly always be designed for the congenital amputee whether for the upper or lower extremity. Lambert and Novotny,[41] state that they rarely require surgery, except for the occasional removal of tiny finger or toe buds, or possibly the amputation of a gross hand or foot deformity.

DEVELOPMENTAL AND ADAPTED PHYSICAL EDUCATION

It should be apparent to the reader that exercise plays a rather important role in the total rehabilitation program of the amputee. By exercise, the patient may be prepared pre-operatively by a series of general conditioning activities, often very successfully administered in bed, and may strengthen specific muscle groups that will bear the burden of prosthetic management after amputation. If such a pre-operative program can be executed, the patient will be well advanced in his rehabilitation and the psychological advantage gained will be considerable as well. The amount of adjustment to his handicap achieved by the individual before actual amputation may bear directly on his emotional response to the post-operative treatment and may affect his acceptance of developmental and adapted physical education.

Obviously, all amputations cannot be anticipated. Some will result from injuries, and others from medical reasons that will permit very

---

[40] Nathan Farber, "The Child Amputee," *Journal of the Association for Physical and Mental Rehabilitation,* 11 (March-April, 1957), p. 56.

[41] Lambert and Novotny, *op. cit.*

little time to elapse between the moment of decision and the operation itself. Furthermore, very little use is made by physicians of pre-operative conditioning, and even less by anyone in physical education. However, one of the authors, as a physical educator with adapted background observed and participated in an excellent hospital reconditioning program designed for just this type of patient. However, it is not the objective of this book to suggest therapeutic treatment procedures for the teacher of the developmental and adapted program; rather, it is our purpose to make known the total picture of medical management of these patients and to suggest courses of action that may be appropriate in such situations.

The success of the developmental and adapted program for any amputee student will depend on a number of factors, including his psychological adjustment to the handicap, the recency of limb loss as well as the extremity amputated, and the site of election on the extremity. For the leg amputee, ambulation restrictions may limit the extent to which running and jumping will be possible, so other activities must be substituted that provide vigorous physical conditioning. The physician should be consulted before this program is begun, but one of the fine exercise modalities for the single-leg amputee is riding the stationary bicycle. The foot can be kept in place by a simple strap arrangement, and the intensity and duration of the ride can be varied so that a progressive conditioning takes place. In addition, a wide variety of other exercises for both upper and lower extremities as well as the trunk can be performed by a person with this type of disability.

A problem frequently encountered with the amputee is his reluctance to be seen in the shower by other students. The obvious immediate solution would seem to be to excuse him, and this may well be the best procedure, especially at first. However, it must be recognized that this is circumventing the fundamental issue, and the student should realize that the more normal thing to do is to take the shower, as everyone else does, after the exercise period. Some have used the activity of swimming to bridge this gap, for, aside from getting in and out of the pool, immersion in the water permits a modicum of protection. In addition, it is possible for even the most severely disabled amputee to learn to swim, the type of stroke modified to his physical limitations, and with primary emphasis on balance and the ability to navigate with complete freedom in deep water. A successful teaching progression may then include instruction in diving, and often by this time the student has adjusted sufficiently to be no longer hesitant about revealing his handicap. In addition, the new skill learned may accord him a certain group status, a situation that may have lasting social benefits. Progress along these lines affords an excellent indication of general adjustment.

For the lower-extremity amputee, and particularly one who must wear an above-knee prosthesis, the gait during walking becomes a very important part of his daily life. Unfortunately, large numbers of such individuals have not had sufficient training from physical medicine and rehabilitation specialists to master the rather detailed skills of walking and may not have achieved the semblance of nonchalance that is desired. In this respect, the teacher of developmental and adapted physical education may help by correcting faulty habits and pointing out deviations of posture and ambulation that may be responsible. Although there may be multiple factors involved in any single deviation, the more common gait abnormalities are the following: lateral bending of the trunk toward the prosthesis; dipping the pelvis on the opposite side when swinging the normal leg through; circumducting the prosthesis in a laterally curved line; rising on the toes of the normal leg in a vaulting movement in order to swing the prosthesis through; and permitting an increase in lumbar lordosis when standing on the prosthetic leg.[42] The causes have been variously linked with such factors as a prosthesis which may be either too long or too short, poor balance, socket discomfort, muscular weakness, contractures of the stump, uneven step length, and fear of stubbing the prosthetic toe.

It is obvious that if the prosthesis itself does not fit properly, due to a fault in its length or to errors in design of the socket, the amputee must compensate in some manner when walking. If it is suspected that this is the case, immediate referral to a medical specialist should be made and steps taken to help in establishing a prosthetic reappraisal for that student. If muscular weakness is responsible for gait abnormalities, it may be possible in the developmental and adapted class to strengthen those muscles by use of progressive resistance exercises. Instruction in walking can be enhanced by having the student walk before a full-length mirror so as to be more consciously aware of his ambulation technique, and perhaps enable him to correct his own faults.

The upper-extremity amputee is capable of a wide range of conditioning exercises, and should be encouraged to so participate. Running is especially important, and a number of other activities can be applied to this student. For a person who must change handedness because of the loss of the preferred one, the various games requiring catching and throwing may help to develop skill in the use of his remaining hand. It is likely that this training will be highly specific, so it should not be anticipated that he will develop greater co-ordination for writing, eating, or other daily activities. Besides, it is important that he develop the use of his prosthesis so as to become somewhat ambidextrous.

It is very desirable that the amputee be encouraged to participate as normally as possible in the various team activities of the regular class,

---

[42] "Evaluation of the Gait of Unilateral Above-the-Knee Amputees," Prosthetic Devices Study, Research Division, College of Engineering, New York University, November, 1951.

and to do this as soon as he seems ready or able. Generalizations are difficult concerning those who could be most readily eliminated from the developmental and adapted class, but certainly the minor amputations of digits would form one group, and it might also be possible to include the below-knee amputee. When the latter student wears his prosthesis, many of the activities and games available to the normal pupil are within his capabilities. Each student must be evaluated separately; with proper medical guidance, an adequate schedule can be established that will lead to a proper personal and social adjustment, one that will ensure meeting his physical needs through a vigorous conditioning and activity program.

SUMMARY

The various orthopedic disabilities have been presented in this chapter. The medical management has been discussed and the role of the developmental and adapted physical education program in schools and colleges has been set forth. In general, an attempt has been made to define the manner in which these students may increase their physical fitness through vigorous conditioning exercises and other activities that can be adapted to their use. In addition, there must be awareness of the problems of personal and social adjustment that many of these students may encounter; the utilization of games involving group participation can frequently lead to increased resocialization.

Injuries to bones and joints constitute a large single group of orthopedic disabilities. Many of these respond well to medical treatment and leave very little residual handicap; these include the various strains, sprains, dislocations and fractures, where primary consideration must be given to the prevention of permanent impairment. The developmental and adapted program may be helpful during the convalescent period and later specific exercises may hasten the return of strength to a normal level.

Joint inflammations, including rheumatoid arthritis and osteoarthritis, can severely limit activity for students. In such cases, medical direction is needed to plan a program of activities that can be performed successfully and safely. During the less severe stages of illness, more intensive exercises may be approved. The same is true for bone disorders, where some individuals may have to avoid weight-bearing on certain extremities, and may face rather long periods of restriction. For many of these, certain activities, notably swimming, may be utilized.

A physical disability that has become more noticeably prevalent is the ruptured intervertebral disc, often called the intervertebral disc syndrome. Resulting from a variety of factors, a herniated disc is apt to cause considerable pain, locally in the back, and often radiating down the leg. Conservative treatment, consisting initially in the more severe cases of bed rest and later by exercise, is indicated, but surgical intervention is often necessary in cases of persistent disability. The application of exercise in developmental and adapted physical education may play a preventive role; and posture training may be important in maintaining proper low back alignment.

The loss of a limb represents a severe physical loss, and such an impairment may carry with it an emotional shock of considerable proportions. Emotional and social adjustment of the amputee is extremely important as is his proper physical rehabilitation. The fitting of the prosthesis first includes the healing and shaping of the stump as well as the application of strengthening exercises. Improper instruction in the use of prosthetic appliances may lead to their early abandonment by the patient, but adequate training may provide the necessary tools for an early and rapid adjustment. In the developmental and adapted program, activities may be selected and adapted which will lead to the student's improved physical fitness; skill instruction and game participation may enhance his personal and social well-being.

SELECTED REFERENCES

Anderson, Thomas P., Ernest Sachs, Robert G. Fisher, and Robert M. Krout, "Postoperative Care in Lumbar Disc Syndrome," *Archives of Physical Medicine and Rehabilitation,* 42 (March, 1961), 152.

Armstrong, J. R., *Lumbar Disc Lesions.* London: E. & S. Livingstone Ltd., 1958.

Cyriax, James, *Text-Book of Orthopaedic Medicine.* Vol. I, *Diagnosis of Soft Tissue Lesions.* London: Cassell and Company Ltd., 1957.

Grantham, Everett G., and R. Glen Spurling, "Ruptured Lumber Intervertebral Disks," *Medical Clinics of North America,* 31 (March, 1953).

Huddleston, O. Leonard, *Therapeutic Exercises.* Philadelphia: F. A. Davis Company, 1961.

Klopsteg, Paul E., and Philip D. Wilson, eds., *Human Limbs and Their Substitutes.* New York: McGraw-Hill Book Co., Inc., 1954.

Knocke, Frederick J., and Lazelle S. Knocke, *Orthopaedic Nursing.* Philadelphia: F. A. Davis Company, 1951.

Lambert, Claude N., and Albert J. Novotny, "Amputations and Amputees; Adult and Juvenile," *Surgical Clinics of North America,* 37 (February, 1957), 120.

Licht, Sidney, ed., *Therapeutic Exercise.* New Haven, Conn.: Elizabeth Licht, Publisher, 1958.

Mazet, Robert, Craig L. Taylor, and Charles O. Bechtol, "Upper-Extremity Amputation Surgery and Prosthetic Prescription," *Journal of Bone and Joint Surgery,* 38-A (December, 1956), 1185.

Mixter, W. J., and J. S. Barr, "Rupture of the Intervertebral Disk with Involvement of the Spinal Canal," *New England Journal of Medicine,* 211 (1934), 210.

Watson-Jones, R., *Fractures and Joint Injuries.* Baltimore: The Williams and Wilkins Company, 1943.

10

Neurological Disabilities

T HE GROUP OF DISABILITIES PRIMARILY AFFECTING THE nervous system is known collectively as neurological disabilities. Perhaps no disorders are more insidious or more devastating than these, for often they come without warning, cause severe crippling and in some cases are progressive and terminal. When affecting a child, a neurological involvement will very likely bring grief to the whole family and may leave a pronounced physical loss to the patient. Most of these conditions are irreversible, and the extent of involvement will range from being very slight to a wholesale loss of nervous function. It is for the student whose disability will permit attendance in school or at college that this chapter is written.

It must be recognized that the more severe cases, or the more disabling phases of certain diseases, may require institutionalization or may perhaps cause the patient to be confined to bed at home. Many will attend school after the disease and may become eligible for the developmental and adapted physical education program. An understanding of these conditions is very important to the teacher who must be fully aware of the problems of medical management and have some knowledge of pathology. Only then can he plan a program for these students that is designed to meet their needs and yet is consistent with their capabilities.

PARAPLEGIA

Paraplegia, by definition, is a paralysis of the legs and lower portion of the body. Both voluntary motion and sensation are affected, and, because it does not abate nor become progressively more severe, the person must adjust and manage with remaining muscular function. Because a large number of these cases result from some traumatic incident, the sudden total loss of leg function presents a number of problems. Brought to public attention during World War II, great strides in the rehabilitation of these individuals have since been made. Although during the war about five times as many civilians became paraplegic as did servicemen, the military hospitals and medical services led the way in the effort to return the patient to home and job. Today rehabilitation begins with the onset of illness and injury and continues until the patient has resumed his place in society or has regained his earning capacity; for the younger person, return to home may mean return to school.

ETIOLOGY

The cause of lower extremity paralysis may arise from several different sources. Abramson[1] cites the following six: bone atrophy, soft tissue ossification, bone erosions, osteomyelitis, sacro-iliac fusion, and pathological fractures. For the purpose of simplicity, however, discussion here will be limited to persons suffering traumatic paraplegia, thus avoiding reference to other diseases.

NEUROLOGICAL ASPECTS

When severance of the spinal cord occurs, the patient loses conscious cerebral control of the lower part of his body, but his intellectual resources are unaffected. Thus, the impulses from the lower part of the body which ascend to the brain and help the individual to orient himself in space, in position, and in relationship to the different parts of the body, are cut off. Similarly, the descending impulses originating in the brain, the cortex, and the deeper centers, all of whose functions are excitatory, inhibitory, or regulatory, are cut off from having their normal, natural influence on the lower trunk and legs. The severity of this neurological impairment is dependent upon the level of the lesion, for the resultant impairment of function is more severe if the cervical cord is involved than is the case if the lesion is in the lumbo-sacral region. For purposes of developmental and adapted physical education, only those patients with lesions at the level of the third thoracic segment or lower

---

[1] Arthur S. Abramson, "Bone Disturbances in Injuries to the Spinal Cord and Cauda Equina," *Journal of Bone and Joint Surgery*, 30-A (October, 1948), p. 98.

will be included in this discussion. In this condition, full normal use of both arms is assured, a factor that may very well be extremely important in determining the person's ability to attend school or college.

Immediately following the injury, loss of motor power with complete flaccid paralysis develops; sensation is interrupted so that there is loss of feeling of all types, whether of touch, temperature, pinprick, cotton touch, deep position sense, etc. Other problems arising include pain, spasticity, the pressor reflex, and ureteral reflux with repeated urinary tract infections. The autonomic activities of the central nervous system, including bowel and bladder control and the vasomotor control, are all severely affected immediately following cessation of function.

PHYSIOLOGICAL ASPECTS

After a few weeks following injury, various metabolic changes occur in the patient, demonstrating the value of the spinal cord in maintaining the physiologic capacity of the individual. As Millen[2] points out, the cord functions by aiding in control of protein breakdown and reserve in the body, also in producing blood changes that may result in anemia for the patient, as well as disturbing his normal water and electrolyte balance. Also, the lack of neural activity in the lower body disturbs the heat regulation and sweating mechanisms, and interrupts the sexual functions. In terms of pulmonary ventilation, the level of spinal cord lesion dictates the amount of vital capacity and maximum breathing capacity of patients; the higher the level, the more severely are these functions impaired.[3] The metabolic aspects of ambulation will be discussed later.

MEDICAL TREATMENT

A number of serious problems confront the paraplegic during the rehabilitation process; fortunately, most of them can be cared for satisfactorily with careful medical handling. A discussion of the medical management and the steps to be followed in physical medicine and rehabilitation will be presented.

Care of bladder and bowels. The lack of bladder and bowel control which is present at first is very vexing to the patient and can be a source of acute embarrassment. However, in most instances, a well-trained reflex mechanism can be developed whereby the patient will have adequate bladder capacity, will void without artificial drainage, and, in general, will develop reasonably good control of urination. Dysfunction

---

[2] Francis J. Millen, "Neuropsychiatric Aspects of Paraplegia," *Journal of the Association for Physical and Mental Rehabilitation*, 7 (May-June, 1953), p. 68.

[3] Allan Hemingway, Ernest Bors, and Richard P. Hobby, "An Investigation of the Pulmonary Function of Paraplegics," *Journal of Clinical Investigation*, 37 (May, 1958), p. 773.

of the bladder can lead to bladder and renal calculi, urinary tract infections, renal insufficiency, uremia, and even death. The importance of genito-urinary diseases is pointed out by Dietrick and Russi,[4] who found them in one form or another in about 90 per cent of 55 paraplegic autopsies. Training of the bowels, on the other hand, frequently precedes bladder control, and even though both functions can be reinstated in the patient, careful nursing attention is required in order to achieve complete independence.

Pressure sores. There is a tendency among paraplegic patients to develop pressure sores or decubitus ulcers on the surface of the body, especially on such places as the sacrum, buttocks, trochanters, and heels. This is the result of his inability to recognize excessive pressure because of the loss of normal sensation; thus, when lying or sitting, he will not feel the need to move or to shift his position. The situation becomes even more severe if the skin is allowed to become moist and remain so, for the combination of both of these conditions interferes greatly with local blood circulation. In order to avoid the decubiti, the accepted procedure is to avoid pressure and to keep dry, which is accomplished by frequently turning or moving the body when in lying or sitting positions. Because of the rather inadequate circulation, treatment of these open sores becomes difficult and lengthy, frequently requiring plastic surgery for their closure.[5]

Spasticity. One of the primary problems arising in the chronic stage of paraplegia is spasticity. Sensory impulses carried to and stimulating the anterior horn cells which remain in the spinal cord cause a reflex spastic contracture in the paralyzed muscles. When severe, this may impede satisfactory bracing and interfere with the patient's self-care and routine activities. The withdrawal from activity increases the spasticity, which in turn encourages the further development of contractures. In addition, inactivity favors the formation of decubiti as well as impeding their treatment. Among the procedures that lessen the severity and frequency of spasms, Newman[6] cites the elimination of any infections, the removal of renal and bladder calculi, the prevention of bowel and bladder distention, and the employment of physical exercise. When the

---

[4] Ronald B. Dietrick and Simon Russi, "Tabulation and Review of Autopsy Findings in Fifty-five Paraplegics," *Journal of the American Medical Association,* 166 (January 4, 1958), p. 41.

[5] H. Conway and B. H. Griffith, "Plastic Surgery for Closure of Decubitus Ulcers in Patients with Paraplegia: Based on Experience with 1,000 Cases," *American Journal of Surgery,* 91 (June, 1956), p. 946.

[6] Louis B. Newman, "Rehabilitation Potentials in Spinal Cord and Cauda Equina Injuries," *Journal of the Association for Physical and Mental Rehabilitation,* 7 (May-June, 1953), p. 67.

spasticity is unusually severe, it may require an anterior rhizotomy in order to improve general well-being.[7]

Pain. Even though paraplegic patients experience marked sensory deficits, it is usual for many of them to experience pain, especially in the lower extremities, in the acute stage or during the first year after injury. Quite probably, the recognition of pain is a result of abnormal stimuli or even the absence of normal stimuli from a certain area, and not because of activity of the normal pain mechanism.[8] If pain interferes with the process of rehabilitation, neurosurgical intervention may be recommended.

Pressor reflex. The pressor reflex is the result of certain stimulation of a reflex nature which is quite significant, particularly in spinal cord lesions above the mid-thoracic level. Some of the manifestations include severe headache, a rise in blood pressure to uncomfortable and even dangerous levels, profuse sweating, slow pulse, and shortness of breath.[9] It has been found that in most cases the stimulus for this reflex can be traced to the pelvis, generally to a distended bladder or rectum.[10] Once again, severity of symptoms may dictate the treatment; in severe cases neurosurgery may be indicated.

PHYSICAL MEDICINE AND REHABILITATION

Today, patients with thoracic and lumbar lesions of the spinal cord enjoy a favorable prognosis with respect to meeting the demands of daily living. With increased knowledge of proper methods of bracing as well as in the techniques of ambulation, patients who formerly were condemned to a slow death in bed by pulmonary or renal infections now are actively engaged in earning a living and taking care of their individual needs. The rehabilitation process for these patients begins as soon after hospitalization as possible, and deals with such problems as self-care, crutch walking, psychological and social adjustment, home responsibilities, employment, and education.

Self-care. The typical paraplegic with thoracic or lumbar lesions has the full use of his shoulders and arms and can perform the various tasks

---

[7] D. Munro, "Rehabilitation of Patients Totally Paralized Below Waist, with Special Reference to Making them Ambulatory and Capable of Earning their Living; Anterior Rhizotomy for Spastic Paraplegia," *New England Journal of Medicine,* 233 (December 13, 1945), p. 731.

[8] Herbert S. Talbot, "Understanding the Paraplegic," *Journal of the Association for Physical and Mental Rehabilitation,* 9 (November-December, 1955), p. 186.

[9] C. D. Scheibert, "The Role of Neurosurgery in Rehabilitation of the Paraplegic Patient," *Journal of the Association for Physical and Mental Rehabilitation,* 7 (May-June, 1953), p. 74.

[10] Talbot, *op. cit.*

required of him for a normal daily existence. His first problems arise when he must move from one place to another. In bed he must be competent in sitting up and turning over; he must be able to reach his feet from a sitting position in order to dress, undress, and put on his braces. Once these maneuvers are accomplished, most of his activities will take place out of bed; the paraplegic must master the techniques of getting from bed into wheelchair, and must maintain a sitting position there without falling. Other normal daily needs include the ability to move from the wheelchair to various other implements such as the chair, toilet, tub, and even the automobile. It is obvious that the performance of any of these tasks involves a muscular capacity of the arms and shoulders far beyond that of the normal individual. An understanding of the role of exercise as it relates to ambulation training is therefore important to the teacher of developmental and adapted physical education.

Pre-ambulation exercise. Before a successful program of ambulation and self-care activities can be carried out, the paraplegic must be conditioned with a series of exercises designed to increase the strength of the unaffected muscles of the upper trunk, shoulders, and arms. These exercises should be started while the patient is still confined to bed, inasmuch as his first strenuous movements will take place there, as he attempts to change position, sit up, and, eventually, arise.

As soon as the patient becomes ambulatory in a wheelchair, an intensive program of exercises performed on a mat will prove valuable as a prerequisite for crutch walking. Inasmuch as much greater than normal strength is required to carry and support the body by the arms, these exercises should stress progressive resistance training using both body weight and conventional weights. Deaver and Brown[11] suggest that emphasis be placed on the following muscle groups considered most important in crutch walking: shoulder flexors for moving the crutches forward; elbow extensors for holding the body weight when it is raised from the floor; the hand-gripping muscles for grasping the crutches; wrist dorsiflexors for holding the hands correctly on the hand pieces; and the shoulder girdle depressors and downward rotators used to stabilize and hold the body when it leaves the floor during that phase of the crutch gait.

Principles of bracing. Adequate bracing is essential for the successful rehabilitation of the paraplegic. Braces serve as supports for the lower extremities so that they may serve in a weight-bearing capacity for the body during ambulation. For example, all long leg braces have a supporting bar that extends on one or both sides of the legs parallel to the longitudinal axis of the extremity. Made of surgical steel, these bars stabilize the joints at the ankle, knee, and greater trochanter by joining

---

[11]G. D. Deaver and M. A. Brown, "The Challenge of Crutches," *Archives of Physical Medicine and Rehabilitation,* 26 (August, 1945), p. 515.

each other with semi-circular bands, generally fashioned of sheet metal. Finally, the entire appliance is attached with a stirrup connection to the patient's shoe. If the extent of disability is sufficient, other special equipment may be prescribed, such as spinal braces, pelvic bands, and leg spreaders, which may help provide additional support necessary for encouraging better balance and stability. In general, the majority of patients with a lumbar or cauda equina lesion will not need a pelvic band, but will be able to ambulate with just the long leg braces. On the other hand, thoracic lesions may require the use of a pelvic band, and frequently a spinal brace for additional trunk stability may be required.[12]

Ambulation training. The program of crutch walking for paraplegics is designed to serve a two-fold function: first, to improve or maintain the health of the patient by reducing complications, such as urinary infections, and decubiti, as well as maintaining the physiological balance of bone and muscle; and, second, to provide a means of locomotion for the performance of daily tasks. The entire effect is to counteract the debilitating influence of prolonged bed rest and ensure the patient's continuous and healthful independency.

The initial approach to ambulation for the paraplegic is to learn balance and to develop the ability to move from one place to another without the use of crutches. For this purpose, rehabilitation clinics frequently have available parallel bars some six or more feet long, and approximately three feet high. If necessary rather sturdy chairs placed back to back can suffice in lieu of more elaborate equipment. Activities that must be learned include moving from wheelchair to parallel bars, locking and unlocking braces, and learning to balance on both feet in the standing position. Inasmuch as all movements begin and end in the standing position, the crutch walker must be able to maintain it with ease. Finally, moving forward and backward must be accomplished, utilizing the various crutch gaits.

The same activities must next be performed with crutches. Beginning with learning to arise from the sitting position in a wheelchair, the paraplegic must master the techniques of balancing and then moving forward and backward. He must also become proficient in changing direction and moving on uneven surfaces, and he must learn to ascend and descend stairs and steps of varying heights. Most of these skills will demand many hours of work and practice before he is able to move freely without assistance.

Crutch gaits. There are several types of gaits that are variously employed for ambulation by crutch walkers. To a great extent the particular method selected will be dictated by the ability of the patient to adapt

---

[12] Harold Dinken, "Physical Treatment and Rehabilitation of the Paraplegic Patient," *Journal of the American Medical Association*, 146, No. 3 (May 19, 1951), p. 232.

to ambulation, as well as by the characteristics of the terrain that must be navigated. A shuffling gait, for example, requires a smooth surface, whereas a swinging one does not. Similarly, the swing-through gait may prove too difficult for one person, yet another may possess the necessary balance and co-ordination which makes its performance possible. The following techniques of crutch walking have been suggested by Dening, Deyoe, and Ellison[13] as applicable to the paraplegic and commonly employed by him.

1. Shuffle gait. The crutches are placed forward four to six inches and the hands assume a great portion of the body weight as the body leans forward. The feet are drawn in a sliding motion along the floor to a position next to the crutches. A very slow and exhausting gait, especially for patients with low cervical lesions, it nevertheless is a practical method of moving over short distances.

2. Swing-to gait. Utilized frequently as preparation for the more difficult swing-through gait, it is similar to the shuffle gait, with the exception that the crutches may be placed slightly farther forward and the feet are elevated from the floor when moved even with the crutches. This gait is also slow, but is rather easily learned and allows the paraplegic with high thoracic lesions to walk as effectively as possible.

3. Swing-through gait. This gait is the most difficult for the patient with paralysis of the hips and lower extremities to perform; still, its rhythmical movement enables the patient to walk with minimum effort while permitting maximum speed. The feet are swung through the crutches some six to eight inches before being placed down. The maintenance of balance is extremely important in this technique, and practice with the aid of an instructor should precede any solo attempts utilizing this procedure.

4. Four-point gait. Sometimes described as a four-point alternate gait,[14] this method follows a simple procedure. The subject first advances his left crutch forward, then his right foot, followed by the right crutch and then the left foot. Patients who cannot voluntarily flex the hips to move the legs, must raise the hip and then use a slight rotating movement of the body to place the foot in the desired position.

5. Two-point gait. Resembling the normal walking pattern more than the other crutch gaits, this procedure involves advancing the right crutch and left foot simultaneously, and then the left crutch and right foot.

---

[13] Kenneth A. Dening, Frank S. Deyoe, and Alfred B. Ellison, *Ambulation: Physical Rehabilitation for Crutch Walkers* (New York: Funk and Wagnalls Company, 1951), chap. VII.

[14] Vincent J. Bruno, "Ambulation for Paraplegics," *Journal of the Association for Physical and Mental Rehabilitation,* 3 (April, 1949), p. 21.

The High Cost of Ambulation

Generally, physiatrists recognized that patients vary greatly in their prognosis for ambulation. The level of spinal cord lesion, the age, the general physical ability and co-ordination as well as the desire of the paraplegic all play important parts in his ability to master the techniques of crutch walking. Obviously, the older the individual the more difficult it will be to teach him to become independent on crutches and to maintain this type of activity, except for very brief periods. Also, many persons lack the general co-ordination to perform a satisfactory gait without assistance, and seem to ambulate always with a great deal of exertion and physical discomfort. One of the most significant reasons for inability to perform ambulation techniques is the level of spinal cord lesion.

As mentioned previously, the musculature available for development in crutch walking is directly related to the place on the cord where injury has taken place. The higher the lesion the fewer the muscles that respond to normal nervous control. Hemingway and associates[15] also found that the lesion site had a direct bearing on the vital capacity and maximum breathing capacity; patients with lumbar lesions were normal in this respect, while those with lower cervical lesions had lowered vital capacities of approximately two-thirds and maximal breathing capacities of about one-half. The resultant restriction of muscular endeavor is apparent.

In recent years, there has been some reflection on the advisability for practical reasons of teaching crutch ambulation to all paraplegic patients. Gordon,[16] for example, feels that since World War II, many months and even years may have been lost in drills for ambulation that for all practical purposes were unwarranted in many patients. Heyl,[17] himself a paraplegic, believes that perhaps crutch walking is overemphasized in the program of rehabilitation, inasmuch as the average person must use a wheelchair to earn a living. In one of the few studies dealing with the physiological aspects of paraplegic ambulation, Gordon and Vanderwalde[18] present data supporting the belief that crutch walking is extremely hard work and should be very carefully prescribed. For some patients, the metabolic activity increased to as much as six times

---

[15] Hemingway, Bors, and Hobby, *op. cit.*

[16] Edward E. Gordon, "Physiological Approach to Ambulation in Paraplegia," *Journal of the American Medical Association*, 161 (June 23, 1956), p. 7.

[17] H. L. Heyl, "Some Practical Aspects on the Rehabilitation of Paraplegics," *Journal of Neurosurgery*, 13 (March, 1956), p. 184.

[18] Edward E. Gordon and Herbert Vanderwalde, "Energy Requirements in Paraplegic Ambulation," *Archives of Physical Medicine and Rehabilitation*, 37 (May, 1956), p. 276.

that at basal level, a situation impossible to maintain for very long. With a limited muscle mass, patients with relatively high lesions face a rather unfavorable prognosis with respect to crutch ambulation, but are capable of carrying out wheelchair activities for extended periods without undue physical stress.

DEVELOPMENTAL AND ADAPTED PHYSICAL EDUCATION

The rehabilitation of the paraplegic must not end with his discharge from the hospital; the thoroughness of his early training and medical care will in large part determine the success of his future endeavors. That is why nothing must be overlooked in making him as independent as possible prior to his return home. Moreover, consideration should be given to counselling the family on the role they will play, and to offering effective vocational counselling so that future job opportunities can be sought that are consonant with the patient's abilities. Returning to school or college to resume his interrupted education should be possible for the paraplegic; when this is the case, a program of developmental and adapted physical education may be available to him.

Careful medical guidance must be sought when dealing with students with such an extensive handicap, but it is hoped that the teacher of developmental and adapted physical education will possess sufficient information concerning the nature of this disability that he can intelligently plan the program of activities. Many paraplegics drive their own cars equipped with special hand controls, and are adept at moving from the vehicle into their wheelchairs. Most schools will make special arrangements for parking and many are now equipped with ramps for wheelchair use and even elevators to make possible attendance at classes on upper floor levels. At times special help may be required to navigate stairs or particularly rough ground. The ease of access to the gymnasium should also be considered as part of the planning for these students.

The most propitious time for a paraplegic to attend the developmental and adapted class might very well be near the middle of his school day when it can offer him a chance to vary his routine in a manner that might be particularly beneficial. If he has been sitting for long periods, the opportunity to stand erect and ambulate with crutches would seem appropriate, and the activities he participates in may be as diversionary as they are conditioning. Other school officials may be consulted if scheduling becomes a problem.

Knowledge of the techniques of crutch walking on the part of the teacher is especially important if the student has some difficulty in performing with crutches. If the physician feels that such instruction is necessary, it should be taught as one would teach any potentially dangerous activity, with all possible safety precautions taken. A fall taken during the early stages of ambulation can not only destroy self-confidence, but the force of such an accident could cause severe physical damage. It is well known that abnormal porousness of bone, called osteoporosis, occurs when function becomes limited, thus increasing the possibility of fracture from a fall.[19] This is true in paraplegia. Therefore, correct spotting is essential, and special care should be taken not to interfere with the arms or crutches or the position of the feet when moving. As the paraplegic becomes proficient, he may achieve the desired independence, a situation that may be enhanced if he knows how to fall in an emergency. Inasmuch as the teacher of developmental and adapted physical education is not a therapist, it is not recommended that he attempt the initial instruction in crutch walking to a paraplegic; rather, competent help should be sought from a corrective therapist, a physical therapist, or some other rehabilitation worker who has had experience with such cases.

As muscular strength plays a dominant role in the ambulation and other activities of the paraplegic the maintenance and development of strength in the developmental and adapted class should be possible. As mentioned, the muscles of the arms and shoulders must be exceptionally strong for him to move his body and maintain rather long periods of activity; failure to acquire and maintain adequate strength severely retards the paraplegic's independence and restricts his activities. Systematic and progressive conditioning should be a regular part of this person's daily routine.

Other activities available to the paraplegic student may be performed in the wheelchair if necessary, although care should be taken to prevent his falling forward and out of the chair. Strapping him in place is advisable if a vigorous movement might dislodge him. A racket game, such as badminton, might be adapted to his use; shooting baskets with a basketball is another activity used very successfully. Considerable publicity about basketball played by all-wheelchair teams has been seen in recent years, and this sport affords an excellent example of the vigorous manner in which such games may be played. In fact, sports and games have been so successfully developed for paraplegics that a "paraplegic Olympics" was held in Rome shortly after the 1960 regular Olympic games. With some ingenuity, even one such case in a school or college physical education program can be worked into the activities of the normal class.

The swimming stroke most easily taught is some form of backstroke, be used for the paraplegic if someone is available to work with him during the time he is immersed. One of the little known facts about such individuals is that while the lower extremities are dead weight on land,

[19] Arthur S. Abramson and Edward F. Delagi, "Influence of Weight-Bearing and Muscle Contraction on Disuse Osteoporosis," *Archives of Physical Medicine and Rehabilitation*, 42 (March, 1961), p. 147.

they become extremely buoyant in the water and will float easily. This change in density of muscle and bone creates a favorable opportunity for teaching swimming strokes; eventually, this activity can be used to develop circulatory-respiratory endurance. Experiencing movement that is free of crutches or wheelchair is most rewarding to the student, and, if the water temperature is raised, it can be most relaxing as well.

The swimming stroke most easily taught is some form of backstroke, but care must be taken to ensure that the student does not lose his balance in the water and turn over. The extra buoyancy of the lower extremities tends to force the head and shoulders down; if the spinal cord lesion is fairly high, he may be unable to hold his head high enough in this position. A life jacket or some type of water wings may be needed at first, but these may eventually be discarded. It is also extremely important for the paraplegic to avoid chilling, as a simple cold may lead to further upper respiratory infections of a serious nature. In addition to having an instructor present with the student in the water, other attendants may be needed to assist him in and out of the pool as well as for help in drying and dressing.

Instructions from a physician are imperative in determining the exercise program and the precautions that must be followed for paraplegic students. The effort taken to meet their needs in developmental and adapted physical education may provide lasting benefits and lead them to experience a more vigorous and satisfying life.

CEREBRAL PALSY

Cerebral palsy may be defined as a neuromuscular condition caused by lesions of the motor area in the brain resulting from damage before birth, at birth, or during infancy and childhood. The manifestations of this disability include motor incoordination, weakness, spasticity, athetosis, rigidity, or other signs of motor disturbance; also, mental retardation, speech difficulties, and assorted sensory difficulties may be associated with this condition.

Rusk[20] has estimated that in approximately one of every 200 births a child is born with brain injury, and further, that there are approximately 550,000 persons in the United States with cerebral palsy, nearly half of whom are under 21 years of age. For the child with cerebral palsy, the help required is not a matter of rehabilitation in the sense of acquiring skills that once were normal; on the contrary, the vast majority of these individuals never performed adequately in many of the tasks of daily living, and, consequently, must be taught motor and speech skills that to them are abnormal. The child who has a congenital disability

---

[20] Howard A. Rusk, *Rehabilitation Medicine* (St. Louis: C. V. Mosby Company, 1958), p. 409.

may never have learned control of the bladder and bowels, self-care, or ambulation, nor developed patterns of movement. Thus, the program is one of learning and habilitation, whereas in the adult it is one of re-learning and rehabilitation.

ETIOLOGY

Usually, three classifications of etiologic factors are recognized.

Prenatal. Prenatal factors occur between conception and the time of labor; these may involve maternal infections, anoxia in the fetus, cerebral hemorrhage, hereditary diseases, and the Rh factor.

Natal. Injury may occur between the onset of labor and the birth of the baby; the involvement may be anoxia from binding or obstruction of the cord, asphyxia resulting from some obstruction of the normal breathing, cerebral hemorrhage or mechanical injury to the brain during labor or by forceps delivery, prematurity, or deficiency of vitamin K.

Postnatal. Cerebral palsy may also occur at any time after the birth of the child; it may be caused by injury, especially to the skull with resultant damage to the brain and higher centers, infections such as meningitis and encephalitis, hemorrhages or other vascular trauma, or anoxia from any cause.

The great majority of cases of cerebral palsy occur either before or during birth. Illness and injury after birth may interrupt the normal functioning of the higher motor pathways and give rise to symptoms described as cerebral palsy; however, the main difficulties seem to occur as the child leaves the confines of its prenatal resting place and passes through the birth canal. Any oxygen deficiency is quickly felt by the brain; if deficiency occurs for an extended period, the injury that results may be permanent.

CLASSIFICATION OF CEREBRAL PALSY

Quite general agreement exists concerning the classifications under which the various manifestations of cerebral palsy may be grouped. The general categories are as follows.

Spasticity. Pyramidal tract lesions result in muscular hyper-irritability, causing an increased response to the stretch reflex which leads to spastic muscular response. The observable signs include muscular stiffness, reflex resistance to passive stretch, and clonus.[21]

Athetosis. Damage to the basal ganglia permits aberrant, involuntary stimuli to the muscles bringing about the condition known as athetosis. Some twelve different types of this condition have been identified; how-

---

[21] Julio P. Roasenda and Paul M. Ellwood, "A Review of the Physiology, Measurement and Management of Spasticity," *Archives of Physical Medicine and Rehabilitation,* 42 (March, 1961), p. 167.

ever, in general, patients exhibit movements that are slow, involuntary, unpredictable, and purposeless.

Ataxia. Damage to the cerebellum causes ataxia and is distinguished by loss of balance and equilibrium. Disturbance of kinesthetic sense makes it difficult for ataxic patients to perform co-ordinated movements, as they experience a lack of a sense of body position.

Tremor. The principle symptom of tremor is readily recognizable as involuntary, uncontrollable motions that act reciprocally and are regular in rhythm.

Rigidity. Generally, diffuse brain damage results in a condition of rigidity in the limbs of the body. Movement of the part has been referred to as a sensation of "bending a lead pipe," as there seems to be continuous resistance of the agonist and antagonist muscles.

In addition to the symptoms of muscular impairment and subsequent difficulty in ambulation and the performance of co-ordinated movements, approximately 50 per cent of these patients may have other symptoms of brain damage which will require treatment. Included among these are blindness, deafness, speech difficulties, convulsive disorders, disturbed behavior, and mental retardation.[22]

MEDICAL CARE

From the standpoint of medical care of the cerebral palsied, the etiology is relatively unimportant, for treatment and rehabilitation are based primarily upon the extent of the patient's disability and in knowing whether the disease process is improving, stabilizing, or worsening. In this way, proper objectives may be set up. It is also important to prevent any secondary disabilities or emotional problems from developing. Medical treatment generally centers about the following procedures.

Bracing. Braces are used for a different purpose in the treatment of the cerebral palsied than is true for most other disabilities. Rather than providing complete support, as would be true in paraplegia, they are employed mainly as an aid in teaching joint function. By locking one joint with braces, the function of another may be emphasized alone. Their use in ambulation training is similar, as frequently unwanted knee movement, for example, may interfere with proper hip function. In addition, they are often used to prevent deforming contractures. As the child grows, however, braces must be lengthened accordingly or a new set provided if they have been outgrown completely.

Drugs. The use of drugs in cerebral palsy to control abnormal movement, such as athetosis and spasticity, has not proved to be of much value, although in individual instances certain types of convulsions have

---

[22] R. E. Bruner, "Cerebral Palsy and Brain Damage in Pediatric Practice," *Journal of the Iowa Medical Society,* XLIV (December, 1954), p. 558.

been relieved. Medical authorities generally agree that some clinical experimentation is important in the administration of drugs to patients with cerebral palsy.

Surgery. Occasionally, surgical procedures on muscles, tendons, bones, and nerves are beneficial in correcting deformities that impede or prevent the rehabilitation of the patient with cerebral palsy. In a follow-up study of 242 patients who underwent some form of orthopedic surgery, Phelps[23] found some procedures were generally more successful than others. For example, in children, the vast majority of muscle and tendon surgery failed due to their rapid rate of growth; and neurectomies were quite unsatisfactory because of nerve regeneration. However, osteotomies and arthrodeses resulted in improvement in 90 per cent of the patients; Phelps concluded that tenotomies of the adductors and hamstrings were the most valuable non-osseous surgical procedures for adults.

Rehabilitation. The vast majority of treatment procedures for the cerebral palsied employ the use of physical means by various specialists in the field of rehabilitation. Chief among these is the use of physical modalities as a means of retraining and co-ordinating muscular response. The therapeutic approach is different with each individual case and several different modalities may be employed on a single patient. In general, attempts are made to reduce the severity of symptoms, to counteract the effects of disability, and to prevent secondary complications. Muscle re-education and relaxation, the development of neuromotor skills, speech correction, visual-perceptual retraining, and adequate social-emotional guidance are certainly high on the list of items important in the rehabilitation of the cerebral palsied child.

DEVELOPMENTAL AND ADAPTED PHYSICAL EDUCATION

More so than is true with most diseases, the person with cerebral palsy must actively be prepared for his future formal education during his pre-school years. The first phase of this program is carried out by the parents, who will train these children not only in the activities of daily living, but in matters of personal and social adjustment as well. Thus, the child with a motor handicap at birth will not naturally develop patterns of movement and, therefore, must be taught to perform in a manner that is apt to be foreign to him. This contrasts sharply with the individual who contracts a disability later in life but retains the essential memory patterns that favor the eventual success of any program of re-education. For the cerebral palsied child, no time should be lost in proceeding with his general education, including participation in nursery

---

23 W. M. Phelps, "Long Term Results of Orthopaedic Surgery in Cerebral Palsy," *Journal of Bone and Joint Surgery,* 39-A (January, 1957), p. 53.

school and continuing through the appropriate levels of academic instruction.

During the early years, every effort should be made to determine the intelligence of the child, and thus, hopefully, to rule out the possibility of mental retardation as a complicating factor to his success in school. Special classes or a home program may be required for those who are mentally deficient, as well as for those with a severe motor handicap, even if they have good intelligence.[24] Medical and educational guidance is necessary in making this decision. In the event the cerebral palsied child does attend public school or college, he may become eligible for the developmental and adapted physical education program. There should be a wide variety of activities available to this child or young adult that are compatible with such disability as he may have.

One of the first objectives that should be considered by the developmental and adapted teacher is that of successfully integrating the cerebral palsied student into group activities in order to help him gain approval among his peers. This adjustment is important for the child as well as for the other pupils, who often react unfavorably to the odd facial grimaces or aberrant physical movements that are so frequently characteristic of cerebral palsy. Uncontrollable muscular activity is apt to interfere with purposeful action and may make simple tasks rather complicated for this individual. It may be necessary, therefore, to teach such elementary skills as catching and throwing as well as running and jumping before more complex games are undertaken. As he becomes more successful, balls may be varied in size or in weight and greater distance added at intervals.

During participation in group activities it may be necessary to modify the rules. When students with a variety of disabilities play together, special changes may be necessary for more than one person; in a game of volleyball, for example, the net may be lowered, but additional limitations of playing space or the manner in which the ball is returned may be adopted for specific individuals. In this instance, it may be perfectly legal to catch the ball and then hit it over the net, or perhaps catch the ball and throw it back. Most activities are capable of modification in some way and the teacher must correctly analyze the situation and make such allowances for individual differences.

Special exercises may be given the cerebral palsied child, but only upon prescription of a physician if he feels the need for them; therapeutic exercises should not be attempted unless specifically requested by the physician. In some cases, he may recommend a general conditioning program; but, once again, any contraindications must be known.

---

[24] Eric Denhoff, "The Child With Cerebral Palsy," in *The Child With A Handicap*, Edgar D. Martmer, ed. (Springfield, Ill.: Charles C. Thomas, 1959), pp. 128-149.

One of the most relaxing forms of activity for these students is swimming; and, if the water is heated, it may help to control spasticity and ease general muscular tension. Under such conditions certain movements may be performed that under ordinary circumstances would be difficult or impossible. Also, it is possible to increase the amount of activity and thereby maintain a regular progression in the conditioning program. Necessary precautions must be taken to ensure the student's safety at all times.

For the individual who has associated handicaps, special help may be needed before he can successfully participate in a wide variety of activities. The teacher of developmental and adapted physical education should be aware of these complications and plan the program accordingly. The presence of speech, hearing, visual, or perceptive disorders may require elementary instruction to help the student develop compensatory skills and learn to adjust to varying distances, speed of moving objects, or other factors. In addition, the medical history should be noted to determine if convulsive disorders have been present and if there is any likelihood that the child may have a seizure while participating in class activities. The limitations for these persons will be similar to those for epilepsy, which will be discussed below.

EPILEPSY

Epilepsy, historically referred to as the "Sacred Disease" and the "falling disease," has been known to exist before language itself was established. Its early associations, as its early name, were linked with religion, and this spiritual or mystical concept has remained with us, in many respects, to this day. Hippocrates made the first real description of epilepsy as he associated it with head injuries and observed that it ran in families. It was not until the middle of the last century that English neurologists decided that the brain was indeed the site of the seizure.

Few diseases of modern man have been so consistently misunderstood by the public. The average layman views the sudden and sometimes violent seizures with fear and mistrust, ignorantly associating them with some manner of mental derangement; teachers and employers have frequently believed half-truths or been ignorant of this condition, so that they become apprehensive in the presence of an epileptic. Fortunately for most epileptics, however, the medical understanding of this disease, especially during the last 40 years, has grown to such an extent that the majority of those so afflicted actually have few, if any, seizures.

Whenever possible, modern education calls for the continued and uninterrupted schooling of those suffering from epilepsy. Not only will their education be better than that usually obtained at home but the socialization resulting from living amongst their peers can be of incalculable value. Only through continued efforts can the public be made aware of the nature of this disease, and only through this awareness can true understanding take place.

The magnitude of this problem has largely been masked by the fact that many epileptics have sought to conceal their condition, especially if it hinders employment. Recent estimates are that approximately 1,500,000 persons throughout this country suffer from epilepsy.[25] The teacher of physical education and the teacher of the developmental and adapted program should know how to safeguard the student who has epilepsy and how to plan an effective activity program for him.

ETIOLOGY

There are two types of epilepsy: idiopathic (of unknown cause), and symptomatic. In the latter category, many precipitating causes of seizures have been identified, including brain scars following head injury or birth injuries and brain damage due to infections such as encephalitis, meningitis, high blood pressure, or degenerative disease. Bona fide seizures, indistinguishable from idiopathic epilepsy, may occur as a result of these conditions, and probably account for 30 to 40 per cent of all cases.

For idiopathic epilepsy, there seems to be no precipitating cause. Approximately 65 per cent of cases which fall in this group have a predisposition to seizure for reasons yet undetermined, although there is a moderate tendency for it to run in families.

PATHOLOGY

Since epilepsy represents a syndrome rather than a specific disease as such, most cases of idiopathic epilepsy fail to reveal specific pathological changes when examined histologically.

CLASSIFICATION

On the basis of clinical findings, the following types of seizures may be described.

Grand mal. Preparatory to a grand mal seizure, the patient may receive a preliminary warning of impending attack; described as an "aura," it is usually specific to the individual. It may consist of a sensation of nausea, numbness, an odor, image or memory. Loss of consciousness generally ensues and as a result the patient may fall to the floor, sometimes emitting a cry, and perhaps incurring a bodily injury. Convulsions usually follow; the patient lies stiff and mildly rigid for as long as a

---

[25] National Health Education Committee, *Facts on the Major Killing and Crippling Diseases* (New York: The National Health Education Committee, Inc., 1959).

minute or two, with the muscles in a state of mild tonic contraction. The stage that follows consists of rhythmic, severe, synchronous, convulsive movements of the body, frequently with incontinence of bowels and bladder. Injuries to the tongue from biting are common, and bone fractures may occur from the violence of the movements. A period of stuporous sleep, variable in length from approximately one to four hours, follows this phase; upon full recovery the patient is aware of sore muscles, but little else.

Petit mal. Misconstrued in the past as just a minor grand mal seizure, the petit mal seizure is now recognized as being qualitatively and not just quantitatively different from grand mal.[26] Assuredly, however, this form of epileptic seizure is not as severe as the grand mal. A disease mainly of children, it is possible to incur several hundred attacks per day. There is a momentary or transient loss of consciousness, so fleeting or disguised in ordinary activity that neither the patient nor his associates may be entirely aware of it. These attacks are not associated with falling or convulsions, although activity is often arrested. Outward signs may consist of staring or rhythmic flickering of the eyelids.

Psychomotor seizures. These epileptic seizures cause states in which the patient exhibits a behavioral disturbance rather than the classical convulsion. Rather bizarre psychic manifestations occur such as feelings of familiarity or unfamiliarity, dreamlike experiences or irrational fear; the individual may even run about or search for something. He has no memory of these happenings. Treatment may be difficult because of the variety of such responses. In some cases, electroencephalograms give evidence of the presence of a temporal lobe focus of spike wave abnormality.

Jacksonian epilepsy. The Jacksonian seizure is characterized by an uncontrollable tic or jerking of muscles on one side of the face or mouth, or in an arm, hand, or leg, and gradually spreads and involves all of one side of the body. The focal irritation is in a portion of the motor cortex. This type of seizure is more commonly associated with organic lesions such as brain tumor.

Status epilepticus. This is ordinarily a serious condition and is characterized by the development of a succession of severe seizures with relatively short or no intervals between them. The patient becomes exhausted and frequently hyperthermic; a fatal outcome may result.

Myoclonic seizure. Myoclonic seizures are characterized by an embarrassing sudden single jerk of the head, the limbs, or the trunk without losing consciousness.

Thalamic and hypothalamic. These forms of epilepsy are suggested

---

[26] Donald J. Simons, "Epilepsy and Rehabilitation," in *The Handicapped and Their Rehabilitation,* ed. Harry A. Patteson (Springfield, Ill.: Charles C. Thomas, 1957), chap. 15.

by attacks of dizziness, pain, sweating, heart palpitation, vomiting, and other such bodily disturbances.

Febrile convulsion. Repeated convulsions with febrile illnesses usually begin in infancy, but rarely continue beyond ten years of age.

DIAGNOSIS

The diagnosis of epilepsy is made on the basis of the history of recurrent seizures and the observation of a typical seizure. Physical examination, neurological examination, and laboratory studies including skull x-ray, cerebrospinal fluid manometrics, cell and protein studies, and air studies are rarely helpful, but are frequently done in the hope that some clue may be disclosed. Electroencephalography has become a useful tool in the diagnosis of epilepsy, although it is not an absolutely reliable test. Wisely used, the percentage of diagnostically positive electroencephalograms is very large, so that this, together with his clinical judgment, permits the physician to make a reasonably objective diagnosis.

TREATMENT AND PROGNOSIS

Medical. The prognosis of epilepsy varies with the type that is present; however, in general, treatment with current medications is successful in substantially reducing both the frequency and severity of seizures to socially acceptable levels. Frequently, the violent, disturbing seizures can be stopped altogether, permitting the individual to enjoy a normal and natural life if he follows a few reasonable precautions.

Epileptic attacks can usually be materially reduced in number and severity by use of such drugs as phenobarbital and dilantin. Other anticonvulsant drugs which have been developed recently include tridione and paradione, mesantoin, and phenurone.[27] An important aspect of current research has been the development of medicines that lessen or even eliminate some of the side reactions, such as drowsiness, dizziness, or irritability that used to accompany such treatment.

Surgical. The development of new surgical techniques for the removal of affected areas of the brain, if used carefully, can also be beneficial in controlling seizures. Obviously, surgery cannot restore an incomplete, defective, or seriously damaged brain, but wise prescription may benefit the patient who is seriously afflicted with seizures. Some 10 per cent of the people with epilepsy are so incapacitated as to require institutional care; of these, only a relatively few require neurosurgery.

Psychological. A variety of stimuli may bring on seizures, including certain drugs, poisons, injuries or strong emotional experiences. A mind and body relationship is recognized by medical authorities; thus con-

---

[27] "Education for all American Children," National Epilepsy League, Inc., 208 North Wells Street, Chicago.

vulsions may be related to the power of unconscious emotional stress in precipitating a visceral or somatic physical response; in addition, the problems imposed by the fact that society may not readily accept these persons provides a further psychological burden. The obvious treatment in this respect is to provide educational and vocational counselling, together with psychological guidance, so that the epileptic gains ability to channel his hostility into constructive outlets. As these conflicts are lessened, such patients generally experience fewer seizures.

DEVELOPMENTAL AND ADAPTED PHYSICAL EDUCATION

The trend in education today is to treat the epileptic as normally as possible and not to segregate him from his classmates. Thus, it may be best to plan a program so that the student may participate as much as possible in the regular physical education class. This attitude is entirely warranted because of the success of the newer drugs in reducing and even eliminating the severe seizures. When a careful medical program is followed, nearly all of these children will be able to attend school and remain free from the uncertainty that the imminence of an attack may bring.

The director of the developmental and adapted program should be aware of any student who has a history of epilepsy, so that he may be observed carefully during his class participation for any sign of an impending seizure. If he is taking part in the regular program of physical education, that teacher should be acquainted with his background and should know what to do in an emergency. Consultation with the physician is necessary to evaluate effectively the student's prognosis, to discuss his activity program, and to learn of any performance limitations that should be imposed.

No single activity or exercise will overcome the seizures of epilepsy, but it is true that general activity is beneficial, partly because of the psychological therapy that play can provide and the physiological benefits of conditioning. If certain rather hazardous events are avoided, such as the flying rings, rope climb, and stunts, on the high bar or trapeze, there should be no objection to physical education class participation.[28] The general rule that should be followed for any epileptic who is subject to the grand mal seizure is to avoid activities that might result in injury should he lose consciousness. To this list, then, might be added swimming alone or in deep water, although it may not be necessary to rule aquatics out altogether if proper supervision can be provided. Once again, these are matters that require medical guidance.

Conditioning activities are helpful to the epileptic, as physical work seems to lessen the likelihood of seizures. However, they should not

---

[28] Donald J. Simons, *op. cit.*, p. 327.

be carried to the point of exhaustion, nor should there be attached stress-provoking or highly charged emotional overtones. Probably, competitive athletics, particularly the body-contact sports, are contraindicated; especially hazardous are football and boxing, which may cause a rather severe jarring of the head, a situation that should be avoided for these persons. Skin diving is another type of activity which is usually not recommended. When epileptics have achieved good control of their seizures, certain sports may be open to them if the physician and coach feel that they can compete successfully.

The onset of epilepsy usually occurs early in life; the majority of epileptic children will have experienced a seizure prior to the age of six years. However, during these early years, many may only be suspected of having epilepsy, so the teacher will have the additional responsibility of observing and recording any information that might be of interest to the physician in making a differential diagnosis. Aside from the major seizures, other symptoms of abnormal behavior should be recognized. In much the same way, the student who is currently taking drugs to control his seizures must be carefully watched for possible unfavorable side reactions; any observed aberrant behavior should be reported to the school health service.

The question of higher education for the epileptic must be answered on an individual basis, as many limiting factors are involved, not the least of which is the reluctance of some colleges and universities to admit such persons. However, suitable activities could be provided by the director of developmental and adapted physical education, which would be within the capabilities of these students; these activities could offer an acceptable outlet for their energies and could provide skills and conditioning exercises for their general benefit.

If a student suffers a grand mal convulsion in class, the physical educator should remain calm and should instruct the other students to do likewise. It is not necessary to call a physician or rush the student to a hospital, as the seizure will usually end of itself after a few minutes; however, if it does continue for 15 minutes or so, medical assistance may be required. If given sufficient warning, the person's head may be lowered to the floor. A piece of cork, rubber, or cloth may be placed between his teeth to prevent tongue and cheek biting; never use a hard metal object for this purpose and do not attempt to restrain the convulsive movements nor administer liquids if the individual is unconscious. Do not leave the epileptic alone when the seizure has subsided, as he may be confused for a while and may require rest or sleep. Intelligent management of the seizure in class may be very helpful in gaining the full confidence of the epileptic, which in turn may further his interest in the program that is presented in developmental and adapted physical education.

ANTERIOR POLIOMYELITIS

Epidemic poliomyelitis has been a disease primarily of the twentieth century, although instances involving groups of cases have been described during earlier periods. For example, in this country, description of poliomyelitis occurred in 1841 in Louisiana; in 1894, Vermont experienced an epidemic involving 132 cases; and New York City had a rather severe epidemic in 1907 when over 2,000 persons contracted the disease. Since that time, hardly a year has passed that some locality has not suffered an epidemic of major proportions.[29]

Poliomyelitis occurs throughout the world, both in endemic and epidemic forms. In temperate climates, the occurrence is principally in late summer and fall, although sporadic cases and occasional epidemics are seen at other seasons. Outbreaks are less frequent in the tropics than in the temperate zone. The advent of the Salk vaccine has materially reduced the danger of further serious outbreaks of this disease, but there is still some question as to whether it can be eliminated entirely. Reluctance to obtain preventive immunization, either through laxity, ignorance, or poverty, has greatly interfered with effective control of polio in this country. Indications suggest that there will continue to be thousands of cases each year, at least until complete population immunization is attained. Therefore, the new cases each year combined with the children and young adults who retain a residual disability, present a sizable number of people of school and college age who may be eligible for developmental and adapted physical education.

ETIOLOGY

The etiological agent of poliomyelitis is a neurotropic filterable virus. This virus may be transmitted to mice, monkeys, and chimpanzees, in whom relatively specific reactions occur pathologically and immunologically. There is some question as to the exact manner in which infection occurs, although experimentally, infection via the gastro-intestinal and upper respiratory tracts can be effected; multiplication of the virus in the gastro-intestinal tract may continue for weeks or months after the acute infection.

Regardless of how the virus gains entrance to the body, one of its principal portals of exit is from the alimentary canal. The virus is detectable in throat washings only in the first few days after the onset of acute symptoms, but may be found in the feces more easily and for longer periods of time, even up to ten weeks. Healthy individuals who harbor the virus in their intestinal tract have often been identified.

---

[29] "Facts and Figures about Infantile Paralysis," The National Foundation for Infantile Paralysis, 120 Broadway, New York, 1947.

PATHOLOGY

Once the virus has reached the central nervous system, it produces characteristic changes. There is predilection for gray matter damage to occur, and changes in ganglion cells occur, varying in severity from mild to severe degeneration, especially in the anterior horn cells of the spinal cord. The lumbar and cervical enlargements of the cord are most affected. The lesions consist of destruction of the neurones, neuronophagia, and perivascular and interstitial round cell infiltration; in the brain, lesions occur in the medulla, motor cortex, vestibular nuclei, and cerebellar centers.

CLINICAL FEATURES

The clinical forms of poliomyelitis are abortive, paralytic, bulbar, and encephalitic. Injury to the central nervous system at different levels during different stages of a single attack is not uncommon.

Prodronal Stage. In the prodronal or preparalytic phase, this disease resembles many other mild infections. One usually cannot predict which of a group of ill patients will develop the severe permanent paralysis and which ones will never be severely affected. During this phase, irritability, drowsiness, diarrhea, abdominal distress, headache, and fever of mild degree may be present. The cerebrospinal fluid examination at this time indicates a mild increase in the number of cells.

Paralytic Stage. The paralytic phase may come on soon after, and may be accompanied by severe general symptoms, collapse, coma, and fever of 103 to 105 degrees F. Usually one to three days after severe symptoms have been present, the fever drops and motor paralysis is apparent. Stiff, painful, and retracted neck muscles and a positive Kernig sign are present early. In the acute phase, there may be tenderness of muscles, with painful contractions precipitated by movement or exposure to cold. Retention of urine is common in the earlier acute phases, but soon disappears. When paralysis of muscles occurs it may be severe and generalized and function returns slowly during the following weeks.

Convalescent Stage. With the disappearance of pain and tenderness, poliomyelitis passes into the convalescent phase, which may last from 3 to 12 months, or occasionally longer. It is during this period that maximal recovery of muscle power occurs.

Chronic Stage. When there is no longer improvement in involved muscle groups and residual deficiencies have become stationary, the patient enters the chronic phase.

Differential Diagnosis

The diagnosis of acute anterior poliomyelitis frequently cannot be made in the early phases of the disease. It is suspected, however, whenever flaccid paralysis is found associated with fever and without loss of sensory function. Other diseases are often confused with it, particularly meningitis, diphtheria, and Guillain-Barré syndrome.

Prognosis

The prognosis of poliomyelitis varies for different epidemics and localities. In the individual patient, the degree of functional recovery cannot be predicted in the acute phase. The early return of a mild or very slight degree of function in a muscle is a good prognostic sign for that particular muscle. In general, with treatment, muscles will recover by the end of three months about half the strength they will eventually recover. During the next three months, recovery is much slower; at the end of the first year, about 75 per cent recovery will have been achieved. Further return may take place, so that by a year and a half after the onset of the disease, severely involved muscles, under a good treatment program, will achieve the maximum results possible. This is not an absolute rule, and, of course, some muscles recover completely immediately after illness, while others may retain their original flaccid condition.

Treatment

There is no specific treatment of poliomyelitis. Treatment is symptomatic and related to the manifestations of the individual case. The principles described are general in nature and are not stated for the purpose of rigid standardization.

Acute Phase. The acute phase begins with onset and lasts until fever, headache, and gastro-intestinal symptoms have subsided. In abortive attacks the disease terminates abruptly without the appearance of paralysis. This phase usually runs its course in three to seven days. Rest, support, and symptomatic relief are the important aims of therapy during this period. Absolute bed rest is considered essential, with particular attention given to maintaining muscles tension-free. Stretching of a paralyzed muscle may cause permanent injury. Application of heat to the involved muscle groups is desirable for relief of pain, tenderness, and hypertonicity, and can be conveniently applied by hot, moist packs of flannel cloth; this type of heat, or any other physical agent, has no curative effect on the paralysis. If there is paralysis of the intercostal muscles or diaphragm the use of the mechanical respirator may be indicated.

Subacute Phase. The subacute phase begins when the acute illness has subsided; when fever, headache, and gastro-intestinal symptoms have disappeared and the general malaise has lessened. In addition to the measures inaugurated for the acute phase, treatment is generally directed to protection of the affected muscles and the institution of movement. In this stage, contractures may develop, producing deformities. Rigid fixation of paralyzed or weakened extremities in splints is discouraged, but appropriate physical procedures are initiated to prevent deformities and to maintain physiological position. At this time, muscle tests are given as a guide to treatment; range of joint motion and circumference of extremities are also measured and recorded. During this period when muscles are tender, painful, and hypertonic, selective exercises are carefully begun under medical supervision. The joints are put through their maximum degree of painless, passive motion daily; the amount of exercise is gradually increased as muscle tenderness and hypertonicity becomes less and muscle strength becomes greater.

Convalescent Phase. With the disappearance of pain and tenderness, poliomyelitis passes into the convalescent phase, which, as mentioned, may last for 3 to 12 months, or occasionally longer. During this period, maximal recovery of muscle power occurs. Every measure should be adopted that will enhance recovery. These procedures may include mechanical support or bracing of the affected parts, heat applied in the form of hot packs, and the use of radiant heat or other conventional measures. Therapeutic exercise progresses from assistive-active and full active movements to exercises of graded resistance. Walking is usually encouraged as soon as possible with careful supervision being given to the development and maintenance of proper gait.

Chronic Phase. When there is no longer improvement in involved muscle groups and residual deficiencies have become stationary, the chronic phase begins. It is during this phase that poliomyelitis patients will be found in public schools and colleges; these individuals will exhibit a wide range of disability involvement. Some will have received thorough and sound rehabilitative treatment during the course of the disease, while others may reflect inadequate care both physically and psychologically.

DEVELOPMENTAL AND ADAPTED PHYSICAL EDUCATION

While the Salk vaccine is important in developing immunity to the virus of poliomyelitis, it has no effect on the residual paralysis of those who have already contracted the disease; and, as mentioned, many thousands of people have not been protected against future attacks by such innoculation. Great hope is held that an oral vaccine, the Sabin preparation, will circumvent some of the objections many have to receiving injections. However, once the chronic phase has been reached, many boys, girls, and adults will seek to further their education; thereby, if they are to be as physically active as their condition permits, they will become the responsibility of the developmental and adapted physical education program.

Disabilities resulting from poliomyelitis will vary with the extent of residual paralysis and with the part of the body affected. Those who incur an abortive attack will have no handicap and will consequently have no limitation for exercise; they should be able to participate in the regular physical education program. The exception to this general statement might be that, immediately upon returning to school after an illness of this sort, the medical advice might call for a progressive conditioning program designed to offset the effects of extensive bed rest. When his former level of conditioning has been regained, the student may then join his regular class. The same may be true for those whose residual paralysis is slight enough as to offer no real handicap to normal vigorous exercise. Consultation with the physician should bring to light any complications or limiting factors.

Many students with severe lower extremity paralysis may be treated in a manner similar to the paraplegic; with respect to his ambulation, he may appear to have the same problems. Use of the wheelchair and walking with long-leg braces and crutches must be dealt with in the same way, although careful analysis may reveal some differences. For example, the post-polio individual may retain some residual strength in certain muscle groups of either leg that might help him in walking or moving about and give him additional stability and confidence. Such strengths and weaknesses must be known before a program of activity can be successfully planned for him. Similarly, the extent of upper-extremity involvement must be evaluated.

At the beginning of the developmental and adapted program, it should be determined if conditioning activities are likely to create a muscular imbalance by strengthening one group of muscles (agonists) at a faster rate than the opposing muscle group (antagonists). This is a matter of great concern during early convalescent care, for excessive activity can cause a loss of strength rather than an increase if not carefully graded. Particularly susceptible are the gastrocnemius-soleus muscles that bear such a burden during weight-bearing. If such a situation exists, extra care must be taken to providing a well-balanced series of exercises that seeks to provide the proper conditioning of all muscle groups.

Adapted physical educators have long been interested in the problem of posture, but perhaps the posture of no group of students deserves more critical observation than those who have had poliomyelitis. Strength imbalance of the muscles in the back can lead to rather serious scoliosis; if not checked in time, it can be progressive and deforming and can lead to further difficulties including an unsightly appearance. A tendency toward a lateral curvature or any other postural change should be reported to the physician who may request certain corrective exercises or may wish to make further diagnostic tests.

In designing activities and games for the post-polio, every effort should be made to take advantage of his capabilities; however, because of the highly intricate nature of this handicap, generalizations become difficult. If they must use crutches for their ambulation, these students should develop and maintain a high degree of shoulder and arm strength; furthermore, they must either avoid activities that involve running or participate in them from a wheelchair. Similarly, upper-extremity paralysis may limit the use of arms and rule out some exercises which demand their use. When motor function is only partially impaired, participation in activities on a modified basis may be possible, the selection depending upon the type of involvement. As was true for other serious disabilities, swimming can be an excellent form of exercise for these students. Whatever is decided, the transition to activity can be a very significant phase in the adjustment of the post-polio student to his handicap; moreover, the student will be provided with new skills and abilities of considerable importance to his physical and psychological well-being.

MULTIPLE SCLEROSIS

Multiple sclerosis is an unpredictable and chronic neurological disease, usually progressive and crippling in nature, that generally strikes persons between 20 and 40 years of age. It is unlikely that many such individuals would be found in elementary schools, although some may attend secondary schools; however, there are relatively more of such individuals in our colleges and universities. Indeed, it is rare for symptoms of multiple sclerosis to appear before the teens and rather unusual for them to occur after the age of 50 years.

Although no really reliable figures are available concerning the incidence of multiple sclerosis, an estimate of 250,000 patients annually has been made, with a possibility that this figure may be higher.[30] It is a disease in which early diagnosis is extremely difficult; thus, undoubtedly, thousands of cases are missed. Possibly, an additional 250,000 have other related demyelinating diseases, including diffuse sclerosis, Schilder's disease, acute disseminated encephalomyelitis, Balo's disease, neuromyelitis optica, melachromatic encephalopathies, post-infectious encephalomyelitis, acute allergic encephalomyelitis, Binswanger's disease,

---

[30] Russell N. Dejong, "Multiple Sclerosis," *Today's Health,* 34 (December, 1956), p. 26.

amyotrophic lateral sclerosis and polyneuritis, both toxic and metabolic forms.

ETIOLOGY

The specific etiology of multiple sclerosis is unknown, although attempts have been made at one time or another to link it to infections, intoxications, nutritional deficiency states, lead poisoning, thrombophlebitis, as well as other causes.

PATHOLOGY

Multiple sclerosis is characterized by destruction of the myelin sheath which covers the nerve fibers. This may occur in many areas of the brain, brain stem, and spinal cord; such "placques" are scattered indiscriminately throughout the central nervous system. This demyelination causes either complete stoppage of nerve impulses or their alteration or enfeeblement to such an extent that their function is impaired.

CLINICAL FEATURES

The signs and symptoms of multiple sclerosis frequently undergo remission following their initial appearance, but ultimately there is progression and exacerbation of the clinical features. Among the symptoms that may occur are diplopia, ataxia, and vertigo, numbness of parts of the body, nystagmus, slurred speech, intention tremor, extreme weakness, emotional disturbances, and urinary and fecal incontinence. Any of these, in various combinations, may be common first symptoms, and the onset and progress of the disease may be slow or rapid. Important to developmental and adapted physical education is the fact that there is gradual loss of power of the legs, a disturbance of the ability to maintain equilibrium in walking, and an apparent incoordination of the arms.[31]

The patient generally becomes progressively more disabled and is apt to develop some infection which may prove fatal, such as pneumonia or a urinary infection. Involvement of the medullary or hypothalamic areas by placques generally hastens the demise of the patient.

PROGNOSIS

The illness is not nearly so grave as some of the earlier observers believed. In fact, the life expectancy is not much less than that of the general population; some 25 years and longer in some instances may elapse after the symptoms first make their appearance. During this

---

[31] Henry H. Kessler, *The Principles and Practices of Rehabilitation* (Philadelphia: Lea and Febiger Company, 1950), p. 315.

time, however, these individuals will experience varying amounts of disability.[32]

MENTAL AND EMOTIONAL DISTURBANCES

Early writers on the psychic status of the patient with multiple sclerosis generally noted that it was common to find him euphoric. Recently, however, more intensive and comprehensive interest has been shown in the personality structure of these patients, with the result that it is more appropriate to state that, in general, "the individual reacts to his disease in a manner which is to some degree dependent upon his personality make-up."[33] In other words, the individual's reaction to his illness is dependent upon his pre-morbid personality structure; his psychological characteristics, however, cannot be considered as predisposing the person to the disease.

There is, perhaps, a tendency for patients with multiple sclerosis to become very dependent in their relationship to the physician. This reaction to a frightening situation seems natural, and the early patient-physician relationship can be important in encouraging the expression of fears and in helping to further emotional growth.[34]

TREATMENT

No specific treatment procedure is available for multiple sclerosis. Various treatments based upon the etiology and pathology in favor at various times have been tried with rather disappointing results. Among the more common of these therapies have been fever therapy, antiluetic therapy, protein shock, histamine desensitization, and blood anti-coagulation therapy, as well as treatment with antibiotics, vitamins, and hormones. However, this does not mean that no treatment is beneficial to the patient. On the contrary, many forms of therapy are helpful in teaching the patient how best to live with his disabilities, aiding him in utilizing his residual capacities to the fullest extent possible. In this respect, certain treatment procedures can be employed "so that the patient's life may be productive; if not productive, self-dependent; and if not self-dependent, at least tolerable."[35]

The fact that patients generally recover from the various acute episodes

[32] Howard A. Rusk, "The Problems of Rehabilitation in Multiple Sclerosis," *Association for Research in Nervous and Mental Disease,* 28 (1950), p. 595.

[33] Francis J. Braceland and Mary E. Griffin, "The Mental Changes Associated with Multiple Sclerosis," *Association for Research in Nervous and Mental Disease,* 28 (1950), p. 450.

[34] William H. Soden, ed., *Rehabilitation of the Handicapped* (New York: The Ronald Press Company, 1949).

[35] Edward E. Gordon, *Multiple Sclerosis* (New York: National Multiple Sclerosis Society, 1951), p. 5.

of the illness for varying lengths of time provides an opportunity to inaugurate a developmental and adapted or rehabilitation program designed to meet the broad objective of maintaining physical function at the highest level possible. Activity, aside from the obvious practical values, may also be helpful in the prevention of secondary infections that prolonged inactivity may foster. Further exacerbations of the patient do not reflect failure of the treatment program, but should be attributed to the development of new lesions of the central nervous system, a situation which cannot be altered by external manipulations. Adequate nutrition, avoidance of undue fatigue, and emotional support are highly important in lessening the intensity of symptoms.

The various dysfunctions manifested in persons with multiple sclerosis can generally be improved with the use of physical modalities, medically prescribed. The most common measures of rehabilitation for these symptoms can be grouped about the dysfunctions as follows.

Spasticity. Severe spasticity can be contained by the use of braces or splints, so that purposeful movement may be permitted. Massage, heat, and electrical stimulation have been recommended; and, passive stretching has proved beneficial in many cases, as well as the use of heavy resistance exercise.[36]

Muscle weakness. Because of the tendency for patients to be inactive with multiple sclerosis, muscle atrophy often accompanies the disability. In order to lessen the variety of physiological and biochemical changes that tend to take place and to gain greater functional muscular control, exercise is important. Carefully prescribed and carried out, resistance exercise can be beneficial in counteracting the various complications mentioned.

Contractures. The prevention of contractures is actually the best treatment for them; this necessitates moving each joint daily through its range of motion as well as maintaining it properly at rest so that it does not remain long in a fixed position. Also, if there is muscular imbalance around a joint due to spasticity and weakness, muscle shortening will result. When contracture deformities are present, however, stretching of the involved muscles is required.

Incoordination. Disturbances of the posterior tract and cerebellum, common in multiple sclerosis, result in varying degrees of loss of coordination. Exercises requiring integrated motor patterns, such as reaching, grasping, and reciprocal motion of the lower extremities, form a basis for the developmental training of the multiple sclerosis patient.

---

[36] H. Kabat, "Studies on Neuromuscular Dysfunction, X: Treatment of Chronic Multiple Sclerosis with Neostigmine and Intensive Muscle Re-education," *Permanente Foundation Medical Bulletin,* V (March, 1947).

DEVELOPMENTAL AND ADAPTED PHYSICAL EDUCATION

Because multiple sclerosis is a disease primarily of older people and young adults, it has obvious limitations for developmental and adapted physical education. While it may be encountered in the public schools, it is more apt to be found in colleges and universities. The incidence of the disease is rather widely dispersed; thus, very few cases, if any, may be enrolled in a university at a given time. However, the presence of only one such case indicates the need for understanding the medical entity and, ultimately, for learning the manner in which such individuals may be helped through physical activities.

The serious nature of multiple sclerosis makes it mandatory that medical guidance be provided the adapted physical educator whenever such students participate. The amount of activity must be carefully prescribed to conform to their limitations and capabilities and their tolerance for exercise; these will depend upon the length of time the individual has had the disease and the extent that it has retrogressed. During the early phases, it will be possible to perform more vigorously; if left until later, a number of restrictions may be imposed.

The disease is characterized by relapses which are followed by periods of partial and sometimes complete recovery. It is during these so-called steady states that most activity will be possible, and the physical fitness program will be most effective. The physician may feel that increasing strength and endurance will delay the onset of handicapping conditions, although it must be recognized that any change here in no way constitutes a cure. Part of the rehabilitation of such persons involves the continued efforts to maintain strength and the ability to perform activities of daily living at as high a level as possible. This concept should be furthered in the developmental and adapted program.

The general health of these individuals should be safeguarded at all times, as relapses can follow certain predisposing conditions. Therefore, care is taken to avoid undue fatigue, to prevent illness or injury, and to minimize emotional upsets. The relaxed atmosphere created by the teacher will foster emotional stability and permit exercises and games to continue at a satisfactory pace. The use of progression in all activities will ensure adequate control of these factors, and the instructor can observe any signs portending physical or psychological distress. Medical approval should be given for all activities undertaken by students with multiple sclerosis and rechecks should be made at regular intervals.

There is no reason why persons with mild or moderate multiple sclerosis should not continue in school until their educational objectives have been achieved, for they may expect to enjoy many fruitful years of successful employment. The conditioning and activity program may well be beneficial in furthering this aim and in restoring some of the self-confidence needed in future years. In this respect, emphasis on carry-over activities such as archery, golf, bowling, dancing, and others play a rather important role and should be taught whenever possible. Skills such as these create an atmosphere that fosters greater social acceptance and improves the morale and general feeling of well-being, which in turn promotes the individual's acceptance of his physical disability and encourages greater personal independence.

PROGRESSIVE MUSCULAR DYSTROPHY

Muscular dystrophy is a chronic, non-contagious, progressive disease, characterized by weakness and atrophy of the skeletal muscles with increasing disability and deformity. By conservative estimates, more than 200,000 men, women, and children in the United States are suffering from this disease, although statistically it is difficult to account for all cases inasmuch as it is not reportable on a national basis at present.[37] The apparent reluctance of the victims or their parents to seek medical advice often results in a delayed or inaccurate diagnosis, which further contributes to a rather unreliable census of the annual incidence of muscular dystrophy. Approximately two-thirds of the cases of the childhood type involve children between the ages of three and 13 years. Other types, however, more frequently affect adults; these are classified primarily on the basis of the age at onset and on the muscle groups first involved.

ETIOLOGY

The cause of muscular dystrophy is unknown, although it is generally agreed that there may be a hereditary predisposition toward all types of the disease. Genetic patterns may be of a sex-linked, simple recessive or dominant type. Of importance recently has been research directed toward the study of enzyme system or other biochemical reactions affecting muscle fibers.

CLINICAL FEATURES

There are several clinical forms which will be described, although all are variations of a single disease, differing only in the muscle groups affected and the age at onset. Although there are numerous classifications of muscular dystrophy, only the more prevalent ones will be discussed here.

Pseudohypertrophic form. This form of the disease is most commonly encountered and has its onset generally before six years of age. It is

---

[37] "Muscular Dystrophy—The Facts," Muscular Dystrophy Associations of America, Inc., 1790 Broadway, New York.

characterized at first by muscular pseudohypertrophy (false swelling) and later by atrophy. In the youngster there is noticed a rather pronounced lordosis and gradual weakness of the lower extremities, with increasing waddling gait and frequent falling. Upon attempting to rise from the ground, one of the most characteristic signs is observed as the patient brings his hands successively to his calves, knees and thighs and pushes his body to the upright position by literally "climbing up his legs." Gradual helplessness eventually ensues with all muscles of the lower extremities, spine, pelvis, and shoulder girdle becoming atrophic. Sometimes large subcutaneous deposits of fat help maintain body contours, but in other cases there is marked wasting. Contractures and skeletal deformities result.

Facioscapulohumeral form. The onset of symptoms in this form of muscular dystrophy generally occurs between 10 and 18 years of age; it is the second commonest type. The muscles of the face are frequently affected first, particularly the orbicularis oris and orbicularis palpebrarum, with the result that the patient becomes expressionless and masklike and unable to close his eyelids, lift his eyebrows or wrinkle his forehead. Later involvements of the triceps, biceps, deltoid, infraspinatus, and supraspinatus muscles are noticed; weakness gradually appears in abdominal, pelvic and hip musculature. In most cases, however, lower-extremity involvement is not so severe as in the pseudohypertrophic form. Dystrophy in these patients is usually very slowly progressive; indeed, some live virtually a normal life span.

Juvenile form. This type of the disease has its onset usually at puberty or in early adulthood. It is slowly progressive with a history of long remissions. The muscles of the shoulder girdle are affected first, with winging of the scapula resulting from atrophy of the serratus anterior and trapezius muscles. Said to be hereditary, males and females are equally affected.

Mixed types. A group of conditions having their onset between the ages of 30 and 50 years are grouped under the category of mixed types.[38] Initial involvement may occur in the shoulder or pelvic girdle. Pseudohypertrophy may occur, and present is the typical lordosis, waddling gait, and girdle wasting. Muscular decline varies, but usually the patient is severely disabled with death occurring in from 5 to 10 years.

PATHOLOGY

Muscle fibers vary markedly in diameter, with large, small, and atrophic fibers scattered throughout the muscle; an accumulation of nuclei is found along the sarcolemnal sheath. Late in the disease, con-

---

[38] *Ibid.*

nective tissue replaces most of the muscle, with only a few small, degenerative fibers observed. In pseudohypertrophic dystrophy the large deposits of fat in the calf muscles give the false appearance of being quite well developed, whereas the muscles themselves are actually very weak. The disease is also accompanied by increased urinary creatine, but decreased urinary secretion of creatine and diminished concentrations of creatine, glycogen, and potassium in the muscle. These and other biochemical defects have been noted but not fully understood in their relationship to the disease process.

DIAGNOSIS

The diagnosis of muscular dystrophy generally depends upon the type of disease and the age of onset. Early diagnostic feaures include a history of falling frequently and the inability to keep up with peers, waddling gait and difficulty in climbing stairs, the characteristic method of arising from a supine position, hypertrophy of the calves, typical facial appearance in the facioscapulohumeral type, and the occurrence of the disease in other members of a family. A number of neurological and metabolic diseases are sometimes confused with progressive muscular dystrophy, all of which exhibit a certain degree of muscular weakness. Some of these include amyotonia congenita, Werdnig-Hoffman disease, progressive neural muscular atrophy, and polymyositis.

PROGNOSIS

The disease is progressive, as the name implies. Nothing now known will permanently arrest the disease once it starts, and the prognosis for the pseudohypertrophic form is grave. Death usually occurs within five to ten years after the onset, few patients surviving the period of adolescence. As the muscles gradually weaken, the patient has greater and greater difficulty in ambulation, with resultant helplessness. The cause of death is usually the result of some intercurrent infection, although in certain rare instances involvement of the cardiac muscle may bring about myocardial insufficiency.

TREATMENT

As yet no specific treatment for muscular dystrophy has been developed, although certain preparations have been used without producing any real effect on the course of the disease. These have included vitamins, enzymes, amino acids, proteins, sugars, hormones, antibiotics, and various diets. Orthopedic appliances and surgical procedures which have been employed to correct the contractures that have developed late in the disease have generally proved to be of temporary benefit. Inasmuch as inactivity seems to contribute to development of muscular dystrophy, exercise of functional muscles seems indicated in an attempt to increase strength and permit the patient greater use of his body. In addition, dietary management has proved important in controlling the tendency for these patients to become obese. Excessive weight obviously places a greater burden on the atrophic muscles and thereby tends to hasten the demise of the afflicted individual. In this respect, a satisfactory diet is one in which the relative content of protein is high and that of fat and carbohydrates low.

DEVELOPMENTAL AND ADAPTED PHYSICAL EDUCATION

The grave nature of muscular dystrophy makes therapeutic measures doubly important to the daily routine of individuals so afflicted. No rehabilitation program is complete without the institution of exercises to strengthen weakened muscles and reduce joint contractures and instruction to improve the performance of daily tasks and activities. These tasks should be supervised by therapists, and usually will accompany the management of the more advanced cases. While the child or adult is in school, everything possible should be done to make him better able to continue his studies and to help him enjoy life in general.

Although there is some doubt as to the efficacy of strengthening exercises to increase the muscular strength in the individual with progressive muscular dystrophy, the physician may nevertheless feel that activity should continue as long as possible, and the developmental and adapted program can be planned to permit a well-balanced approach in meeting the student's needs.[39] Once again, it is not expected that the teacher will become a therapist, so in his planning he must thoroughly understand any limitations that may be imposed to safeguard the health of his student, and yet be sufficiently challenging to hold his interest and increase his capacity for further activity.

For the younger student with muscular dystrophy the adjustment to his condition may not be as difficult as it will be for the young adult or older person. Being able to participate in games with the normal students in physical education may be very important initially if the student is capable. A transition can then be made to the adapted program where exercises can be carefully controlled. The emphasis for the elementary school student should be to make the activities as enjoyable as possible, utilizing story plays and mimetics to simulate the movements desired, and employing brightly colored balls and other implements as needed. The heated swimming pool is very appealing to youngsters, and can be used to great advantage for these students if available either in one of the schools or elsewhere in the community. Medical approval must

---

[39] Morton Hoberman, "Physical Medicine and Rehabilitation: Its Value and Limitations in Progressive Muscular Dystrophy," *American Journal of Physical Medicine,* 34, No. 1 (February, 1955), p. 110.

first be obtained and then every care should be taken to ensure protection not only of their safety but of their general health as well. It is always best to prevent infections or colds if at all possible; controlling water and air temperatures and carefully drying after swimming will help in this respect.

For the older student, adjustment to an unfavorable prognosis may be the most difficult part of his illness, especially for the new patient with muscular dystrophy. The inner turmoil and frustration might find no better outlet than through physical activity; the teacher of adapted physical education should take advantage of this fact and provide a variety of interesting games and exercises sufficiently vigorous to occupy the student's attention and energies. Success in this program may create greater self-confidence for him, and the acceptance by his peers of his physical handicap may serve additionally to strengthen his emotional reserves. This program should logically continue until such time as the student is no longer able to continue in attendance at school or until his activity is otherwise restricted.

SUMMARY

A number of disabilities of neurological origin have been presented in this chapter. Because most of these involve children and young adults, they become a social problem with ramifications far beyond the individual family unit. Assuredly, untold grief is caused among the parents and siblings of the affected child, and this is inevitable. However, the widespread incidence of these diseases and disabilities has invoked concern on the community, state, and national levels. Understanding these conditions and learning how exercise and activities can be of help to these students in developmental and adapted physical education has been the aim of this chapter.

Paraplegia may be caused by a number of diseases or from some traumatic incident; the result is a paralysis of the legs and lower part of the body. Aside from certain medical problems, the outstanding limitation is the inability to walk without the aid of long-leg braces and crutches. The rehabilitation of these individuals therefore is concerned with self-care activities and instruction in ambulation techniques, both of which require the development of a high degree of strength in the normal muscles of the upper trunk, shoulders and arms. These concepts should be furthered in the adapted physical education program, where conditioning exercises can continue and where skills may be taught that will help the student to a more vigorous and normal life.

In contrast to paraplegia, which involves the spinal cord itself, cerebral palsy is a neurological condition of the motor area in the brain. As a result, a variety of symptoms becomes manifest, varying in intensity and classification. The resultant disability may cause impairment in ambulation and co-ordination and, in some cases, complications such as sensory disturbances, emotional disorders, and mental retardation. Medical care is concerned with increasing the patient's control of unwanted movement, lessening or preventing contractures, and improving the performance of activities of daily living. In school, the physical activities utilized should assist in developing greater neuromuscular control in running, jumping, throwing, catching, etc., and in striving toward better social adjustment and group integration.

Epilepsy is a syndrome characterized by various types of seizures. Their clinical features, ranging from mere behavorial disturbances to those involving loss of consciousness and massive convulsions, help determine the form of epilepsy the patient may have. Medical treatment has progressed sufficiently so that the majority of seizures can be lessened or even eliminated; annoying side reactions can be controlled as well in the majority of cases. A correction of the unfortunate public misconception of the true nature of epilepsy has long been sought, and this should be furthered in school. General physical conditioning and instruction in a wide variety of activities will help the epileptic student to a more normal acceptance among his peers.

While epidemic poliomyelitis can now be significantly controlled, recent observations show that it may be some time before it is completely eliminated. Various factors contribute to public reluctance to obtain preventive immunization, so that each year a number of post-polio students will be enrolled in public schools. Caused by a filterable virus, characteristic changes occur especially in the anterior horn cells of the spinal cord, which cause paralysis of the muscles to varying degrees. Medical treatment is symptomatic, beginning with absolute bed rest during the acute phase and continuing with measures to help increase the strength of affected muscles as the disease abates. Residual paralysis may involve one or more limbs; and, the extent of disability may vary rather widely among the various muscle groups. For these reasons, the adapted program must be individually planned for each post-polio student, emphasizing careful gradation and progression of exercises and conditioning activities.

Multiple sclerosis is a chronic neurological disease that becomes manifest generally between the ages of 20 and 40 years; as a result, attention to it centers more in the college and university population. While the etiology is unknown, it is characterized by destruction of the myelin sheath of the nerve fibers distributed rather widely throughout the central nervous system, causing a stoppage or alteration of the nerve impulses which control muscle function. The life expectancy after onset may be as much as 25 years, during which time the individual experiences a series of relapses which are followed by periods of partial and sometimes complete recovery. The physician may feel that increasing strength and endurance may delay the onset of handicapping conditions, which should then become the objective of developmental and adapted physical education. In addition, the emphasis on teaching carry-over activities should also be stressed for these students.

Muscular dystrophy is a disease primarily affecting children, and is chronic, non-contagious, and progressive. The cause is unknown and the prognosis is grave. The most prevalent type encountered in children is the pseudohypertrophic form, which generally has its onset before six years of age; its outward manifestations are difficulty in walking, development of a lordotic and waddling gait, and, when arising, literally "climbing up the legs." No specific treatment is effective as yet, although it may be desirable to inaugurate strengthening exercises and activities of daily living in order to make the individual independent for as long as possible. In developmental and adapted physical education, a variety of interesting activities should be presented; for the older student, understanding and adjustment to his handicap may be furthered through increased participation in physical activities.

SELECTED REFERENCES

Deaver, G. D., and M. A. Brown, "The Challenge of Crutches," *Archives of Physical Medicine and Rehabilitation*, 26 (August, 1945), 515.

Dening, Kenneth A., Frank S. Deyoe, and Alfred B. Ellison, *Ambulation: Physical Rehabilitation for Crutch Walkers*. New York: Funk and Wagnalls Company, 1951.

Forster, Francis M., ed., *Modern Therapy in Neurology*. St. Louis: C. V. Mosby Company, 1957.

Kessler, Henry H., *The Principles and Practices of Rehabilitation*. Philadelphia: Lea and Febiger Company, 1950.

Martmer, Edgar D., ed., *The Child With a Handicap*. Springfield, Illinois: Charles C. Thomas, 1959.

Merritt, H. Houston, *A Textbook of Neurology*. Philadelphia: Lea and Febiger, 1955.

McAlpine, Douglas, Nigel D. Compston, and Charles E. Lumsden, *Multiple Sclerosis*. London: E. & S. Livingstone Ltd., 1955.

Pattison, Harry A., ed., *The Handicapped and Their Rehabilitation*. Springfield, Illinois: Charles C. Thomas, 1957.

Penfield, Wilder, and Herbert Jasper, *Epilepsy and the Functional Anatomy of the Human Brain*. Boston: Little, Brown and Company, 1954.

Rusk, Howard A., *Rehabilitation Medicine*. St. Louis: C. V. Mosby Company, 1958.

Soden, William H., ed., *Rehabilitation of the Hanidcapped*. New York: The Ronald Press Company, 1949.

Spencer, William A., *Treatment of Acute Poliomyelitis*. Springfield, Illinois: Charles C. Thomas, 1956.

"Summary Report: Evaluation of 1954 Field Trials of Poliomyelitis Vaccine," *American Journal of Public Health*, 45 (May, 1955).

11

Medical, Sensory, and Surgical Disabilities

A FORMIDABLE LIST OF DISABILITIES COULD BE PLACED UNDER the general classifications of medical, sensory, and surgical. Certain of the more serious ones will be considered here, although this does not intend to minimize the medical significance of other diseases which, naturally, are of considerable importance to the individuals so afflicted. There are certain diseases, however, that influence more directly one's ability to perform vigorous physical activities and seem sufficiently prevalent to warrant close inspection.

The tendency today among physicians and surgeons to encourage an early resumption of normal physical activity following an illness or operation is well known. Indeed, medical practice has shown great progress in aiding recovery from the debilitating effects of surgery by getting the patient out of bed and ambulatory within a few hours after his operation. The intended result is to regain strength and endurance as the wound heals, and to do this as rapidly as feasible, so that the patient's recovery is speeded and he leaves the hospital in as good condition as possible. In hospitals of the armed forces and the Veterans Administration (and occasionally elsewhere), formal exercises of graded intensity are administered to bed patients and to patients who are ambulatory but largely confined to their wards, as a means of further accelerating their recovery. However, this latter practice is seldom found in civilian hospitals and clinics; furthermore, little objective evidence is obtained by physicians relative to the strength and endurance of patients either during their stay in the hospital or upon discharge. Such patients, therefore, must regain their former fitness levels by their own devices rather than through any planned and systematic manner.

This chapter deals with those students who return to school or college following debilitating illness or surgery. Further, consideration will be given to those who have sensory disabilities of sufficient degree to constitute a handicap to their participation in the full physical education program.

CONGENITAL HEART DISEASE

A very small number of children (a fraction of 1 per cent) are born with defective hearts. In fact, only 1 to 2 per cent of all organic heart diseases are congenital in origin, and some 90 per cent of these do not live to school age. Sometimes children are born with heart deformities so severe that they live only a few months or even a few minutes; yet, in other instances, they may have such a mild defect that it is not recognized during the course of a normal lifetime.

Congenital defects occur as a result of improper foetal development, the precise cause of which is usually not known, although infection of the pregnant mother, particularly with German measles during the first three months, may be one precipitating reason. In addition, and unfortunately for the patient, he may frequently possess more than one congenital anomaly, which further complicates the prognostic picture. At any rate, for the majority of children with such problems, continued schooling will be a serious consideration; and these boys and girls will present a wide variety of capabilities and potentialities for the teacher of developmental and adapted physical education.

Recent advances in corrective and ameliorative surgery have played an extremely important role not only in prolonging the life of these patients, but in restoring them to a normal or nearly normal life. Three of the more common congenital heart abnormalities which can often be corrected by surgery are patent ductus arteriosus, tetralogy of Fallot, and coarctation of the aorta.

Patent Ductus Arteriosus

Every baby prior to birth has an open passageway between the pulmonary artery and the aorta, known as a patent ductus. Its purpose during foetal life is to cause blood to bypass the lungs, which are not being utilized, and transport it back to the main circulation by means of the aorta. Normally, at the time of birth or during the first few weeks after birth, this passageway is closed; however, occasionally it remains open, with the result that some of the blood that should go through the aorta is short-circuited to the lungs. This two-way process works to the disadvantage of both pulmonary and general circulations, and may result in a variety of symptoms including shortness of breath, retardation of development, and, perhaps, heart failure. In addition, these patients often fall prey to some bacterial infection or subacute bacterial endocarditis.

In 1939, the first successful surgical correction of the patent ductus arteriosus was carried out; since that time, this process has been developed to the point where mortality is nearly negligible.[1] For the very young child, it may be impossible to ascertain the precise complications that this defect may cause during a lifetime, for obviously some will be affected to a greater degree than others, depending mostly upon the size of this passageway. Therefore, "the mere existence of a patent ductus arteriosus is the indication for surgery."[2] In performing this operation, the patent ductus is ligated and transected, with rather spectacular results for the patient. In most cases he is capable of carrying on a completely normal life.

TETRALOGY OF FALLOT

Tetralogy of Fallot ("Blue Baby") is the name given to a combination of four defects of the heart first identified as early as 1672 by a French physician, Etienne Fallot. Specifically, these abnormalities consist of an opening in the septum between the two ventricles, an abnormal positioning of the aorta to the right, in such a manner that it lies over the defect in the septum to the left ventricle and thence out the aorta artery, and a resultant enlargement of the right ventricle. As a consequence, unoxygenated blood from the right ventricle passes through the defect in the septum to the left ventricle and thence out the aorta and into the systemic circulation. Also, a diminished portion of the blood goes to the lungs for reoxygenation, with the result that the skin and mucous membranes acquire a bluish tinge. The patient is generally breathless upon the slightest exertion and his general development and nutrition are usually very poor.

In 1945, the famous "blue baby" operation was devised for the amelioration of this condition.[3] While not every blue baby can benefit

---

[1] R. E. Gross and J. P. Hubbard, "Surgical Lesion of a Patent Ductus Arteriosus: Report of First Successful Case," *Journal of the American Medical Association,* 112 (1939), p. 729.

[2] Marvin C. Becker, "Rehabilitation of the Patient with Heart Disease," in *Principles and Practices of Rehabilitation,* ed. Henry H. Kessler (Philadelphia: Lea and Febiger, 1950), p. 372.

[3] A. Blalock and H. B. Tausig, "The Surgical Treatment of Malformations of the Heart," *Journal of the American Medical Association,* 128 (1945), p. 189.

by surgery, many of those who have undergone such an operation have gone from nearly complete invalidism to a life that permits moderate physical activity. The operation originally proposed consisted of placing a shunt from the subclavian or the innominate artery to the right or left pulmonary artery, thus providing a channel through which more of the blood can flow into the lungs for oxygenation. While modifications have been made in this process, the fact remains that in certain cases surgery can be extremely important to the individual patient, often creating a much greater exercise tolerance, which is ultimately the important factor.

COARCTATION OF THE AORTA

One other congenital defect that is relatively common is coarctation of the aorta, a condition that has rather severe complications if left untreated. This anomaly consists of a constriction or narrowing of the aorta, generally in the area where the arteries branch off to the head and arms; the natural result is the limitation of blood to the tissues and organs of the body. As a consequence of this resistance to blood flow, the heart is obliged to contract with greater force; as a consequence, a high blood pressure is developed in the upper extremities; and a low blood pressure, in the lower extremities. Eventually, an excessive strain is placed on the vessels of the upper part of the body, frequently precipitating, among other complications, a rupture of the aorta.

Before surgical techniques were developed around 1945, the majority of people with coarctation of the aorta could not hope to reach middle age. The only hope for cure of this disability is surgical intervention, which, in this case, usually consists of excising the constricted portion of the aorta and connecting the ends together. Also, arterial grafts have been developed, which have proved successful in some cases. Normal blood pressure and an apparent cure generally follow recovery from surgery, thus heralding an essentially normal life of activity.

RHEUMATIC FEVER

As a result of medical and public health investigations, rheumatic fever, often the precursor of rheumatic heart disease, has been recognized as one of the most serious diseases with which children of school age may be afflicted. It is probably responsible for two-thirds of all heart diseases among children and usually begins between the ages of six and 12 years. In general, this disease flourishes most in the North Temperate zone; and, in this country, it is especially prevalent in the winter and spring months. The aftereffects on the heart, often leaving it permanently scarred and with diminished efficiency, are its most serious complications.

Inasmuch as young children and young adults are particularly susceptible to rheumatic fever, a close liaison should exist between the classroom teacher and the school medical authority for early detection and prompt care and supervision of the child. Information as to signs and symptoms to be observed and subsequent follow-up procedures are important in early patient care as well as prevention of recurrence. Susceptibility to rheumatic fever appears in most cases to be an inherited tendency. Such conditions as poor diet, inadequate protection from cold and damp, and crowded living conditions that permit the spread of bacteria increase the likelihood of acquiring the disease. Unfortunately, the first attack makes a child more susceptible to future rheumatic fever attacks rather than immune to them; repeated occurrences also increase the possibility of damaging the heart.

ETIOLOGY

The cause of rheumatic fever is not known. Attacks are usually precipitated by a streptococcal respiratory infection, frequently unrecognized or so mild as to receive no medical attention. Infection may follow tonsilitis, scarlet fever, or a streptococcal cold; these usually precede the rheumatic fever by one to three weeks.

CLINICAL FEATURES

Many of the early signs and symptoms of rheumatic fever may be extremely vague, such as a failure to gain weight, poor appetite, pallor, low persistent fever, and frequent complaints of pain or soreness in the arms, legs, or abdomen. Indeed, the most frequent of the symptoms is pain, manifesting itself quite often in the joints, and may, in some cases, be rather severe. The next most common symptom is that of chorea (St. Vitus' dance), which begins with nervousness and awkwardness, and later is manifested in purposeless jerking movements of the arms, legs, and face. In addition, nosebleeds frequently occur without apparent cause. Nodules, small structures about the size of a pea or larger, are present in some 10 per cent of the cases, appearing under the skin at the back of the elbows, the front of the knees, or on the back of the head; these entirely disappear as the disease subsides. Medical examination of the patient with rheumatic fever reveals evidence of inflammation of the heart in the majority of cases, with or without attendant enlargement and characteristic murmurs. Again, these symptoms may disappear with the lessening of the disease.

PATHOLOGY

As a result of this infection, some evidence of permanent heart involvement may appear. Frequently, there is residual damage to the mitral or aortic valve or, less frequently, to the tricuspid valve. As a result of the improper functioning of these valves, leaking or blocking may occur, resulting in enlargement of the heart itself. Over a period of time there is a tendency toward additional scarring of the damaged valves and often rather serious sequelae. This may go on for months or for years.

DIAGNOSIS

Not all children who contract a streptococcal infection will develop rheumatic fever, but a history of such infections will aid the physician in evaluating early symptoms. With a history of previous attack, combinations of symptoms may suggest a recurrence of the disease. There is no specific test for diagnosing rheumatic fever.

PROGNOSIS

Rheumatic fever is a leading cause of death among children 6 to 10 years of age in the United States; the fatality is around three to five per cent in endemic areas.[4] For the vast majority of rheumatic fever patients, however, recovery from the disease itself is complete in a few weeks.

TREATMENT

Acute Phase. The treatment of rheumatic fever is essentially one of bed rest until the signs of illness have passed, which may not be for weeks or months, depending upon the individual patient. Prompt and continuing medical care is essential, and good nursing care is extremely important. The heart should be given as much rest as possible, which is difficult at times because the patient often does not look or feel particularly ill. Difficulty is experienced in knowing when an attack has ended, because the symptoms tend to lie dormant for some time and then to recur even more acutely. Aspirin has, for years, been given these patients for relief of joint pains, and recently cortisone, and its related products have produced rather remarkable results in some patients. However, it remains to be settled whether this relief portends a real influence on the long-term disease complications.

Inactive Phase. Management of the rheumatic fever patient when the active phase has passed, of course, depends upon whether he has suffered permanent heart damage. Inasmuch as further attacks are possible, every effort should be made to improve the health of these individuals, which should include maintaining a proper diet and getting

---

[4] *Control of Communicable Diseases in Man* (New York: American Public Health Association, 1955).

ample rest, exercise, and sunshine. Protection against contracting colds or other respiratory infections from others and the prevention of chilling and getting wet are also important precautions to observe. Undoubtedly, strict parental supervision and guidance of the young child are essential if these measures are to prove successful. In addition to these procedures, continued and constant prophylactic chemotherapy is usually prescribed by the attending physician. Penicillin or a sulfonamide drug is usually given the rheumatic fever patient, possibly throughout life, but at least to age 18 years or for five years from the last attack.

Surgical Treatment. Perhaps the most spectacular method of rheumatic heart treatment developed in recent years has been the use of surgery to repair heart valves that have become damaged by scar tissue. These new techniques, however, have limitations depending largely on the nature of the individual patient and the judgment of the cardiologist. Surgery of the mitral valve to relieve mitral stenosis (blocking of the mitral valve) has been highly successful, but procedures to relieve mitral regurgitation (leakage of the mitral valve) and aortic stenosis and regurgitation are still in developmental stages, with strict reservation concerning their general applicability.[5]

DEVELOPMENTAL AND ADAPTED PHYSICAL EDUCATION

The question of how much and what kind of exercise to provide an individual with a history of cardiac disease is a complex one, which makes generalization difficult. If the student is enrolled and is pursuing a normal course of study in school or college, the assumption may be justified that he has medical approval for a certain amount of activity. The more severe cases of heart involvement will not permit such freedom; these may vary from complete bed rest to exercise which is limited and seldom prescribed in any formal manner. For any student with a history of heart disease, medical supervision and prescription are necessary before he begins a program of developmental and adapted physical education.

For persons who are recovering from rheumatic heart disease, physical activity is gradually resumed during convalescence to the limit of their capabilities. For some, this may merely eliminate them from competitive athletics in school, while for others restrictions may be imposed on running, stair climbing, or any vigorous activity. By the time these individuals return to school, such limitations should be fairly well decided by his physician, who should then communicate them to the school health authorities. Obviously all teachers of this student must under-

---

[5] Richard J. Clark, "The Patient with Heart Disease," in *The Handicapped and Their Rehabilitation*, Harry A. Pattison, ed. (Springfield, Ill.: Charles C. Thomas, 1957), chap. 7.

stand these problems and co-operate to protect and supervise his daily routine so as to maintain his health at the highest possible level.

The tendency in schools today is to give the cardiac student a blanket excuse from physical education whenever his condition requires any exercise limitations in order that he will not participate in the vigorous actvities of the regular program; if there are no provisions for an adapted program, this is quite right. However, if an adapted program is available, physical activities can be provided that are within his capabilities and these can be sufficiently controlled to meet his needs. In fact, many cardiac pupils will be able to perform fairly vigorously for short periods without undue stress; for them, participation in activities such as swimming, modified basketball, volleyball, or a limited form of conditioning exercises may be possible. Whatever is decided by the physician obviously must be strictly observed by both the student and the adapted physical educator.

Introducing a number of recreational activities of a carry-over nature will be helpful to both the high school and college student who must remain on a restricted exercise regimen after his education has been completed. Many of these, including golf, bowling, dancing, archery, swimming, and others, may provide him with skills that can be enjoyed throughout his lifetime and be a source of great personal satisfaction to him. Most medical authorities agree that cardiacs should participate on a restricted basis, rather than discontinue exercise and slowly become more and more sedentary, which, in turn, may ultimately be detrimental to their cardiac health.

The physical activities selected for heart cases should be taught with dual purposes in mind: to present skills correctly, including proper understanding of the rules and nuances of strategy; and to inculcate a realization of each student's personal restrictions of play. These purposes are more difficult to achieve if the student is young, as in elementary school and junior high school physical education, where youthful enthusiasm for sports is apt to overcome good judgment. Part of the teaching of activities should include instruction of the individual on what not to do; when he understands these limitations and accepts them, he must be watched carefully to see that he enforces them on himself. Perhaps alerting his classmates to some of these factors may increase their appreciation of the situation, thus, engaging their willingness to help the cardiac student maintain a safe level of performance.

The student who has had one attack of rheumatic fever is not immunized against future ones; thus, inasmuch as they may be precipitated by a respiratory infection, he should make every effort to prevent getting chilled or wet or to be exposed to other contagious diseases. Periodic medical examinations are important; these children should be carefully watched for symptoms of impending illness, as well as for such other factors as failure to gain weight, loss of weight, irritability, poor appetite, pallor, repeated colds and sore throats, and muscle or joint pains. For a person with a history of rheumatic fever, these signs become doubly important, necessitating referral to the school medical service. Likewise, the exercising cardiac student must be carefully observed for any appearance of distress, such as shortness of breath when resting or on exertion that usually causes no breathlessness, swelling of the ankles and feet, blueness or dizziness, or unusual pain in the chest.

DIABETES MELLITUS

Joslin[6] has estimated that there are 1,600,000 known diabetics in this country and probably as many as 800,000 unknown cases. Diabetes was the eighth leading cause of death in the United States in 1954. Although the percentage of the populace that are carriers remains the same, the number of persons developing the disease seems to be constantly increasing. Thus, diabetes has become a significant public health problem.

Although no age period is immune from the development of diabetes, the disease is essentially one of later life; approximately half of those who have diabetes are over 60 years of age, while only 10 per cent are found among children or young adults. With increased life span and improved diagnostic procedures, an early, more precise diagnosis can be made, with the result that control of this disease can be facilitated for many patients.

Diabetes mellitus is defined as "a complex metabolic disease, the trait apparently transmitted as a Mendelian recessive characteristic, in which the ability to oxidize carbohydrate is faulty, due to diminished production or effectiveness of insulin secreted by the beta cells of the islands of Langerhans of the pancreas."[7] Persons most likely to develop diabetes are those who have blood relatives with the disease, are over 40 years of age, or who are overweight.[8]

ETIOLOGY

It has been known for centuries that diabetes is inherited. Because of its association with a recessive genetic factor, difficulty is experienced in recognizing carriers, or those who do not necessarily develop diabetes but carry the trait and may transmit it to their offspring. Mating of diabetics to either non-diabetics or diabetics is likely to produce the

---

[6] E. P. Joslin, *Diabetic Manual* (Philadelphia: Lea and Febiger, 1954).

[7] U.S. Department of Health, Education and Welfare, *Diabetes Program Guide* (Washington: U.S. Government Printing Office, 1956), p. 1.

[8] U.S. Department of Health, Education and Welfare, *Taking Care of Diabetes* (Washington: U.S. Government Printing Office, 1958), p. 8.

disease in the first or second generation, according to the Mendelian hypothesis. For this reason, the disease adopts a certain socal significance with respect to marriage and parenthood.

Certain secondary factors are apparently capable of provoking the onset of diabetes in a person who is hereditarily predisposed. Between 70 and 90 per cent of diagnosed diabetics have had a history of obesity; inasmuch as these people usually eat a high percentage of carbohydrates and fats, this tends to put an excessive strain on an already weakened pancreas. In addition, "infections, various endocrine imbalances, mental trauma, and sedentary life may at times appear as precipitating factors in the onset of diabetes."[9]

CLINICAL FEATURES

Frequently, few symptoms of diabetes are present in the early stages of the illness. During advanced stages, classical symptoms include hunger, thirst, the passage of large quantities of urine, and the loss of weight and strength. In addition, other accompanying symptoms include intense itching of the skin, especially about the genitals, diminished acuity of vision, boils, carbuncles, ulcers, and gangrenous sores. The onset may be sudden or very gradual, the former applying particularly to younger patients. Those in whom the symptomatology is gradual are generally the middle-aged, overweight patients, whose diagnosis may be accidental, often coming as part of a routine physical examination.

PHYSIOLOGY

Insulin is normally produced in the body in varying amounts depending upon the food intake and the needs of the body. It is principally concerned with the metabolism of carbohydrates, and also of some protein and fat. Its primary function is to help maintain the blood-sugar level within normal limits, regardless of a high or low caloric diet. Insulin is required in the form of glycogen, which is derived largely from the carbohydrate portion of the diet and which is vital as an energy source in muscular contraction. Half of this glycogen is stored in the liver, where it can be converted to sugar and released into the blood stream when some dietary insufficiency occurs. In a non-diabetic, the ingestion of excessive amounts of carbohydrates causes the secretion of an abundance of insulin which once again converts the food into glycogen. The plight of the diabetic person can be appreciated when it is realized that during his illness there is an insufficient amount of insulin in the body, so that glycogen is not being formed from the carbohydrates. Instead, this excess sugar accumulation in the blood

---

[9] Joseph T. Beardwood and Herbert T. Kelly, *Simplified Diabetic Management* (Philadelphia: J. B. Lippincott Company, 1947), p. 4.

stream is eliminated from the body in the urine. Without glycogen, physical activity is impossible, as is life itself.

DIAGNOSIS

While the clinical symptoms of diabetes are important in diagnosing the disease, a knowledge of the blood-sugar level is essential. Quite frequently, early detection and treatment are accomplished by early laboratory examinations of the blood and urine. Urinalysis, while simpler and less expensive, is not as valid and reproducible as the blood-sugar test. In both instances, sensitivity and specificity ratings are medically valuable in helping the physician make his diagnosis.

PROGNOSIS

Since the discovery of insulin in the treatment of diabetes, the prognosis for these patients is very good; before this time, the diabetic had a much shorter life span than the non-diabetic. However, there are certain serious complications of diabetes that must be detected and given early care. These inculde ketosis, arteriosclerosis, impaired vision, and gangrene and lesions of the lower extremity. In this latter instance, there are still many patients for one reason or another who become candidates for amputation surgery; as such, they will come under an additional rehabilitation service when fitted for a prosthesis and trained in procedures of ambulation. These individuals usually are treated by both the internist and the orthopedist.

TREATMENT

The treatment of diabetes is essentially threefold: first, there must be rigid control of the diet, as prescribed by the physician; second, insulin or oral hypoglycemic agents are administered to provide for the amount not produced by the pancreas and; third, there should be participation in exercise which may help stimulate pancreatic secretion. A balance between all of these factors will result in adequate treatment, although diabetes may be controlled by diet alone in a significant percentage of patients. Continued medical follow-up is essential for a successful prognosis.

There are two main complications associated with these treatments of which all diabetics must be wary; these are diabetic coma and insulin shock. Diabetic coma can be prevented entirely, and when it occurs, is usually the result of neglecting to take prescribed insulin injections. Although there are other precipitating causes, the result is an excess of sugar without enough insulin in the blood, which causes the loss of consciousness. Insulin shock, on the other hand, results from too little sugar in the blood brought about by an imbalance in the dosage of

insulin and the amount of carbohydrate consumed in the food. A variety
of symptoms of this state may be present including nervousness, sweating, hunger, weakness, and even unconsciousness. This condition may
also follow fatiguing exercise. The immediate administration of a carbohydrate, such as a lump of sugar or a glass of orange juice, usually
causes these symptoms to disappear.

DEVELOPMENTAL AND ADAPTED PHYSICAL EDUCATION

As indicated earlier, a number of diabetics are found among the
younger age groups even though the disease is primarily one that affects
older people. For this reason, it is important for the teacher of developmental and adapted physical education to understand the medical
treatment as well as to have knowledge of the physiological mechanisms
underlying the disease entity. He should know of any diabetic student
in school or college so that a proper program may be planned for
him, based upon his capabilities and interests and guided and supported
by the physician.

The exercise given to the student with diabetes, of course, should be
prescribed by the physician and faithfully carried out by the student.
At first, exercise may begin rather slowly and continue for short periods;
later, it may be possible to increase gradually his exercise tolerance while
at the same time carefully controlling the amount of insulin taken.
Particularly high levels of endurance have been achieved by some
diabetic individuals; these accomplishments stand as spectacular proof
of the efficacy of the treatment process. The responsibility for maintenance of any medical treatment or drug prescription must ultimately
remain with the student, although he may be encouraged by the teacher
to stay on schedule so that any difficulty or complication can be avoided.

Whenever possible, the diabetic should engage in sports or recreational activities. The question of participation in certain interscholastic
or intercollegiate athletics will require careful consideration by the
physician. In the developmental and adapted class, many diabetics are
able to learn most of the skills necessary for successful participation in
a wide variety of activities both in school and out of school; obviously,
however, the amount of such participation must be within the tolerance
of the individual at all times.

When the diabetes has become well controlled and when the patient
has achieved an adequate level of physical fitness, he may be able to
return to the regular physical education class. The teacher should be
made aware of his health and exercise status so that he can be observed
for any signs of difficulty or discomfort associated with either diabetic
coma or insulin shock or other complications. On the other hand, a
diabetic student may have to remain on a restricted exercise regimen,
and will stay in the adapted class where his program can be more

carefully controlled and where he can learn to regulate his physical activity and become adjusted to his disease and treatment program.

BLINDNESS

The American Foundation for the Blind[10] estimates from a survey conducted in 1953 by the World Health Organization that there are about 6.6 million blind people in the world today. The actual figure may be twice as high as this, because of difficulty in obtaining reliable statistics on the incidence of blindness. Furthermore, the lack of an internationally acceptable definition of blindness results in some confusion when compiling such estimates.

In this country, a blind person has been defined as an individual whose central visual acuity does not exceed 20/200 in the better eye with correcting lenses, or whose visual acuity is greater than 20/200 but is accompanied by a limitation in the field of vision such that the widest diameter of the visual field subtends an angle no greater than 20 degrees.[11] This definition is applied not only in this country but in Canada and Great Britain as well. By contrast, other countries recognize as blind only those who have total loss of vision. More simply stated: "A person is said to have visual acuity of 20/200 if at a distance of 20 feet he can recognize symbols and objects which a person with normal vision can recognize at a distance of 200 feet. It may also happen that an individual has practically normal visual acuity, but the field of vision is so restricted that he can see only a very limited area at a time and can make very little practical use of his vision."[12]

In the United States alone, based on this definition, there are approximately 350,000 blind persons, about 10 per cent of whom are under 21 years of age and 50 per cent of whom are over 65 years. In addition, 1,500,000 Americans are blind in one eye only. Industrial accidents account for 300,000 eye injuries annually.[13] A serious visual disability at any age demands an immense personal, economic, emotional, social, and vocational adjustment on the part of its victims. As a consequence, a sizable problem exists in the treatment and rehabilitation of the blind or visually handicapped person.

ETIOLOGY

There are many etiological factors responsible for blindness, including infectious diseases, injuries, and various prenatal causes. Growing aware-

---

[10] "Blindness. Some Facts and Figures," (New York: American Foundation for the Blind).

[11] "Income Tax Exemption for Blind Persons," (New York: American Foundation for the Blind).

[12] "Blindness. Some Facts and Figures," *op. cit.*

[13] "Preventing Blindness. For More Than Half a Century," (New York: National Society for the Prevention of Blindness).

ness of and increasing public responsibility for the blind have resulted in great progress in controlling eye injuries, although it is estimated that there are still 122,000 eye accidents to children every year.[14] Limitations in the use of air rifles, fireworks, and other potentially harmful toys have contributed to the eye safety of children; industrial membership in the Wise Owl Club attests to the efforts of business to further the prevention of blindness.[15] Following are a number of diseases of the eye of significance to this discussion.

Ophthalmia Neonatorum. Ophthalmia neonatorum is an acutely infectious disease of the conjunctiva which is caused by certain bacteria, notably gonococci, at birth. Unless treated immediately, complications, including corneal ulceration, may result; if left unattended, blindness is the usual end result. At the present time, this disease has become nearly non-existent due to efforts to control its incidence. Legislation in every state now requires that a 1 per cent solution of silver nitrate be administered to the eyes of every newborn child, as well as the antibiotic treatment of those few cases that do occur.

Retrolental Fibroplasia. Another condition that has been brought under control as a cause of blindness among infants is that of retrolental fibroplasia. In the treatment of premature babies, this condition results from the use of oxygen over too long a period or too much oxygen in too short a period of time. Eventually, this leads to a retinal overgrowth due to a proliferation of the vascular portion of the retina. Apparently, a high concentration of oxygen causes vasoconstriction of blood vessels of the retina which are not completely developed in the premature child. Therefore, the controlled proper use of oxygen in the treatment of prematurity has largely prevented the occurrence of this eye involvement.

Cataract. Cataracts are generally recognized to be the leading cause of blindness among adults, partly because of their prevalence among older persons who are now living longer and consequently are susceptible to this eye disease. However, it is by no means limited to the aged; it may be present at birth or may develop during infancy or adolescence. A cataract is an opacity of the lens or its capsule, which brings about a gradual loss of vision. It can develop from other diseases of the eye or from certain metabolic disturbances such as diabetes and parathyroid insufficiency; furthermore, it may be transmitted to the fetus if the mother has German measles during the first three months of pregnancy. Cataracts of both eyes that cause reduction in vision below 20/50 are frequently removed, although the question of surgery is complicated by many factors to be assessed by the ophthalmologist.

Retinitis Pigmentosa. A chronic, progressive degeneration primarily

---

[14] Virginia S. Boyce, "The Prevention of Blindness Program. Its Objectives and Scope," (New York: National Society for the Prevention of Blindness).
[15] *Ibid.*

of the rods of the retina is characteristic of retinitis pigmentosa, with accompanying atrophy and deposits of star-shaped pigment on the inner layer. Gradually, the visual field diminishes, night blindness occurs, and, finally, sight is lost in the central region. Cataract is often a terminal complication.

Detached Retina. A detachment of the retina may result from severe myopia, trauma, or retinoblastoma. Diminished vision occurs with a limitation in the field of sight. The retina is gray and a hole or tear may be seen. Operative treatment may be effective, although in children the prognosis is generally poor.

Interstitial Keratitis. Interstitial keratitis is a chronic cellular infiltration of the deeper layers of the cornea, which leads to clouding and vascularization, usually in both eyes. Most cases are the result of congenital syphilis, although some stem from tuberculosis. Vision may be greatly reduced, and the patient may experience pain, lacrimation, and intolerance to light (photophobia). Pencillin will combat the syphilis and the keratitis, although local application of hot compresses and atropine may be important. When treatment is effective, the cornea will clear in a year or so.

Uveitis. Uveitis (endophthalmitis) is usually a blood-borne infection with involvement of the vitreous and the uveal tracts. The disease may occur with meningitis, scarlet fever, measles, or subacute bacterial endocarditis. The end result is usually blindness.

Glaucoma. It has been estimated that one million Americans over 40 years of age have glaucoma, half of whom are not aware of it.[16] In this disease, the cornea becomes enlarged, thin, bulging, and sometimes cloudy. There is increased intraocular pressure and consequent enlargement of the eyeball. This disease usually progresses slowly to blindness, although some cases spontaneously recover and retain moderately good vision.

PREVENTION

Probably the most important step in the care of blindness is its prevention. Early diagnosis of eye diseases leads to early treatment and in many cases the eye involvement may be prevented or the visual loss minimized. Protective legislation previously mentioned and industry's awareness of its role in accident prevention have helped to lessen eye injuries; the efforts of the public schools to screen students with apparent visual difficulties have also been important measures. In education, such factors as sight-saving classes, adequate lighting, size of type in textbooks, color-ease paper and blackboards, etc. have been instrumental in maintaining normal vision for the vast majority of children. Medical

---

16 "Preventing Blindness," *op. cit.*

referral and follow-up procedures contribute to the control of visual difficulties, as do laboratory and clinical research into the fundamental nature of blinding eye diseases.

VISUAL DISTURBANCES

Hyperopia. The human eye is generally too short at birth; as it develops, the lens gradually assumes its proper place. The power of the lens system to focus an object on the fovea correctly in a single eye is known as accommodation. Measurement of this power is in diopters. At birth the average accommodative strength is 14 diopters; in hyperopia (farsightedness), a strength of over 4 diopters is considered abnormal. This is contrasted with the adult lens system which has a strength of approximately 57 diopters. In hyperopia, the focused image falls posterior to the retina; in order for the visual image to be placed properly on the fovea, the ciliary muscles must be constantly in use, which, in slight cases of hyperopia is sufficient to supplement the refracting power. However, headache and ocular discomfort may result and may lead to nervousness, irritability, and lack of interest in reading. If other visual difficulties are involved, such as corneal distortion or astigmatism, the entire learning process may be impeded. Proper lenses are needed to correct this difficulty and to prevent fatigue.

Myopia. Myopia (nearsightedness) is the opposite of hyperopia. The child is born with an eye that is longer than the average so that the focused image falls short of the fovea; consequently, he does not see distant objects well. The accommodation is constantly relaxed; the ciliary muscles do not develop progressively and, with the exception of objects close at hand, he does not see. Proper lenses must be worn constantly and the eyes continually re-examined.

Astigmatism. Astigmatism consists of a difference in the refractive power of the various areas of the eye, giving a distorted or blurred image. Symptoms include headache, eye pain, fatigue, nervousness, and conjunctival irritation. Slight astigmatism may not require the use of corrective lenses, and a moderate condition may require that they be worn only when using the eyes for extended periods. However, severe astigmatism requires that glasses be worn constantly.

Strabismus. Strabismus (cross-eye) is the result of an imbalance of the extraocular muscles which cause one or both eyes to diverge. The individual therefore tends to see a double image. In order to prevent this, he concentrates his vision on the good eye and eventually may suffer a permanent loss of sight in the deviating eye from disuse. In addition, the impaired vision may cause the behavior pattern of the child to be seriously affected; he may fall, over-reach or appear awkward, or may become fussy and irritable. It is therefore highly important that treatment begin early. Correction of the strabismus may enhance the cosmetic effect, as the obvious eye deviation often presents a somewhat unsightly appearance. Glasses may help in the correction of the divergence, as well as the use of muscle exercises; those who do not respond to this treatment may require surgery.

Binocular vs. Monocular Vision. It might be thought that a child born with one good-vision eye and one poor-vision eye would have a rather serious disability and be at a considerable disadvantage in reading and playing. This has not been found to be the case, as such children learn readily and can get along in most situations as well as individuals with two good-vision eyes. However, correction with glasses is necessary as both eyes must work together for effective functioning. The deleterious effect of poor, uncorrected binocular vision on the learning process of youngsters cannot be overstressed.

SOCIAL, EMOTIONAL, AND EDUCATIONAL FACTORS

A great emotional shock is usually experienced by the newly blinded person, especially if it happens suddenly as the result of some traumatic incident, or if he learns of an unfavorable prognosis concerning some eye disease. Socially, he feels isolated from his environment and friends and consequently tends to withdraw from his personal relationships. If he is an adult, the loss of earning power deprives him of his chief source of independence, placing him at a disadvantage vocationally and creating a serious obstacle to rehabilitation. When the blind person is a child or adolescent, one of the most important considerations concerns the attitude of his parents toward his disability; ignorance and superstition frequently play a prominent role in their reaction to such a situation. A resultant rejection by them can be the cause of severe emotional problems experienced by the child. On the other hand, acceptance of the handicap by the parents can be a leading factor in his early adjustment.

The educational objectives for the blind student are generally the same as for other students, although there may be a change in emphasis necessitated by his handicap; it is hoped that he will take his place with other children as quickly as possible. Special schools for the blind have provided an environment and the individualized instruction necessary for his education. The child in this situation will generally have vision in the better eye of 20/200 or less, with correction; for attendance in sight-saving classes, the requirement is usually that vision in the better eye be less than 20/70 and better than 20/200.

DEVELOPMENTAL AND ADAPTED PHYSICAL EDUCATION

In dealing with students who are blind or partially sighted, a new approach must be adopted in conducting a program of physical activity. While the blind person has a sensory disability of severe proportions, he should not be considered physically disabled and permitted to retire from a vigorous and active life on the basis of his lack of vision alone. He is able to continue his education to the point of obtaining higher degrees, and may even become a teacher and scholar himself. He is entitled to the guidance and help of the developmental and adapted physical educator.

Theoretically, there is no limit to the amount of conditioning exercises that a blind person may perform; for this reason, a very vigorous program of strengthening and endurance activities should be planned for him so that he progresses systematically. Considerable thought must be given to the indiviudal's safety so that he does not stumble over equipment, wander into the path of other students, or otherwise endanger himself during the class period. Many exercises can be demonstrated verbally so that he understands the directions, while others may require more careful presentation before they can be performed correctly. There is no reason why the blind student should not participate with the other members of the developmental and adapted class; indeed, one of the most important objectives in his rehabilitation is the resocialization and increase in self-confidence that can be achieved through the acceptance and approval of his peers.

For the younger child of elementary school age, the selection of activities may be different than for the high school or older student, although the objectives sought are very similar. A great deal of enthusiasm for mimetics and story plays may be elicited, and a large variety of activities may be taught that can be of interest to the blind child. Games of low organization are possible, although in some instances certain special precautions may be needed, such as lines to guide the pupil in certain running events. These may be fashioned by attaching ropes between volleyball standards erected along the path the student must follow; if a lead-in cord is tied to a ring circling the rope, he should be able to reach his destination safely. In other instances, verbal instructions may help him in making correct decisions in locating objects, for which the co-operation of other students may be essential.

When the student is older, his level of activity and performance is much greater and his attention span longer so that he may become interested in a wider variety of skills and wish to become more expert in the execution of the ones he does select. Weight lifting may be employed, as he can perform the exercises and change the weights with a high degree of independence after the initial period of instruction. If the weight room is to be used by blind students, the instructor must insist on the meticulous care and replacement of all equipment by other students, so that the blind pupil can locate the proper weights without undue difficulty, and without danger of tripping over barbells or other items that might be carelessly misplaced.

A number of individual activities may be successfully learned by the blind student that afford him an opportunity to experience a great deal of physical mobility and independence and achieve rather remarkable success. High on this list are apparatus and tumbling stunts; these have reached a prominence of some note and can be performed by the totally blind individual. Especially efficacious are the horizontal and parallel bars, where the blind student can "feel" his position; various routines of tumbling and balancing can be performed separately or in groups. These activities illustrate the co-ordination and body control such a person can successfully achieve.

Wrestling has long been an activity that blind students have enjoyed, and some have achieved significant results in interscholastic and intercollegiate competition. This skill can be taught in the manner it would be presented to other students, except that more verbalization, or other means of illustrating desired movements, will be necessary. Swimming can also be taught and enjoyed by the blind, although special care should be taken to familiarize them with the pool and its surroundings as well as the route to and from the shower and locker rooms. Running, especially the dash events, can be handled too, if some device is provided to assure safety. Such exercise is excellent for conditioning purposes and should be exploited whenever feasible. Other activities can be adapted to use by the blind student, including dancing, bowling, golf, horseshoe pitching, etc., although some of these may require special procedures before successful participation is realized.

When the student is partially sighted, a wider range of physical activities will be available to him, depending upon the amount of vision he retains. When he sees shapes and changes of light, and can tell direction and even estimate certain distances, he may enjoy more vigorous participation, and may even enter group games. His assistance in working with the totally blind is also very helpful to the teacher, as he can often anticipate problems that may arise and help in certain phases of instruction. Usually such students wear corrective glasses and their safety must be assured, although advances in design have made them less breakable, and the more recent use of contact lenses is even more helpful.

It is important that the teacher of developmental and adapted physical education know the medical history of any blind or partially sighted student so that he is familiar with the manner in which the handicap occurred and may also be made aware of the prognosis. If there are any contraindications for exercise or special safety precautions imposed by the physician, these must be very carefully followed to ensure the blind student's continued good health. His gradual familiarity with the surroundings of the gymnasium and the other students in class may be instrumental in promoting an over-all adjustment to school and his handicap and contribute greatly to his enjoyment of life. The blind student should be treated as naturally as possible and should be accepted wholeheartedly into the physical education program; his appreciation and performance will reflect this treatment.

DEAFNESS

Accurate statistics of the number of people in this country who are deaf or hard of hearing are unobtainable, although it is likely that more than 15 million have some degree of hearing loss.[17] Even when deafness is not total, it can be a very severe handicap; the safety of the individual, his earning power, and enjoyment of life are threatened by this disability. In addition, the child who is born deaf faces an additional problem in learning to speak, because one normally learns to speak a language as he hears it spoken.

Hearing loss is measured in terms of decibels (db). A five or six db loss is considered within normal limits. A loss of 20 db or less in the better ear should not cause an impairment of the use of speech; such a child may occasionally pronounce certain words incorrectly, but a seat near the teacher should suffice to obviate the necessity for special help. A 20-40 db loss in the better ear is considered mild; these individuals will acquire speech normally except for certain sounds that will require special help and additional amplification. A loss of hearing of 40-60 db is considered a moderate deficiency; these children will detect only excessively loud speech without amplification, and may require special training before they can attend school with normal children. Between 60 and 90 db, the loss in hearing is severe; such children will require special training, although, with a hearing aid, they may acquire a fairly intelligible vocabulary and understand part of what is said. If no residual hearing exists, however, children may be taught to speak by special methods limited to lip reading or speech reading.

The two kinds of hearing loss that are generally recognized are perceptive (also called sensory, or nerve) and conduction deafness. Perceptive deafness is caused by an involvement of the sensory nerves somewhere between the cochlea and the temporal lobe of the brain and is usually a serious condition that is difficult to treat medically. Conduction deafness is caused by a middle ear involvement and may well respond to treatment if begun early enough. Early diagnosis and treatment of ear disorders are extremely important measures in the prevention of hearing loss, which in young children is made more difficult because of the difficulty of communication. The U.S. Department of Health, Education, and Welfare[18] estimates that 80 per cent of early

---

[17] "Facts About the American Hearing Society," (Washington: American Hearing Society).

[18] "How to Protect Your Hearing," U.S. Department of Health, Education, and Welfare, Public Health Service, Health Information Series, No. 53, 1960.

deafness occurs before the age of five years, and states that, "Proper care and protection of the ears, prompt and adequate medical treatment of injuries or infections are our best safeguards for the maintenance of sound hearing and the prevention of deafness."

CONGENITAL DEAFNESS

Hearing loss in infants is very difficult to detect accurately, for during the first two or three months they behave as normal youngsters; it is not until six or seven months of age that inability of the deaf child to respond to sound is noticed. Furthermore, at the age of 12 to 16 months, when other children are beginning to talk, the congenital deaf child will be vocalizing even less than before.

ACQUIRED DEAFNESS

When the child has developed speech and has learned to hear and interpret sound stimuli, the problems that are encountered with an acquired hearing loss are quite different. In most cases the impairment will not result in a total loss of hearing, so the residual patterns of speech can be utilized to a considerable extent. With proper amplification, normal development will ensue. In severe cases, benefit will be gained by lip-reading instruction, speech training and, in some cases, perhaps, psychological guidance. Acquired deafness may result from middle ear infection and from diseases such as tuberculosis, syphilis, scarlet fever, meningitis, encephalitis, measles, influenza, and mumps.

DEVELOPMENTAL AND ADAPTED PHYSICAL EDUCATION

The inherent difficulty encountered by the deaf student in taking part in physical activities is the danger of being injured when he does not hear directions or anticipate moving objects. If he has no other physical impairment, there are very few activities or exercises that are not open to him. Whether or not this takes place in the developmental and adapted program or during the regular class period will be a matter for individual consideration. It is certainly agreed that he should have every opportunity to develop physically and socially to the highest degree possible in physical education through the media of sports and exercise.

With a deaf person in class, visual demonstration of a new skill or activity will be necessary so that there will be no doubt in his mind what happens next, unless he has mastered the technique of lip reading. These students are apt to pay rather close attention to the teacher in order not to miss anything; some instructors even use hand signals similar to those used in baseball to communicate certain basic instructions such as "ready" or "go" or "stop," etc., with a reciprocal arrangement for the student in the event he fails to understand directions. In a special school for deaf children, the physical educator would probably consider learning formal "sign language," in order to communicate more effectively with these students and to gain more insight into their problems. The extent of this need will depend upon the number and extent of speech difficulties these students have. Furthermore, the physical educator's use of hand communication will improve his rapport with deaf students, as he is more apt to gain their respect and confidence when he can "talk their language."

Damage to a human ear may cause a disturbance in balance for the deaf student, so this factor must be evaluated by the teacher of developmental and adapted physical education before an activity program may be safely prepared for him. This does not mean that all of these individuals will have balance difficulty; actually, this factor may be vastly overrated, for the great majority can participate in skills involving a good deal of co-ordination. Gymnastic events, including the use of apparatus, tumbling, and certain balancing activities, can be taught and performed rather well; and, group games of all types can be played by both boys and girls.

Physical activity can be an excellent means of integrating the deaf student into social situations where he can achieve some success and group approval in situations where ability speaks for itself. This relationship should be cultivated by the adapted physical educator; he should guide the student into activities for which he is prepared developmentally and in which he has expressed some interest. Not only will this counteract any tendency to withdraw socially, but will help the deaf or hard-of-hearing student to develop naturally his special talents and abilities.

POST-SURGERY AND ILLNESS

The harmful effects of bed rest have been discussed in Chapter 5, and it has subsequently been pointed out that current medical practice favors early ambulation for patients recovering from illness and surgery as a means of preventing or alleviating some of the severe physiological complications resulting therefrom. During World War II, and subsequently in hospitals of the armed forces and the Veterans Administration, active hospital physical reconditioning was conducted, which emphasized the importance of an exercise program for surgical and medical patients confined to bed or chair; these programs were expanded more fully when the patients became ambulatory. Such a service performed by developmental and adapted physical educators will not be feasible in schools and colleges. However, physical reconditioning may still be indicated for students returning to school who are still convalescent from debilitating illnesses, injuries, or operations before permitting them to participate fully in the vigorous activities of the regular physical education program.

Because injuries to the knee are so prevalent, they will be singled out for an example of the type of program that can be utilized in recovery following surgery or an extended period of inactivity. The experience of physicians, therapists, and others familiar with knee disabilities is that atrophy of the muscles of the leg, particularly of the quadriceps and hamstring groups, leaves a rather sizable imbalance in strength that may persist for some time if not counteracted with exercise. Initial measurement of knee extension and knee flexion strengths should be made bilaterally in order to determine quantitatively the difference, and to serve as a base line against which future tests may be compared. The use of cable-tension tests (described in Chapter 4) at this time may also help in assessing the starting weight to be used in progressive resistance exercise.[19,20] Klein[21] has suggested that such a program continue for several weeks. Although hamstring weakness accompanies quadriceps deterioration, the hamstrings apparently do not advance in strength as quickly as do the quadriceps muscles. The addition of double-leg exercises and running are also important procedures when strength returns sufficiently to permit such activity. When residual ligamentous weakness follows injury or is present after surgery, Klein[22] found no change in such stability after an exercise regimen, and suggested that the students be taught compensatory static contractions of the leg muscles to provide greater security.

The success of any exercise program following severe illness or surgery will depend upon conscientious follow-up procedures in developmental and adapted physical education with the active co-operation of the physician who must first approve such a program. It is anticipated that reconditioning following surgery or illness would be largely temporary as most students would quickly respond to strengthening and conditioning efforts and would then move on to participate in the regular program of physical education. In some instances, limitations to full participation in physical education activities, including competitive athletics, may be

---

[19] David H. Clarke and E. L. Herman, "Objective Determination of Resistance Load for Ten Repetitions Maximum for Quadriceps Development," *Research Quarterly,* 26 (December, 1955), p. 385.

[20] David H. Clarke and Robert N. Irving, "Objective Determination of Resistance Load for Ten Repetitions Maximum for Knee Flexion Exercise," *Research Quarterly,* 31 (May, 1960), p. 131.

[21] Karl K. Klein, "Progressive Resistive Exercise and its Utilization in the Recovery Period Following Knee Injury," *Journal of the Association for Physical and Mental Rehabilitation,* 10 (May-June, 1956), p. 94.

[22] Karl K. Klein, "A Group Comparison of Post Operative and Post Injury Cases in Progressive Resistive Exercise," *Journal of the Association for Physical and Mental Rehabilitation,* 13 (September-October, 1959), p. 145.

imposed by attending physicians; in such instances, the student may well be a regular member of a developmental and adapted physical education class.

OTHER MEDICAL DISABILITIES

Other medical disabilities deserve special mention because of their prevalence and because of their long-term effect on physical activity. Some may become chronically disabling and others may respond well to medical treatment so that eventual recovery will lead to continuation of normal participation. These and any other conditions must be individually evaluated by the physician and exercise planned in co-operation with him so that satisfactory progress can be made toward realistic goals.

IRON-DEFICIENCY ANEMIA

There are a number of diseases of the blood that commonly affect children and adults; perhaps one of the most common is anemia, especially the iron-deficiency form. In such a condition, the red blood cells are smaller than normal and are deficient in hemoglobin pigment. The deficiency in iron may result from its inadequate intake, loss, or perhaps poor utilization in the synthesis of the hemoglobin for the red blood cells. This form of anemia is most frequently associated with inadequate nutritional intake, whereby the child obtains a deficient amount of iron in the diet, as well as from acute chronic infection or chronic bleeding; it has also been seen in infants born of mothers suffering from a similar anemia.

Some of the clinical symptoms of iron-deficiency anemia include skin pallor, loss of appetite, irritability, fatigue, and general weakness. Laboratory findings indicate a reduction in red cells as the hemoglobin deficit becomes more pronounced; effective diagnosis includes analysis of possible underlying causes of the iron deficiency. These conditions must be remedied before treatment can be completely effective. Specific treatment of the anemia requires the oral administration of iron which brings about rather prompt recovery.

The physician may feel that an anemic student should not engage in very strenuous activity during the early part of recovery, and the student himself may be sufficiently tired that he will be reluctant to do so himself. If he is in attendance at school during this period, some quiet games in developmental and adapted physical education may be provided. Later, when activity is permitted, he may be able to participate in some of the more recreational activities, such as horseshoe pitching, bowling, archery, and others. For the elementary school student, reliance may be placed on the more inactive mimetics, story plays, and games of low organization. As recovery continues, the pace may quicken until a normal level of performance is reached whereupon the student may be able to return to his regular class.

BRONCHIAL ASTHMA

The cause of asthma is not known, except that it is the result of some allergic phenomenon; it is characterized by spasm of the bronchial musculature and edema of the mucus membrane, which cause obstruction to the flow of air in the lungs. As the attack continues, a thick mucus fills the bronchial tubes; as the patient exhales, he produces a characteristic wheezing sound. These episodes may last for a few minutes or may persist for two or three days; upon subsiding, mucus will be coughed up. Asthmatic attacks may be precipitated by a variety of circumstances, including vigorous exercise or exposure to cold air, smoke, or mildly irritating gases, or from some pollen or other allergy-producing substance. Death is extremely rare as a result of bronchial asthma; however, the disease can be most uncomfortable. Treatment is aimed at the elimination of desensitization of the responsible allergens and the administration of epinephrine during an attack. Exercises designed to help in breathing may help restore the confidence of the patient and lessen his fear during an attack.[23]

In developmental and adapted physical education, the danger of precipitating an attack through exercise and vigorous activity should be assessed; the same should be done for environmental factors in the gymnasium which might be responsible for such attacks. The physician should make specific recommendations or impose certain restrictions for exercise as he sees fit; perhaps, too, he should give the teacher instructions concerning specific first aid if any such student should experience asthmatic difficulty while in class. Strengthening and other conditioning activities are indicated for the general fitness of these persons; and, instructions in a wide offering of skills would provide a means of socializing which may be helpful as a form of supporting therapy. The older student who has trouble in participating in extended endurance activities and finds that asthmatic attacks follow running or vigorous games should be allowed to adopt his own pace as he learns to deal with the bronchial congestion; this may also include provision of a longer time to recover from exercise. As the allergy is effectively controlled, the student will probably find that his attacks are less frequent and less severe; under these circumstances, he may increase his exercise dosage, perhaps in the regular physical education class.

---

23 Robert J. Walsh, "Corrective Breathing Exercises for Patients With Bronchial Asthma and Obstructive Pulmonary Emphysema," *Journal of the Association for Physical and Mental Rehabilitation,* 12 (November-December, 1958), p. 194.

INFECTIOUS HEPATITIS

There are actually two forms of hepatitis (catarrhal jaundice), infectious and serum, which are different etiologically, but are indistinguishable both pathologically and clinically. In infectious hepatitis, the virus agent is transmitted naturally; in serum hepatitis it is transmitted artificially by administration of plasma or blood or of vaccines made from human serum. The disease produces varying degrees of destruction of the liver cells, which lasts for three weeks or more, although there is an incubation period which is variable for the two forms. Clinical symptoms may include fever, malaise, headache, and chilliness, with loss of appetite frequently followed by nausea and vomiting. The presence of bile in the urine usually precedes the outward yellow appearance which characterizes jaundice. The prognosis is good, as complete recovery can be expected; relapses are uncommon.

During the illness, rest is important, because activity aggravates the symptoms. The convalescent period may last for several months, during which the activity level of the student must remain fairly minimal. During this time, the physician may indicate that certain less vigorous activities should dominate the selection in developmental and adapted physical education. Fatigue should be avoided, so vigorous conditioning and exhausting exercises should be postponed until the student has returned to normal. At this time, the activity load may be increased until he is once again able to join the regular physical education class.

PULMONARY TUBERCULOSIS

Pulmonary tuberculosis probably requires little introduction to most readers, as, for decades, an excellent public relations program has heightened public awareness of this disease. That it has neither been eliminated nor made extremely rare may only attest to the tenacious nature of the disease and the basic difficulty in establishing completely effective preventive measures. A diagnosis of tuberculosis is made when the tubercle bacilli are present in sputum, or in material taken from the lungs, or in gastric contents. The use of chest X-rays and the cutaneous reaction to tuberculin are also very helpful. The prognosis is excellent for recovery from the primary infection; many may be unaware of its presence during the active phase; reinfection may result in chronic tuberculosis. The mortality rate is high when the disease is present during the first years of life and, again, during adolescence and early adulthood.

Modern treatment includes the use of appropriate antimicrobial agents, such as streptomycin and its derivatives. Also, bed rest is a most important factor in the treatment of progressive tuberculosis. This is probably best accomplished in an institution, because of the extended period of time that such restriction of activtiy may require. Home care is feasible if rigid sanitary procedures are carried out, the parental attitude is receptive, and the individual can be given proper care. During this period, too, a home program of school work may be possible; and, as the patient recovers from the illness, gradual physical activity may be included in his daily routine. Fresh air and sunshine are usually indicated; and, special attention is given to the protein, mineral, and vitamin content of the diet. Surgical treatment, including certain excisional procedures, may be indicated in the management of tuberculosis after preliminary chemotherapy has resulted in maximal reversible benefits.

Many months or even years may elapse before tuberculosis is completely cured; during the entire course of the illness, every care is taken to ensure the continuous and uninterrupted recovery of the patient. For this reason, exercise is carefully controlled, and restrictions are placed on the amount of time out of bed. Later, the patient will gradually resume physical activity until finally he is able to carry out a relatively normal routine. It is now recognized in physical medicine and rehabilitation that these patients often profit from a very limited but effective amount of exercise involving no movement and little cost in energy.

One of the problems often experienced by tuberculous patients is their inability to relax after the first weeks of rest; they begin to exhibit characteristics of nervous tension, such as irritability, trembling, rigidity, restriction in breathing, cold hands, sweating, palms, insomnia, etc. Learning to relax involves learning to differentiate a feeling of tension from one of relaxation. As Kuitert and Templer[24] illustrate, the exercise regimen requires that the patient actively and systematically contract various muscle groups without movement; then relax them by degrees beyond the point of apparently complete relaxation. These "exercises" can be moved progressively from one body segment throughout the major muscle groups, including those about the eyes and mouth; they should be followed by sleep when possible. Gradually, the patient learns to control his tensions and will be able to apply these exercises by himself when he is unable to sleep or is unable to relax.

When ambulatory, the activity content of the daily lives of the tuberculosis patient becomes much greater; eventually he should be able to follow a normal way of life, although for many months there may be restrictions placed by the physician upon formal exercise. During this time, quiet recreational activities may be in order; shuffleboard, dart-throwing, and miniature golf are among those that the physician might approve. When the student returns to school, all activities must be care-

---

[24] John H. Kuitert and Robert C. Templer, "Relaxation in Disease and Disability: An Orientation," *Journal of the Association for Physical and Mental Rehabilitation,* 7 (January-February, 1953), p. 3.

fully prescribed and carried out until he regains strength and endurance and can eventually rejoin the regular class. In the meantime, a number of recreational activities and sports skills can be taught that will help smooth the way for his early social integration with his classmates.

SUMMARY

This chapter dealt with the nature, diagnosis, and treatment of several medical, sensory, and surgical disabilities; program suggestions for developmental and adapted physical education were made. One of the most important of these disabilities, both from the standpoint of incidence and its effect upon one's ability to perform exercise, is rheumatic fever. Because it so frequently leaves residual cardiac lesions, rheumatic heart disease, the medical treatment is carefully prescribed and followed and the patient examined repeatedly during convalescence and beyond. The cause is unknown, although it is usually precipitated by a streptococcal infection, and the clinical features are varied. Joint pain is quite common and evidence of heart inflammation may be present. During the acute phase, bed rest is indicated. When the illness becomes inactive, the patient must still be careful of his general health because recurrences are common; if there is scarring of the heart, severe limitations may be imposed upon his physical activity. In developmental and adapted physical education, physical activity may be gradually resumed, but, usually, within restrictions imposed by the physician. It is generally considered important that the cardiac be taught to resist the tendency to adopt a completely sedentary life; thus, learning certain physical skills and activities may provide an acceptable outlet for him.

Diabetes mellitus is a metabolic disease of the pancreas, in which the ability to effect the oxidation of carbohydrates is impaired by the insufficient secretion of insulin by the beta cells of the islands of Longerhans. Although it is more likely to affect persons over 40 years of age, children and young adults develop the disease as well. Hereditary factors are recognized in its etiology; obesity seems also to play a part. Blood and urine examinations form important elements of the diagnosis, although the blood-sugar test is the more valid of the two. The discovery of insulin has changed the entire prognosis of diabetes; it is now possible and usually advisable for the individual to engage in some exercise. The amount and nature of physical education that can be planned for this student will depend on a number of things; however, the ceiling for such activity is much less limited than in the days before the disease was so well controlled.

Blindness is a severe sensory disability with definite limitations for participation in physical education as well as nearly all other activities. The law defines a blind person as one whose central visual acuity does not exceed 20/200 in the better eye or whose field of vision at its widest diameter does not subtend an angle greater than 20 degrees. The causes of blindness are many, including the two general categories of accidents and disease. Great strides have been made in controlling eye diseases, especially by attending to factors of prevention; efforts by industry to protect the eyes of workers have played important roles as sight-saving measures. This disability involves certain social and emotional problems which are often deep-seated and form obstacles to rehabilitation. Developmental and adapted physical education should reflect concern for these problems and introduce a variety of activities modified for these students in addition to a general conditioning program.

The loss of hearing may result in a severe handicap impeding one's ability to participate in vigorous activity. Because the deaf person does not hear, he may not anticipate suddenly changing events, understand instructions, or perceive directions; thus, he may be susceptible to serious injury. His tendency to withdraw socially can be successfully countered in developmental and adapted physical education through group participation in games, and his conditioning needs may be met through vigorous exercise.

Suggestions for the physical participation of students recovering from surgery or serious medical conditions are also presented as a guide for the teacher of developmental and adapted physical education.

SELECTED REFERENCES

American Public Health Association, Committee on Child Health, *Services for Children With Heart Disease and Rheumatic Fever.* New York: American Public Health Association, 1960.

Beardwood, Joseph T., and Herbert T. Kelly, *Simplified Diabetic Management.* Philadelphia: J. B. Lippincott Company, 1957.

Buell, Charles E., *Sports for the Blind.* Ann Arbor, Michigan: Edwards Brothers, Inc., 1947.

Daniels, Arthur S., *Adapted Physical Education.* New York: Harper & Brothers, 1954.

Lowenfeld, Berthold, *Our Blind Children.* Springfield, Ill.: Charles C. Thomas, 1956.

Morkovin, Boris V., and Lucelia M. Moore, *Through the Barriers of Deafness and Isolation.* New York: The Macmillan Company, 1960.

Pattison, Harry A., *Rehabilitation of the Tuberculous.* New York: Livingston Press, 1949.

Rathbone, Josephine L., *Teach Yourself to Relax.* Englewood Cliffs, N. J.: Prentice-Hall, Inc., 1957.

12

Psychologic Disorders

Deviant behavior is the subject of considerable interest among lay and professional people of all kinds. Stories of irresponsible acts fill our newspapers and magazines, and various forms of antisocial conduct are exploited daily on television and in motion pictures; indeed, the results of the conduct of disturbed persons in high positions of power and authority have been recorded throughout history. Mental illness is widespread and deserves the attention of students of developmental and adapted physical education if there is to be proper understanding of all aspects of the handicapped individual and if a more complete study is made of the role of exercise and activity.

Mention has been made repeatedly of the adjustment patients must make following serious injury or disability, a situation calling for every effort on the part of physicians, parents, teachers, and others to see that there is complete acceptance of any handicap. It is to be expected that there will be great individual differences in this adjustment among the normal population, although fortunately most people respond very well after varying periods of time. In fact, those who work closely with patients often express amazement at the durability of human personality when faced with great personal loss.

On the other hand, our mental hospitals and psychiatric clinics are filled with patients without physical handicap whose adjustments to the vicissitudes of life have been insufficient, so that they are unable to live in society. Recent estimates[1] suggest that as many as 17,000,000 people in the United States are suffering from some sort of mental illness, representing one out of every ten individuals. Not all of these need to be hospitalized, but the figures do present a staggering problem not only to psychiatry but to all who deal with people in their daily lives. Especially important are teachers, who may be in a position to know the student and to identify early symptoms of abnormal behavior and, perhaps, to do something about it.

High on the list of teachers is the physical educator. The nature of this program makes it possible to observe students in a wide variety of situations, some of them formal, others informal, in which very revealing behavior may be evidenced. The relationships that may be established by the pupils with the instructor and with other students using physical activity as a medium offers an excellent setting for studying expressions of personality. Experienced physical education teachers are acquainted with the so-called "troublemakers" in school, know something of the background of many of them, and are generally concerned that they receive the full benefits of education. A casual glance at our objectives is sufficient to realize that social, emotional, and psychological benefits have long been advocated by this profession; however, ways of achieving them have frequently been beclouded by generalities and consequently have proven inadequate. In fact, few university or college programs of undergraduate professional preparation have attempted to provide a proper background for such study, leaving the teachers to handle these problems as best they can.

This vast middle ground is the main subject of this chapter, that group of individuals in school who may show abnormal behavior symptoms, who are the "problem cases" in education, who may respond to adult guidance from teachers, to whom physical activities may become the outlet for aggressive or antisocial behavior, or perhaps whose withdrawal symptoms may be counteracted by group participation. It would seem that these needs can be most successfully met only when one understands extreme behavior deviations and gains some insight into their psychiatric treatment. Once again, it is through knowledge of the whole picture, in this case psychologic disorders, that one may successfully fit the pieces together; merely talking about social and emotional adjustment, peculiar behavior, or problem children really does not lead very far toward a deep understanding of mental illness. Unfortunately, space does not permit more than a cursory examination of this subject; consequently, the reader is encouraged to pursue the study of abnormal psychology so as to obtain a more adequate background.

---

[1] "A Survey of Mental Disease in an Urban Population," Baltimore Survey by Commission on Chronic Illness, October, 1956.

TEMPORARY PERSONALITY REACTIONS

The individual's atypical reaction to a sudden physical handicap or other disability or his reaction to continuing stress might come under the general category of personality disorders that are temporary or transient. These are the behavior manifestations of normal people who have reached the end of their physical and emotional tolerance and have broken down in some way. They are a product of one's environment; an abnormal situation, rather than a weakness of personality, is the causative factor.

REACTIONS TO STRESS

In psychological terms, stress is "a situation in which a person's ongoing behavior is altered from its customary pattern, because of continuing pressure from others or from his own reactions."[2] On a minor scale, such situations can be found in education as students prepare for examinations or some imminent recitation, and the pressures increase usually in proportion to the importance of the event. In a similar way, students taking part in athletics know of the stress that competition imposes, and of the emotional adjustment that must be made to meet these demands. Fortunately, most of those involved have had previous experience with such matters and can adjust adequately; that some college students have emotional difficulties at examination time, however, can be shown through student health service records.

The business world, too, has contributed its share of stressful situations; some of these are long continued, while others are related to a specific and immediate crisis. The amount of tension each individual associates with any one of these situations will determine its potentiality for personality distortion, for if a serious penalty is to be assessed for failure even seemingly harmless acts may create anxiety. In a similar manner, wartime annals are filled with illustrations of abnormal environmental conditions that imposed great stress on soldiers in combat.[3] The stakes were often high and, under fire, many were called upon to perform in a highly skilled way. It is interesting to note that many were able to complete such tasks efficiently while others underwent certain behavior changes, affected by the so-called "shell shock" or "battle fatigue" syndrome of past wars.

It should be remembered that such dramatic instances are mentioned only for purposes of illustration. A situation that appears routine for

---

[2] Norman Cameron and Ann Magaret, *Behavior Pathology* (Boston: Houghton Mifflin Company, 1951), p. 44.

[3] F. P. Moersch, "The Psychoneuroses of War," *War Medicine*, 4 (November, 1943), p. 490.

one person may be fraught with anxiety for another, for it is ultimately what the individual himself feels that is most important in determining his reaction to a situation.

REACTIONS TO FRUSTRATION

Frustration involves the thwarting of one's plan or preventing the consummation of certain desires. Ordinarily this takes place over an extended period of time, although the reaction is similar to that produced by stress. The simplest and most easily recognized situation may be found in infancy, when simple frustration of desires brings about an immediate response that is highly predictable. As the child grows older, he conforms to more adult behavior and gradually learns to adjust to such experiences in a mature manner. Once again, there are great individual differences in the extent to which people will endure frustrations, depending largely upon one's own conception of himself and the obstacle. The ambitious young executive may aspire to a higher position only to realize that he is not favored for the advancement; another very common illustration relates to the frustration experienced by minority groups when faced with problems of prejudice. Under these conditions some will experience adverse personality reactions which may affect others in society as well. In a similar manner, the thwarting by society of his sexual needs may produce tensions in the individual that cannot be ignored.

PSYCHONEUROSES

Neurotic traits are more easily recognized in adults than in children, for many of the manifestations often seem childish when exhibited by mature persons. Psychoneuroses may be characterized[4] by a great variety of symptoms, either mental or physical, without any constant organic basis and are usually traceable to some disturbance in the psychologic processes of the individual. They are the result of persistent mental conflicts, and while they do not disturb the intellectual functions or distort the hold on reality, they do represent a failure of adaptation within the personality. The following classification is generally helpful in understanding the variety of reactions of the psychoneuroses.

Anxiety States. Anxiety is probably the most characteristic trait of the psychoneurotic person, although all such feelings do not belong to the neuroses alone. They are rather common occurrences of normal behavior in everyday life, often the result of feelings of fear, helplessness, or the anticipation of unpleasant future events, or others involving forms of negative excitement. In an anxiety neurosis, there is an exaggeration

---

[4] J. C. Yaskin, "The Psychoneuroses and Neuroses: A Review of One Hundred Cases With Special Reference to Treatment and End Results," *American Journal of Psychiatry,* 93 (July, 1936), p. 107.

of the normal anxiety reaction; the individual experiences an intense mental conflict until the exciting factors spread in a generalized fashion so that he becomes anxious in nearly everything he does, whether it be of a serious or trivial nature. He may complain of difficulties encountered in concentration, feelings of tension and strain, a sense of unreality or mental exhaustion, or become irritable, restless, or apprehensive.[5] Often he has difficulty sleeping and may even lose his appetite. He may exhibit a number of other skeletal and visceral characteristics including the dilation of pupils, trembling hands, rapid heart beat, the feeling of faintness; he perspires easily and may have digestive disturbances.

Neurasthenia. Neurasthenic behavior is typically one of withdrawal, in which the individual seems to be defeated by his environment. He appears physically exhausted from the tension and frustration of his daily life, and indeed may well be, although the cause of this condition is primarily mental rather than physical. This preoccupation with his emotional problems often gives the impression that he is daydreaming, and some people do substitute this type of escape for actual adjustment. The neurasthenic is generally isolated socially, which may further increase his withdrawal tendencies, and he may exhibit other symptoms including muscular pains, loss of memory, insomnia, and loss of appetite. The acute exhaustion states of "battle fatigue" may also illustrate this condition.

Obsessive-compulsive Reactions. A person with obsessive-compulsive reactions feels an inner motivation to perform some act and cannot resist it. Mannerisms may be the result of such reactions, the interference of which is annoying and frustrating to the individual. Stepping over cracks in the pavement, always touching a landmark in the same way, or some other repetitive movement or motion are examples, although such tendencies are frequently seen in children. Most of these are not true obsessions, the main difference being that children can usually stop whenever they want; the obsessed person cannot. Compulsive disorders are the more exaggerated and distorted reactions of self-control that a neurotic individual experiences. Anxieties and tensions are expressed by the performance of serial acts, excessive tidiness, or perhaps repetitive gestures; however, such expressions usually afford only temporary relief from anxiety.

Psychosomatic Conditions. Psychosomatic disorders are visceral responses to anxiety reactions. They result from the union of body and mind that has received such attention in recent years, the realization that every part of the body reacts to the inner emotional forces of the individual. This often takes the form of some illness, such as a cold, an upset stomach, or a head or backache, the pain of which may be real but

---

[5] K. Hazell, "The Anxiety Syndrome," *Medical Progress,* 216 (1946), p. 153.

caused by underlying tensions. Indeed, prolonged emotional strain is recognized as being responsible for pathology, as in the case of gastric ulcers; organs of the body can bear certain pressures but not for an indefinite period, for if function is disturbed for too long a time organic tissue may succumb.

Conversion Hysteria. As a small child may have a temper tantrum, so may the older person experience an emotional response, sometimes similar in nature, as a result of incomplete repression. He has failed to inhibit his impulses as anxiety and tensions have mounted; instead of furthering his efforts at self-control, he has converted them into some physical reaction. Sometimes this is merely crying, screaming, or swearing, but in severe cases it may result in hysterical blindness, deafness, or paralysis. Still other examples may include the inability to speak, to eat, or to recall past events (amnesia).

Depressive Reactions. A very common reaction of individuals is that of depression, and it is a perfectly normal response to some irrevocable loss or personal tragedy. The patient who learns of a loss of limb or some residual paralysis may express profound grief, as one would upon learning of the death of some loved one. This may persist for a time, but eventually he responds to the positive efforts of others or to social situations and he recovers. However, behavior that resembles that of the grief-stricken individual but for which the causes cannot be identified, or in which the intensity of the reaction is greater than apparently is justified, is neurotic behavior. Extreme moodiness or an exaggerated sense of guilt characterize this disorder.

Phobias. A phobia may be defined as a morbid fear of some object or situation. The difference between this fear and a normal reaction is that in a phobia the thing that is feared offers no actual danger. When this occurs in an individual, it suggests that the real fear is somewhere else, and that this symbolization is merely a substitution, even though the terror felt may be compelling and intense. Although it does not help explain them, many persons have become enamored of the fancy names given to phobias, so that one who has a morbid dread of closed or constricted places has claustrophobia and one who fears open places has agoraphobia; hundreds of others can be derived, although such nomenclature seems to be gradually disappearing from medical literature.

PSYCHOTIC DISORDERS

The psychoneuroses are generally considered minor psychiatric disorders, although they may be merely the forerunners of more serious mental illnesses. Most neurotic individuals learn to live normal lives, and compensate for their problems in an adequate manner. Indeed, if their accustomed routines remain relatively unchanged and reasonably free of frustration and anxiety, they may become known as merely odd

or unusual and will be largely accepted by society. Few cases of psycho-
neurosis are sent to hospitals for the mentally diseased, which, of course,
accounts for the inability to estimate with any accuracy the extent of
their frequency in the population.

In contrast are the major mental abnormalities known as psychoses.
The distinguishing characteristic of a psychosis is a serious loss of contact with reality; the individual is either unable to take care of himself
or is potentially dangerous to himself or others. In other words, he meets
the legal criteria of insanity and is clearly in need of institutional care.
These patients present a wide variety of symptoms, but in general they
are said to lack insight into their problems; consequently they do not
regard themselves as abnormal. Psychiatrists would probably prefer to
dispense with rigid classification schemes for psychoses, as they may only
be moderately helpful in medical practice. In fact, they have been
altered through the years as information concerning behavior pathology
has changed; in addition, considerable overlapping of syndromes may
occur in any single patient. However, for the purposes intended here,
the following classification may prove helpful.

SCHIZOPHRENIA

Schizophrenia is the most common type of psychosis, perhaps accounting for about 20 per cent of original hospital admissions for mental illness. Although it may appear during childhood, this disorder is more
common during adolescence and later. It tends to defy treatment, which
is the reason neuropsychiatric hospitals may have as much as 50 per
cent of their population at any given time classified as schizophrenic.
Although the term itself is familiar to lay persons a perusal of the patients so designated may well lead one to wonder what it is that they
all have in common. This, of course, emphasizes the fact that there are
great differences within the disorder, and a typical hospital ward might
show these individuals sitting rather listlessly about, or adopting awkward postures, or performing repetitive movements and gestures, or
repeating bits of speech, most of which is done without recognition of
other patients or employees. Patients portray a general picture of
apathy, and respond incongruously to situations, often laughing when
there is no mirthful stimulus, or smiling at something that would normally provoke sadness. They may talk to themselves and appear to be
in a world of fantasy, or have delusions in which they become the central figure, sometimes of a persecutory drama, often of a scheme of
grandeur.

The term schizophrenia actually means a splitting of the personality.
While this definition is common, it really is not too helpful in understanding the problems involved, even though it does emphasize the split
between the world of reality and the world of fantasy. Psychotic dis-

orders are much too complex for such simplicity; schizophrenia itself
may be of several different kinds, based upon certain dominant symptoms. Furthermore, a great deal of overlap exists between each of these
varieties; however, considerable justification may be found for the
convenience of the classification below.

Simple Type. This type of schizophrenia represents a gradual loss
of contact with reality, and patients may have given little indication of
such difficulty in their early history. However, the symptoms suggest
that they slowly experience a loss of interest in their environment, and
that they have become increasingly ineffective in meeting social demands.
They become increasingly derelict in their responsibilities, and gradually withdraw into seclusion, apparently content with a slothful, un-
emotional existence. As patients, they appear contented and reasonably
happy, although there is little outward expression of either enthusiasm
or displeasure. The symptoms that characterize other forms of schizophrenia are apparently absent in these individuals, or at least the
hallucinations and delusions tend to remain suppressed from observation.

Hebephrenic Type. Patients in this category are rather easily identified
as mentally ill because of some of the peculiar mannerisms that they
may display. Although it may not be as clearly defined as other forms,
some of the outstanding symptoms include inappropriate smiling and
laughter, silliness, bizarre disorganized ideas, and incessant talking
frequently spiced with words they may have made up (sometimes called
"word salads," more appropriately termed neologisms). The flow of
conversation appears absurd, incongruous, and flighty; the patient jumps
from one idea to another in a jumbled fashion, and seems only inciden-
tally to return to the main theme. There may be delusions and hallucinations as in other forms of schizophrenia; and, the patient often becomes
untidy in his personal appearance and impulsive in behavior.

Catatonic Type. The catatonic schizophrenic is characterized by some
disorder of posture or muscular tension. He may adopt some odd position
or make curious facial expressions or repeat some other action in endless
succession. Commonly, these individuals resist efforts to move their body
parts by pulling in the opposite way. They may go through stages during
which they enter a state of stupor, mutism or negativism, or the opposite,
a period of great excitement. During this latter phase, they may become
extremely overactive and even violent, in which case they may become
dangerous to themselves or others. More frequently and for longer periods, however, they enter periods of stupor; in the more severe stages,
they become immobile and do not move to care for daily needs including
eating, dressing, and toilet care. Such persons become completely
dependent on hospital wards until such phases pass. At other times, the
catatonic schizophrenic may remain mute and seemingly inattentive,

although there is reason to believe that there is actually a silent mental alertness during such periods.

Paranoid Type. The outstanding characteristic of a paranoid schizophrenic is the presence of delusions. The content of these delusions is generally poorly organized and with no foundation in reality. They are usually changeable, numerous, fantastic, and accompanied by hallucinations, so that not only does he believe that people are persecuting him, he actually hears them plot against him, perhaps sees them "lurking in the wings," or has sensations that convince him of the presence of these enemies. Sometimes they are accompanied by delusions of grandeur, in which case he may claim to be a king, the President of the United States, or even God. As time goes on, these patients experience a growing confusion with gradual deterioration of conduct and thought.

PARANOIA

The form of psychosis known as paranoia must be differentiated from the paranoid type of schizophrenia, inasmuch as it is generally classified separately. The most readily distinguishing feature is the absence of hallucinations but the retention of persistent systematized delusions embodied in clear and orderly thinking. The paranoiac perceives correctly what is happening but misinterprets the events to fit his warped system of ideas. This delusional structure is not casually or hastily built, but is developed over a long period of time and then erected with great care. Except for this, the patient is perfectly normal and well oriented; he retains his interest in the environment and is knowledgeable concerning events around him. This can be quite misleading to the casual observer who hears his story told in all seriousness, not knowing that certain factors are quite false but neatly contrived and presented. Such individuals may become leaders of various movements, or may even be quite dangerous to society, but no matter what evidence is presented to them concerning the fallacy of their delusions, they remain unshaken and their beliefs do not become modified or dislodged.

MANIC-DEPRESSIVE

Next to schizophrenia, the most common form of psychosis is manic-depressive, which may account for as much as 12 per cent of first admissions to mental hospitals. As the name implies, two distinct reactions, one highly excited phase and one extremely depressed phase, are included in this psychosis. The patient's behavior may alternate between these two extremes, or he may manifest one or the other. During the manic phase, he may experience bursts of enthusiasm, hilarity, hyperactivity, or aggressive behavior. This conduct differs from normal elation typically because the patient goes too far. He may prance wildly about,

334   Psychologic Disorders

jump from bed to bed, play aggressive pranks on others, and may build upon certain grandiose delusions. In periods of hyperacute mania, this activity may reach delirious proportions, so that the ceaseless activity leaves sleeping and eating practically ignored; as might well be expected, sometimes this may lead to various physical complications.

The depressed phase, on the other hand, is just the opposite, at least in mood. It may result in complete stupor or just in simple depression, and is an overexaggeration of normal anxiety, mimicking the behavior of one who is grief-stricken. This type of patient is self-condemnatory and given to delusions; he may sit for hours, head bowed, wringing his hands, or performing other actions that portray the extremely depressed. These individuals rarely have hallucinations, but their delusions are persecutory in nature in which they remain the central figure. Until this phase passes, they are usually unresponsive, or are slow in responding to questions; more may be learned from them after their mood has changed.

Mania and depression, while extremes of mood, may not be so dissimilar in other ways. From a biological standpoint, for example, there is evidence to suggest that these two states may have much in common, and that their differences may be due more to the level of activity of the individual rather than his mental state.[6] In their reaction to stress, mania and depression may also be alike, as the same stimulus may provoke either reaction; it is possible, then, for personal tragedy to lead to a manic attack in these individuals. In other ways, too, there appears to be justification for the belief that the two phases have a certain unitary nature. There is an excellent prognosis for this form of psychosis, as happily there is a tendency for spontaneous recovery to occur; when treated, most of those discharged from mental hospitals do not have recurrences severe enough to require repeated hospitalization.

PSYCHOPATHIC PERSONALITIES

The term psychopathic personality, or constitutional psychopathic personality as it has been called, is a catch-all category into which have been placed a number of psychiatric misfits who do not qualify as either neurotic or psychotic. Individuals in this category exhibit rather obvious patterns of personality abnormality and present a history of social maladjustment and social deviation. They typically exhibit a chronic inability to accept an ordered and conformed life socially, frequently coming at odds with the law. One of the main traits exhibited by them is their seeming inability to profit by experience. Many criminals may fit this pattern, and when caught and punished may be released only to commit the same crime once again; a pathological liar persists in his fabrications,

---

[6] N. Cameron, "The Place of Mania Among the Depressions from a Biological Standpoint," *Journal of Psychology*, 14 (1942), p. 181.

often for no obvious reason. There is apparently an inability to forecast consequences of certain impulsive, self-centered action, and a difficulty to establish warm and lasting personal relationships.

It could be interesting but probably not too enlightening to go down the list of cases involving psychopathic personality, taking note of the sadists, masochists, etc., but it would perhaps be more profitable to characterize them as biosocially immature individuals.[7] In this way, one is struck by the similarity in the behavior between the overprotected child who continually evades adult responsibility by certain well-known adjustive techniques, and the behavior of the group in question. In many circumstances, at school, in his "gang," in jail or in hospitals, the psychopath may perform in a manner commensurate with his age, but at other times he may demonstrate juvenile or infantile behavior appropriate to those who have not achieved personal independence. When viewed in this light, reference to the "constitutional," nature of this condition may be obsolete, or at best, inadequate.

DELINQUENCY

A form of social deviation well known to modern society is that of delinquency. This is definitely a problem in public education, as the requirements of school attendance cut directly across populations at early ages. Juvenile delinquency is of major concern to society and to developmental and adapted physical education specifically, inasmuch as there is more frequent opportunity to work with such individuals than with the other forms of psychiatric disorders mentioned in this chapter. In addition, one never knows the future path that delinquent behavior may take, and those who are viewed today as "problem children" may be tomorrow's mentally ill. It should be recognized that every effort must be made for them to channel their social abilities into acceptable outlets.

Delinquency is neither psychotic nor neurotic behavior, nor is it necessarily psychopathic. However, one sees in the delinquent's conduct the type of social deviation found among so-called psychopaths, except that delinquency has certain legal implications. The term is applied to those whose conduct violates the law, or social expectation, providing the legal basis for arrest and punishment; thus one act of abnormal behavior might be termed delinquent and another might not, although the underlying problems might be the same. Immature social behavior is once again exhibited in the actions of the delinquent, although as Healy and Bronner[8] note, the individual may be seeking escape or flight from a stressful situation, and the thrill that accompanies the delinquent be-

---

[7] Cameron and Magaret, *op. cit.,* chap. 7.

[8] W. Healy and A. F. Bronner, *New Light on Delinquency and Its Treatment* (New Haven: Yale University Press, 1936), chaps. 4-7.

havior, especially if performed with a group, gives the act more personal satisfaction and recognition. It may also serve as a test of masculinity or courageousness, as revenge against parental authority, or as a means of alleviating unconscious feelings of guilt by seeking punishment.

PSYCHIATRIC TREATMENT

There can be no doubt that the treatment of patients with mental illness today has progressed far from the days of the eighteenth and nineteenth centuries when very little treatment existed. The increased understanding of psychiatric disorders has produced a diversity of procedures to deal with them, although there is by no means a simple and effective means of recovery which becomes apparent simply by knowing the pathology. Seldom can such a cause and effect relationship be established completely in advance. As has been true with the physical disabilities discussed in previous chapters, discussion of therapy here is intended to lead to better understanding and appreciation of the total psychiatric problem. Through this increased knowledge, it is hoped that a better perspective will be established and that a firm foundation can be laid for future study of the role of exercise and games designed for participation by such persons, as well as leading to a better basis for expecting positive social and psychological outcomes for the normal individual.

The field of psychotherapy is complex; the techniques utilized will vary with the psychiatrist. The therapeutic progress made in recent years is reflected in the increased rate of discharge from mental hospitals as well as fewer disturbed episodes in the wards themselves. This in turn helps to maintain a more healthy atmosphere within the institution for the patients and ultimately helps in their adjustment. One of the former characteristics of such hospitals was the physical deterioration of the patients; this situation has now been largely changed through the inclusion of physical activities in their treatment routines.

Undoubtedly, the variety of disorders presented has dictated the diversity of treatment procedures, and certainly pathological behavior responds slowly to such efforts. The ultimate aim is to change socially deviant behavior to socially accepted behavior, and to this end the active participation of the patient and all others involved is necessary. Today it is common to hear of "total push" therapy;[9] the effort is made to utilize every resource in promoting both the mental and physical health of the patient. Today's modern facilities include such ancillary therapies as occupational therapy, corrective therapy, recreational therapy, educational therapy, and manual arts therapy, as well as the inclusion of self-

[9] A. Myerson, "Theory and Principles of the 'Total Push' Method in the Treatment of Chronic Schizophrenia," *American Journal of Psychiatry*, 95 (1939), p. 1197.

service cafeterias, canteens, and other agencies designed to promote resocialization. These, of course, are in addition to doctors, nurses, other ward personnel, counselors, and social workers, who comprise the main body of hospital personnel. The team approach demands the appreciation of the various modalities employed in the treatment of a patient, but also recognizes that he is to be considered as a whole individual with many interests and capabilities. There is a great need for the individual with psychiatric disturbances to rebuild his capacity to deal with reality; through these agencies, he may relearn this process and establish lost self-confidence and ego strength.

In addition to psychotherapy in all of its related aspects, various methods of shock therapy are available for use. Whereas psychotherapy may be used with neurotic and psychotic patients, as well as with other troubled individuals, shock methods are restricted almost exclusively to disturbed psychotic patients. The initial enthusiasm generated by the reports emanating from the first use of shock as therapy have since been tempered somewhat, although the success that is achieved, especially when combined with other treatment measures, justifies its continued use. The first of these methods is *insulin shock*. The administration of insulin in carefully controlled doses brings about a deep coma, as experienced by diabetics; consciousness is restored by the administration of glucose after a period of time, usually less than one hour. Such treatment is apparently more effective when given to schizophrenic patients, although many of the benefits seem to be temporary.

Injection of the drug metrazol brings about a reaction similar to a grand mal seizure of epilepsy, and is known as *metrazol shock;* this is another technique that has been of value to psychiatrists in the treatment of psychiatric disorders. It has proven more helpful when used with the manic-depressive cases, however, than with schizophrenia. *Electroshock* therapy has likewise proved more effective with manic-depressive patients. This form of treatment also produces a convulsion similar to the grand mal seizure but not so severe as with metrazol; it is the newest and most widely used shock procedure. The frequency with which any of these forms is given to the patient will depend upon the extent of his condition and the success of the treatment; treatments may vary from several per day to a few each week.

Another procedure in the treatment of psychiatric disorders can be listed under the term *prefrontal lobotomy*. Specifically, this involves surgically severing neural connections between the prefrontal area and the thalamus and hypothalamus of the brain. Following the operation, patients recover rather quickly from the slightly stuporous and confused condition that ensues, although certain problems may persist. They may become tactless and outspoken, neglectful of personal appearance, and often develop such appetites that they gain excessive weight. After a few weeks they appear to be functioning as well as before, and interest and enthusiasm for the environment may be even greater. For the patient who was agitated and aggressive, this procedure seems to bring about a change in symptoms, so that he becomes quieter and more easily managed; in such cases, this may definitely be improvement. However, the fact remains that only the more severely ill patients are selected for such drastic treatment.

ROLE OF EXERCISE AND PHYSICAL ACTIVITY
FOR PSYCHIATRIC PATIENTS

Exercise and other physical activities are considered important and now form a part of the treatment program in psychiatric hospitals. Experiences from the second world war in the treatment of psychiatric casualties by physical reconditioning personnel in the theater of combat and in convalescent hospitals led to increased understanding of the role that such physical activity could play in contemporary treatment. Since that time reconditioning, or corrective therapy as it is now called, has become an important part of the Veterans Administration program in neuro-psychiatric hospitals. The effort has been made to gear the activities "to the patient's level and ability, and provide for the channelization of socially unacceptable behavior into acceptable expression of behavior."[10]

Within the framework of games, sports, exercise and other activities, corrective therapy can be expected to perform two major functions in the treatment of hospitalized psychiatric patients. One is to improve or maintain at an optimum level the physical fitness of the individual; the other is to serve as a medium for the communication by which patients may express their thoughts and feelings.[11] To be more specific, such a program, in addition to the obvious fitness benefits, can provide activities adapted to the individual who cannot adjust to group participation; promote greater physical and emotional relaxation; create a diversification and variety of activities to bring to light the patient's interest so that it can be redirected into constructive behavior; aid in he resocialization of the patient so that he may participate with others in activities both in the hospital and later; and provide an emotional outlet for tensions, aggressions, and hyperactivity so that they may be directed into constructive channels.[12]

---

10 Harry B. Dando, "Corrective Therapy," *Journal of Health, Physical Education and Recreation*, 32, No. 8 (November, 1961), p. 35.

11 Lucy D. Ozarin, "Corrective Therapy in the Psychiatric Hospital," *Journal of the Association for Physical and Mental Rehabilitation*, 4, No. 8 (April-May, 1951), p. 3.

12 *Physical Reconditioning*, TM 8-292, Departments of the Army and the Air Force. Washington: United States Government Printing Office, May, 1952, p. 158.

To perform such a function, the corrective therapist, as well as the instructor of developmental and adapted physical education, must use the activities of the gymnasium and playing field and must motivate the patients through a process that is consistent with modern psychiatric treatment. Some of the techniques adopted may resemble the elementary school teacher giving instruction to a group of young pupils whose attention span is short and whose motivation is limited; or the regressed and lethargic actions of a similar group may appear completely noncommunicable and so seclusive that any response is difficult of attainment. On the other hand, manic and excited patients may become wildly enthusiastic and proceed vigorously from one activity to another. Each patient requires special consideration and individual attention for maximum results to be achieved. Treatment is patient oriented; definite steps are followed which assist the patient from the time he enters the hospital until his discharge.[13]

Closed-ward psychiatric patients are generally in need of vigorous physical activity, and can benefit from a planned developmental approach. Occasionally one finds physical as well as mental handicaps in such persons, but ordinarily the physical health will not be a limiting factor to such participation. That the fitness of these patients is generally low is emphasized by two independent reports, which presented the results of the Physical Fitness Index test given to 50 and 42 subjects respectively. Both studies reported scores of approximately 70 for these samples, which is far below the national average of 100 for normal subjects. This would indicate the need for increased efforts at conditioning these patients at the same time other results are sought.[14,15]

As every therapist knows, a treatment program is dependent upon a medical diagnosis and prescription even if certain details of management are left up to the individual worker. No patient should be included in activities until this occurs. Just what activities are to be utilized for a particular individual will vary in general with the degree of psychiatric disability and the manner of symptoms presented. Thus, the schizophrenic patient who has lost the ability to deal with reality may profit from experiences that give him success; such an atmosphere may be readily created in the gymnasium or on the playing field when games are involved. Teamwork, co-operation, and a give and take relationship among patients are sought, leading to therapeutically approved goals

13 Richard G. Hannan and Richard C. Cowden, "PM and R Treatment Aims for NP Hospitals: A Simplification," *Journal of the Association for Physical and Mental Rehabilitation,* 12, No. 2 (March-April, 1958), p. 60.

14 Harry T. Zankel and James M. Field, "Physical Fitness Index in Psychiatric Patients," *Journal of the Association for Physical and Mental Rehabilitation,* 13, No. 2 (March-April, 1959), p. 50.

15 Robert E. Hodgdon and Delilah Reimer, "Some Muscular Strength and Endurance Scores of Psychiatric Patients," *Journal of the Association for Physical and Mental Rehabilitation,* 14, No. 2 (March-April, 1960), p. 38.

and maximum rehabilitation. Many of the specific methods by which these objectives may be achieved are both casual and serious and depend very little upon equipment used or the score resulting from any contest;[16] rather, the activity or game is merely a means to an end. For some negativistic patients there is an attempt to motivate social behavior,[17] while for certain hyperactive ones, the reverse may be true.[18] A careful study of such methods is needed before one attempts to deal with these patients; only a cursory one can be made here. The next task is to examine the role of activities and their social importance to the normal individual.

PERSONALITY AND SOCIAL ADJUSTMENT
IN PHYSICAL EDUCATION

Personality development and the achievement of desirable social adjustment have long been objectives of physical education; historically, as a better understanding of psychology and the nature of play and the role of games was reached, better insight was gained into such programs. When physical education expanded beyond the formalized approach that emphasized gymnastics, calisthenics, and marching, some of the potentialities were recognized for personality development. For example, Tryon[19] studied seventh-grade children's opinions of each other and concluded that the boy who lacks skill and has a distaste for organized games is ridiculed and shunned by the group. Activity of any sort is preferred to inactivity, and skill, leadership, and daring in games are among the attributes most prized. Kuhlen and Lee[20] also pointed out that boys active in games were highly rated in social acceptability.

Jones[21] reported that competitive athletic skills among boys are one of the chief sources of social esteem in the period preceding maturity, and he attributed this not merely to the high premium which adolescents place upon athletic proficiency, but also to the fact that strength and other aspects of physical ability were closely joined to such favorable traits as activity, aggressiveness, and leadership. After studying the physical ability of 78 elementary school boys, he found that boys

---

[16] James M. Field, "An Approach to the Treatment of the Neurotic and Psychotic by Corrective Therapy," *Journal of the Association for Physical and Mental Rehabilitation,* 11 (July-August, 1957), p. 120.

[17] Geraldine L. Hoseason, "Social Motivation of Catatonics," *Journal of the Association for Physical and Mental Rehabilitation,* 15 (July-August, 1961), p. 111.

[18] *Physical Reconditioning,* TM 8-292, *op. cit.,* p. 165.

[19] Carolyn C. Tryon, "Evaluation of Adolescent Personality by Adolescents," *Monograph of the Society for Research in Child Development,* 4 (1939), p. 1.

[20] Raymond G. Kuhlen and Beatrice J. Lee, "Personality Characteristics and Social Acceptability in Adolescence," *Journal of Educational Psychology,* 34 (1943), p. 321.

[21] Harold E. Jones, "Physical Ability as a Factor in Social Adjustment in Adolescence," *Journal of Educational Research,* 40 (1946), p. 287.

superior in strength at the end of adolescence showed a tendency to be tall, heavy, mesomorphic, early maturing, proficient in athletics, high in popularity and social prestige, and well adjusted; and, that biological fitness and social acceptance may be due largely to the tendency of the social group in question to accord a high value to physical superiority.

Rarick and McKee[22] utilized the case-study technique to discover personal characteristics and environmental factors which were common to ten children of high and ten children of low motor proficiency. They concluded that children in the superior motor performance group tended to be active, popular, calm, resourceful, attentive, and co-operative. On the other hand, children in the inferior motor performance group more frequently showed negative personality traits and were more often shy, retiring, and tense.

In a study by Popp,[23] the Physical Fitness Index test was administered to 100 high school sophomore boys. The 20 boys with the highest and the 20 boys with the lowest scores on this test were arranged in a single alphabetical list. Independently, five judges who knew all the boys selected the ten most desirable boys and the ten least desirable boys. Sixteen boys were named by at least one judge in the "desirable" classification; of these, 11, or 69 per cent, had high PFI's and five, or 31 per cent, had low PFI's. In selecting the "undesirable" boys, again 16 were chosen. Of this group, 4, or 25 per cent, had high PFI's and 12, or 75 per cent, had low PFI's.

Clarke and Clarke[24] studied upper elementary school boys on maturity, structural, and strength measures as related to criteria of social adjustment. Results indicated that boys accorded high social acceptance by their peers tended to be stronger and larger in size than those whose social status was low.

In studying the effects of physical training on personality, Milverton[25] studied boys of 14 years of age at the beginning and at the end of a twelve-week period of physical training. A sixteen-item scale which included traits assumed to be influenced by physical training was used. Of these traits, only five (gregariousness, sociability, co-operation, con-

22 G. Lawrence Rarick and R. McKee, "A Study of Twenty Third-Grade Children Exhibiting Extreme Levels of Achievement on Tests of Motor Proficiency," *Research Quarterly*, 20 (1949), p. 142.

23 James Popp, "Case Studies of Sophomore High School Boys with High and Low Physical Fitness Indices," (Master's thesis, University of Oregon, 1959); reported by H. Harrison Clarke, "Physical Fitness Benefits: A Summary of Research," *Education*, 78 (1958), p. 1.

24 H. Harrison Clarke and David H. Clarke, "Social Status and Mental Health of Boys as Related to Their Maturity, Structural Characteristics and Muscular Strength," *Research Quarterly*, 32 (October, 1961), p. 326.

25 F. J. Milverton, "An Experimental Investigation into the Effects of Physical Training on Personality," *British Journal of Educational Psychology*, 13 (1943), p. 30.

centration, and initiative) showed sufficient consistency to the three school masters who served as judges, to be regarded as validly estimated. In a group of boys given a so-called "progressive course" of physical education, improvement was registered in the trait described as concentration.

In order to study the personality traits of college fencers and other physical activity groups, Flanagan[26] assembled a personality inventory designed to measure the following four elements: ascendence-submission, masculinity-femininity, extroversion-introversion, and emotional stability-emotional instability. Results showed differences in the four personality traits between those students who participated in fencing and those who participated in other physical activities. Apparently, groups who spontaneously select one activity in preference to another demonstrate that personality is a factor in making such a selection.

To determine the relationship between body build and social traits and play activities, Bartell[27] administered the Washburne Social Adjustment Inventory, the California Test of Personality, and the Bell Adjustment Inventory, as social adjustment devices, and Van Dalen's Play Inventory as a measure of play activity to 697 high school boys. He concluded that there was a tendency at all levels for the medium build subjects to be better adjusted socially than either the obese or slender subjects.

Hanley[28] conducted a study designed to test the hypothesis that certain sociometrically derived reputation traits of junior high school boys would be found to correlate significantly with components of their mature somatotypes. He found that the traits "good-at-games" and "active-in-games" correlated .48 and .45 respectively with mesomorphy, both being significant at the 1 per cent level of confidence.

Jones and Bayley[29] studied the physical maturity of adolescents as related to behavior. Social behavior ratings were made by staff members of subjects as observed in free play, and the score on a reputation test was decided by classmates. The results indicated that the early-maturing boys were more likely to gain and maintain prestige associated with athletics.

When the sociometric questionnaire is used, positive relationships between peer status and physical measures are obtained. However, when the inventory-type instrument is utilized for "personality" assessment,

---

[26] Lance Flanagan, "A Study of Some Personality Traits of Different Physical Activity Groups," *Research Quarterly*, 22 (1951), p. 312.

[27] Joseph A. Bartell, "A Comparison Between Body Build and Body Size with Respect to Certain Sociophysical Factors Among High School Boys," (Microcarded Ph.D. dissertation, University of Pittsburgh, p. 1952).

[28] Charles Hanley, "Physique and Reputation of Junior High School Boys," *Child Development*, 22 (1951), p. 247.

[29] Mary C. Jones and Nancy Bayley. "Physical Maturing Among Boys as Related to Behavior." *Journal of Educational Psychology*, 41 (1950), p. 129.

the results are likely to be conflicting and frequently contrary to those obtained with the sociometric device.[30] The reason for these differences is primarily speculative at the moment.

Concern over the manner in which a student answers questions posed on an inventory test makes it necessary to evaluate results very carefully, although the prevalance of their use for counseling and guidance purposes is well known. Assessments of peer status by sociometric questionnaires and similar devices may prove to be more beneficial for physical education, although the type of information obtained may be somewhat limited. Peer estimates or adult assessments of pupils give an indication of social adjustment but say very little about the student's internal adjustment and mental health, except that certain aspects of over-all adjustment are reflected in external responses. The indications from the studies reviewed are that ability in games, activities, and physical fitness help to determine an individual's total personality, and that these conditions may be enhanced by such participation, although the question of how long it takes to effect changes is not clear. On the premise that physical activities are helpful to the psychiatrist in counteracting psychiatric disturbances, and their potential value to the normal individual seems assured, the task is next to determine how developmental and adapted physical education may be of value to emotionally disturbed students in schools and colleges.

DEVELOPMENTAL AND ADAPTED
PHYSICAL EDUCATION

The difference between working with emotionally disturbed students and dealing with psychiatric patients is largely one of degree; however, such disturbances among school children are not considered psychotic; even if certain mannerisms or characteristics seem to suggest such a designation. Certainly, emotional and behavior abnormalities have become a problem in public education, brought on by a number of circumstances. For example, mandatory rules of attendance cause many students to remain in school when they would perhaps be happier elsewhere, and any number of home and family problems can cause untold grief among children, resulting in antisocial conduct. There are those who feel that imposing severe penalties for misbehavior does not solve anything but the immediate issue; that such discipline does very little to help the student reach a greater understanding and insight into the reasons for his conduct. The approach to this problem should be mature and logical; long-range objectives to help such students reach solutions for their situations should be paramount.

Concern for boys and girls who have psychological, social, or emo-

---

[30] Clarke and Clarke, *op. cit.*

tional problems in schools and colleges should rest primarily with guidance personnel and psychologists. However, the developmental and adapted physical education program can make a positive contribution to this problem when properly utilized. As stated in Chapter 2, a function of this phase of physical education is to assist with "psychological and social adjustments of 'normal' individuals with atypical tendencies." It was stressed that the physical educator should recognize psychological and social deviates, that physical activities should be utilized to improve their condition, and that efforts should be made to create or recreate a positive mental attitude toward the use of physical activities as a means for further growth and development of the individual. The appealing nature of many of the physical activities can prove to be very important in bridging the gap between the student and the school; the possibilities offered in this area should be understood by everyone dealing with these pupils.

EMOTIONALLY DISTURBED STUDENTS

Obtaining proper medical guidance for dealing with those students possessing physical disabilities has been stressed repeatedly in this book; no less support from qualified school mental health personnel should be expected when teaching emotionally disturbed pupils. The nature of the difficulty, including past histories and other pertinent data, must be made available if maximum results are to be achieved. In addition, a reciprocal arrangement would require that the developmental and adapted teacher keep a record of performances and other information concerning the student's conduct. Behavior expressed in a games setting may be quite revealing, and progress made in all other aspects of the student's school life may first be noticed here. Also, a rapport with the physical educator may be more easily established than with his other teachers in school. All of these factors strengthen physical education as a curricular area that can deal effectively with the disturbed student and help prevent more lasting psychologic disorders.

For emotionally disturbed boys and girls, the game or activity is essentially unimportant; what is important is that they become involved in activities which are engrossingly interesting to them. The difficulty of including these individuals in the regular physical education class comes from the very nature of their problems and their tendency to defy the rules of conduct and shun conformity. On the other hand, the relaxed and congenial atmosphere of developmental and adapted classes is more apt to meet with success, especially when a wide choice of activities is available.

Play activities provide a means for students to express feelings of hatred, fear, or anger, in socially acceptable ways, just as they may be cheerful, joyous, or excited. A free and spontaneous atmosphere is important; this supports the concept that the activity itself is not so vital as the participation. In this manner, the hostile and aggressive pupil may obtain satisfaction in such activities as bag punching, aquatic games, handball, squash, tennis, and badminton, while the student who is negativistic may find group activities and team games more beneficial, especially volleyball, touch football, softball, group calisthenics, and soccer. The physical educator should develop a co-operative atmosphere, utilizing as many gradations of activity as are necessary for the participant to achieve a sense of accomplishment. Many of these students have underlying feelings of inadequacy that are masked behind external bravado. Their real need is for success, and they may easily be overwhelmed in physical activities and be consistent losers. The same need may exist for the timid, or for the poorly skilled person. Realistic goals should be placed before them, so that the accomplishment of objectives is within their grasp. Success experiences are important; physical education activities should be so selected and arranged that the individual has a chance to succeed, and will do so a fair share of the time.

There may be reluctance on the part of some students to participate spontaneously in the program. These are the students who react negatively to any of the school's organized functions. They should be allowed some time in class to become acquainted not only with the instructor but with the other students. Their background in athletics or interest in activities should be ascertained, and every effort should be made to provide the instruction in skills that would be of most value to them. Repeated invitations to join in the activities should be made, but it is probably best not to try to force them into a game until they are ready. Quite frequently the enthusiasm and enjoyment of others are infectious enough to draw the reluctant students into the game; the alert teacher will sense this and adroitly make room for an extra player, quietly seeing to it that he meets with some initial success.

Students with behavior abnormalities will exhibit some of the immature social behavior that is characteristic of them, and become unruly and disruptive in class. It is difficult to know just how to handle each individual case, but no teacher in developmental and adapted physical education should be too surprised when this happens. In general, these students should understand that they are expected to participate in class activities, but, if they reject the ones offered, a permissive attitude by the instructor might be better than an assertive one. If the student gains very little by his unruliness, these episodes may become less frequent and eventually lead to a more acceptable manner of dealing with his emotions.

The teaching of skills is very important in this program as indicated above; however, the underlying basis of physical fitness and developmental activities should still be emphasized for these students. Not only will they be better able to participate vigorously in the other activities offered, but the relaxation and reduction of emotional tensions that this produces may be very important. This type of effort is often enjoyed when presented in groups, as in calisthenics, or some may enjoy the more individual approach that weight lifting offers. The value of these exercises should not be underestimated for the secondary school student who may be concerned about his body image. Body-building exercises may help him increase his self-confidence and create a greater sense of security. This, combined with other activities, may form a very firm foundation for continued emotional stability.

An activity recommended very highly for hospitalized neuropsychiatric patients is aquatics. It provides an excellent medium for physical fitness emphasis, and has the additional advantage of being relaxing and sedative as well as being generally enjoyable, especially for those who can already swim. A similar program can be utilized in school and college developmental and adapted physical education if the facilities are available. In these institutions, however, it may not be possible to heat the water in the pool; however, if a sufficient number of students are involved, including those with emotional disturbances and those with various physical disabilities, it may be justified to raise the temperature of the water, at least for part of the week. The temperature selected is subject to some variation, although success has been found in the past with water as warm as 90 degrees F.; lower temperatures should be used, of course, if the water feels uncomfortably warm to the students.

In addition to swimming instruction, relays and polo are popular water activities; also, other games adapted to water have proven very enjoyable. Placing movable basketball backboards and baskets on either side of the shallow end of the pool creates sufficient equipment for water basketball, played with a rubber volleyball or polo ball. Also, erecting a volleyball net across the width of the pool provides a setting for aquatic volleyball, in which the better swimmers must play on the deeper side of the net. The rules may be modified in any way the instructor thinks advisable, but activities of this sort provide excellent media for enjoyable group participation and for physical fitness benefits as well.

Perhaps not enough has been said about the use of dance in dealing with students in all aspects of adapted physical education. Many forms of dancing have obvious social and recreational values for individuals with physical handicaps. This form of physical activity is recommended for use with emotionally disturbed persons as well. As a nonverbal form of communication, it is very important; for mentally ill patients, it is said to represent "the externalization of those inner feelings which cannot be expressed in rational speech but can only be shared in rhythmic, symbolic action."[31] The use of such rhythmic movement should be explored more fully and utilized when possible with both children and adults in developmental and adapted physical education.

SOCIAL ADJUSTMENT

In this book, social efficiency is defined as the development of desirable standards of conduct and the ability to get along well with others. As presented in Chapter 2, this efficiency involves individual traits, group traits, and their interrelations for the common good. The more extreme social deviates may easily be recognized; examples are the "grandstand" player, the bully with a "chip on his shoulder," the unsportsmanlike player, and the retiring introvert who shuns group participation. Furthermore, the physical educator may use tests, as considered in Chapter 4, to identify those with asocial tendencies. Such tests may be administered by or with the co-operation of the counseling service in the school or college.

Differentiation between the socially maladjusted and the emotionally disturbed is usually not clear cut. In many instances, it may be merely a matter of the degree of involvement. Thus, some boys and girls identified with socially unacceptable traits may be in the early stages of certain psychologic disorders. In any event, it is well to recognize these individuals; by early sympathetic treatment, the course of the involvement may be checked or reversed.

In other instances, the improvement of social efficiency may "merely" be a question of education. The "grandstand" player may be brought to a realization of the importance and satisfaction of team play; the energies and interests of the bully may be directed into socially constructive efforts; the merits of good sportsmanship can be presented as lasting benefits to the individual and to society; and the retiring boy or girl may be led into group and team activities with satisfaction. The developmental and adapted physical educator should perform counseling procedures and generally supervise the situation. These students, however, will usually participate in the regular physical education program. In these cases, therefore, the co-operation of the regular class instructor is essential, and he should be briefed thoroughly on each individual case.

In another book, one of the authors[32] presented a number of procedures that can be utilized by physical educators to improve the social

[31] Marian Chace, Warren Johnson, and Bettie Jane Wooten, "Movement Therapy for Children and Adults," *Journal of Health, Physical Education and Recreation,* 32 (November, 1961), p. 30.

[32] H. Harrison Clarke, *Application of Measurement to Health and Physical Education,* 3rd ed. (Englewood Cliffs, N. J.: Prentice-Hall, Inc., 1959), pp. 412-14.

efficiency of their pupils. These consisted of giving special emphasis to the utilization of team sports, of equating the powers of opposing individuals and groups, of providing opportunities for leadership, and of creating situations whereby success may be experienced. Mere participation in activity, no matter how potentially valuable, however, will not automatically result in desirable social outcomes. The teacher or coach is the key to social education. Social growth is dependent to a considerable degree upon the understanding and ability of the teacher to inculcate these desirable qualities into the lives of boys and girls, especially those with atypical behavior patterns.

TENSIONS

Tenseness occurs not only in a muscle but also in the individual as a whole; the popular concept of the tense person is that he is "high strung," "on edge," "jittery." Rathbone[33] has shown that psychological and physical manifestations of tension are intimately related. "When the psyche is disturbed, the reacting tissues of the body—glandular and neuromuscular—will be affected; when the glands are disturbed in their functioning or the muscles are tense, the 'person' will be apprehensive and emotionally on edge." Rathbone[34] also established that general chronic fatigue and tenseness are not identical conditions but are in many ways related. The fatigue to which she refers is not the fatigue brought on by hard work but rather the fatigue resulting from general lethargy, often caused by lack of exercise, insufficient sleep, boredom, and mental distress. Jacobson[35] has illustrated the presence of nervous and emotional excitability in case studies of acute endocarditis, cardiac asthma, chronic insomnia, compulsion neurosis, mild phobias, and neurasthenia. Moreover, he cited the presence of neuromuscular hypertension in various diseases.[36]

Pronounced tenseness in boys and girls may frequently be identified by such easily recognized manifestations as inability to relax, being constantly on the move, difficulty in getting to sleep, irritability, chronic indigestion, and various nervous mannerisms. However, if these are the only criteria applied, many tense individuals will not be discovered. A technique utilized successfully by Rathbone[37] follows: With the subject lying on his back preferably on a mat or other soft level surface, he is asked to relax his muscles as completely as possible and to remain relaxed during the teacher's manipulations; manipulations consist of

---

[33] Josephine L. Rathbone, *Corrective Physical Education*, 6th ed. (Philadelphia: W. B. Saunders Company, 1959), p. 127.

[34] *Ibid.*, p. 128.

[35] Edmund Jacobson, *Progressive Relaxation* (Chicago: University of Chicago Press, 1938), chap. XX.

[36] *Ibid.*, chap. III.

[37] Rathbone, *op cit.*, p. 143.

raising and releasing some part of the body, such as the wrist, forearm, arm, or leg. Signs of hypertonus are revealed if the student assists the movement, resists the movement, holds a raised position, or gradually lowers the part when released by the tester. Recommended scoring is in terms of negative, slight, medium, and marked hypertonus.

In the treatment of tensed boys and girls, the developmental and adapted physical educator should be aware of the cause or causes of this condition and steps should be taken for their removal or amelioration. This process may well be a part of the case-study approach described in Chapter 6. If psychological and emotional involvements are present or suspected, referral to a specialist will be desirable; if sufficiently serious, adapted programs should be conducted under advisement from these specialists.

Relaxation procedures through adapted physical education may start with cot rest or rest on mats in a quiet place; if possible, this can well be extended to actual sleep. While in a resting position, the child may be taught how to relax his muscles systematically as a significant aid to relaxation. As mentioned in Chapter 11 concerning tuberculosis, an effective way to do this is to tense, holding briefly a given muscle group as hard as possible; then, let go and relax the muscles to the opposite extreme. This process can start with small muscle groups such as the facial and gripping muscles and progress to the larger muscles of the arms and shoulders, neck, abdomen, and legs.

Mild rhythmic exercises are a desirable form for the tensed individual; if these can be performed out-of-doors in the sunshine, additional benefits will accrue. Walking and hiking, eventually building up to jogging and running well within the person's exercise tolerance, are desirable. General conditioning exercises, such as those presented in Chapter 7, are indicated. Until relaxation is achieved, avoidance of competitive situations is recommended, so as not to invoke the extra tension attendant thereon; this recommendation may well be extended to the many classroom situations that employ various forms of competition and other tension-producing conditions.

SUMMARY

This chapter has focused attention on many forms of psychologic disorders, and has presented the point of view that those students in school who show evidences of abnormal behavior can best be understood when viewed in the broad perspective of psychiatric deviations. No program of developmental and adapted physical education is complete until an attempt is made to include activities for these students.

A normal reaction to physical disability may be the temporary breakdown of the individual's emotional barriers, and what ensues remarkably resembles some of the more acute psychotic disturbances. What differ-

entiates this behavior from true mental illness is the manner in which
.most patients respond to time and sympathetic understanding. Our lives
are traditionally filled with many situations that produce stress and
frustration; the extent to which one will endure them will depend largely
upon his conception of himself and the obstacle.

Psychoneuroses are characterized by many mental or physical symptoms which have no constant organic basis but which may usually be
traced to some disturbance in the psychologic processes of the individual.
They do not distort the hold on reality, but are generally a failure
of the personality to adapt adequately to external or internal situations.
Neurotic states have been described as anxiety, neurasthenia, obsessive-
compulsive reactions, psychosomatic conditions, conversion hysteria, depressive reactions, and phobias.

The psychotic disorders entail a serious loss of contact with reality,
and the individual may be unable to take care of himself and others;
he may even be potentially dangerous. He meets the legal definition of
insanity and as a rule requires institutional care. Their symptoms are
varied with considerable overlapping between them; however, the
classification presented is as follows: schizophrenia, with the four categories of simple, hebephrenic, catatonic, and paranoid; paranoia; and
manic-depressive psychoses. In addition, psychopathic personality and
certain phases of delinquency have been discussed.

Treatment of psychiatric disorders includes the wide field of psychotherapy which has proceeded from a better understanding of the disorders themselves. Some of the other techniques utilized include the
use of the ancillary therapies of occupational therapy, corrective therapy,
recreational therapy, and others. Furthermore, newer types of treatment
have been used, such as various forms of shock and certain surgical
procedures. Exercise and a variety of physical activities are now considered important in the total treatment program, with the emphasis
placed upon social and emotional adjustment.

There are indications that ability in games and activities and the
development of physical fitness are helpful in determining a normal
individual's total personality, that those children who are active enjoy
a favored status among their peers. It should be considered that developmental and adapted physical education may be of value to emotionally
disturbed students in schools and colleges, inasmuch as a number of
them may be enrolled but fail to conform to classroom procedures.
In dealing with them, counseling and guidance personnel and others
concerned should be consulted and a program of activities planned to
provide an acceptable outlet for aggressive behavior.

SELECTED REFERENCES

Bennet, Ivy, *Delinquent and Neurotic Children*. New York: Basic Books, Inc., 1960.

Cameron, Norman, and Ann Magaret, *Behavior Pathology*. Boston: Houghton Mifflin Company, 1951.

Chace, Marion, "Dance as an Adjunctive Therapy with Hospitalized Mental Patients," *Bulletin of the Menninger Clinic*, 17 (November, 1953), 219.

Cole, Luella, *Psychology of Adolescence*. New York: Holt, Rinehart and Winston, Inc., 1948.

Cowell, Charles C., "The Contributions of Physical Activity to Social Development," *Research Quarterly*, Part II. Vol. 31, No. 2 (May, 1960), 286-306.

Fait, Hollis F., *Adapted Physical Education*. Philadelphia: W. B. Saunders Company, 1960, ch. 15.

Klein, D. B., *Abnormal Psychology*. New York: Holt, Rinehart and Winston, Inc., 1951.

La Salle, Dorothy, "Mental Hygiene Aspects of Physical Education," *Professional Contributions*, No. 5, American Academy of Physical Education (November, 1956), 30-38.

Physical Reconditioning, TM 8-292, Departments of the Army and the Air Force (Washington: United States Government Printing Office, May, 1952), ch. 7.

Rathbone, Josephine L., *Corrective Physical Education*, 6th ed. Philadelphia: W. B. Saunders Company, 1959.

Scott, M. Gladys, "The Contributions of Physical Activity to Psychological Development," *Research Quarterly*, Part II, Vol. 31, No. 2 (May, 1960), 307-320.

Strecker, Edward A., *Basic Psychiatry*. New York: Random House, 1952.

White, Robert W., *The Abnormal Personality*. New York: The Ronald Press Company, 1948.

Index

Index